Population Health and the Future of Healthcare

Richard K. Thomas

Population Health and the Future of Healthcare

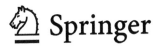 Springer

Richard K. Thomas
University of Tennessee Health Science Center
Memphis, TN, USA

ISBN 978-3-030-83886-7   ISBN 978-3-030-83887-4 (eBook)
https://doi.org/10.1007/978-3-030-83887-4

© The Editor(s) (if applicable) and The Author(s), under exclusive license to Springer Nature Switzerland AG 2021
This work is subject to copyright. All rights are solely and exclusively licensed by the Publisher, whether the whole or part of the material is concerned, specifically the rights of translation, reprinting, reuse of illustrations, recitation, broadcasting, reproduction on microfilms or in any other physical way, and transmission or information storage and retrieval, electronic adaptation, computer software, or by similar or dissimilar methodology now known or hereafter developed.
The use of general descriptive names, registered names, trademarks, service marks, etc. in this publication does not imply, even in the absence of a specific statement, that such names are exempt from the relevant protective laws and regulations and therefore free for general use.
The publisher, the authors, and the editors are safe to assume that the advice and information in this book are believed to be true and accurate at the date of publication. Neither the publisher nor the authors or the editors give a warranty, expressed or implied, with respect to the material contained herein or for any errors or omissions that may have been made. The publisher remains neutral with regard to jurisdictional claims in published maps and institutional affiliations.

This Springer imprint is published by the registered company Springer Nature Switzerland AG
The registered company address is: Gewerbestrasse 11, 6330 Cham, Switzerland

Preface

There is growing interest in the concept of "population health" among health professionals, policy analysts, and government agencies. This interest is driven by, among other factors, the inescapable conclusion that the US healthcare system has become increasingly ineffective at improving community health. Given the system's obvious deficiencies, it has become clear that a different approach is necessary to reverse the increasingly documented decline in the population's health status while containing the continuously growing cost of care.

Efforts to work within the existing framework have not been successful, and it is increasingly clear that a system that impacts one patient at a time is not going to address the health issues we face as a society. We realize today that fewer and fewer health problems result from the characteristics of individuals, but they reflect the characteristics of the groups of which they are a part and the social contexts in which they find themselves.

Despite the growing emphasis on "population health" and the growing number of advocates for this approach, there is considerable confusion over the nature and significance of the model. There is no widely accepted definition of population health, and the attributes of this approach to community health improvement are poorly understood. Those on the front lines of healthcare delivery often fail to recognize the implications of population health for the delivery of care and for the operation of their organizations. Misunderstandings over the nature of population health are common, and the term is more often than not used inappropriately.

This book is designed to provide a definitive explication of the nature and characteristics of a population health approach to community health improvement. Here, as is always the case, the starting point must be an understanding of the

---

It should be noted that this book has been written in the midst of the coronavirus pandemic and much of what is discussed reflects the circumstances that prevailed prior to the pandemic. It is likely that conditions post-pandemic will be much different and thus require the rethinking of many issues discussed in this work.

concept—what it is and is not—and the ways in which the concept can be applied in today's healthcare environment. As will be seen, this approach can be applied at both the micro and macro levels, although its primary impact is expected to be community- or society-wide. The approach can address many practical issues facing healthcare providers today—from more efficient patient management to reduction of readmissions to better control of capitated plan members to the generation of an IRS-acceptable community health needs assessment. At the organizational level, a population health approach can be applied to every area in which healthcare administrators are likely to be evaluated in the future.

The long-term benefit of this approach, however, is derived from its effectiveness in improving community health. There is a growing body of evidence that the US population is actually getting sicker after a century-long run of improving health status. The changing nature of health problems, the societally generated etiology, and the characteristics of patients themselves render the traditional one-patient-at-a-time approach obsolete. An approach that can impact *populations* not individual patients is increasingly needed.

Adopting a population health approach, it must be conceded, is not an easy task. In effect, this approach sets the healthcare system on its head. Health professionals must forget much of what they know about health and healthcare delivery in order to adopt a perspective that supports a population health approach. This will require a different mindset, a mindset that represents a challenge for health professionals but is a requirement for the adoption of a population health model.

An inconvenient truth is that the US healthcare system as currently constituted cannot contribute to community health improvement. Healthcare organizations must transform themselves into the type of organization that can operate within a population health model. This involves an even more radical conversion that in a sense is more challenging since we are advocating changing the direction of an "ocean liner" in a very short period of time. Organizational transformation is already underway at a number of healthcare organizations. Too often, however, this transformation is limited to trying to adapt existing processes to the new environment. Unfortunately, there can be no "business as usual" in the future.

Healthcare organizations are going to have to recreate themselves to survive in the new environment—an environment that emphasizes outcomes over volume, quality over quantity, prevention over treatment, and keeping people out of treatment. As mandated by the Affordable Care Act, not-for-profit hospitals must be accountable for the health status of the entire community and not just their own patients. These types of mandates can be expected to increase in the future as payers, government regulators, and policy makers realize that the only way to improve community health status is through a population health approach.

Memphis, TN, USA   Richard K. Thomas

Contents

✓1 Defining Population Health 1
   Introduction. 1
   Defining Population Health. 2
      Micro and Macro Dimensions of Population Health 6
   Attributes of Population Health 10
   What Population Health is Not. 14
   Summary. 17
   Key Points. 18
   References. 19

✓2 The Road to Population Health: A Changing Society 21
   Introduction. 21
   Changing Population Characteristics 22
      The Changing Age Structure. 24
      The Changing Sex Ratio. 26
      Growing Racial and Ethnic Diversity. 27
      Changing Household and Family Structure 28
      Changing Lifestyles 30
   Changing Patient Characteristics 35
      Changing Disease Etiology. 39
   Summary. 43
   Key Points. 45
   References. 45

✓3 The Road to Population Health: A Changing Healthcare System 47
   Introduction. 47
   The Emergence of Modern Medicine 48
   Emerging Deficiencies 56
   Late-Century Paradigm Shift 62
   The Impact of Medical Science on Population Health 63

	Deficiencies in the "Healthcare" Model	67
	Summary	73
	Key Points	74
	References	75
4	**The Roots of Population Health**	77
	Introduction	77
	The Contribution of Public Health	78
	History of Public Health	78
	The Organization of Public Health	79
	The Functions of Public Health	81
	The Current State of Public Health	86
	The Current Focus of Public Health	87
	Public Health Professional Organizations	90
	The Defunding of Public Health and Its Consequences	92
	Public Health Does Not Equate to Population Health	94
	Why Public Health Cannot Champion Population Health	95
	The Contribution of Demography	97
	The Contribution of Social Epidemiology	99
	The Contribution of Medical Sociology	100
	Summary	102
	Key Points	103
	References	104
5	**Health Status and How to Measure It**	107
	Introduction	107
	Conceptual Issues	108
	Defining "Health"	108
	Defining Health Status	111
	Health Status Indicators	114
	Global Measures	114
	Outcome Measures: Morbidity	115
	Outcome Measures: Mortality/Life Expectancy	117
	Other Outcome Measures	118
	Healthy/Unhealthy Behavior	120
	Environmental Factors	120
	Social/Economic Factors	120
	Cultural/Subcultural Influences	121
	Life Circumstances Indicators	121
	Access/Utilization Measures	122
	Health Status Rankings	122
	A New Approach to Health Status	124
	The Importance of Non-Health-Related Data	126
	Summary	127
	Key Points	129
	References	130

Contents

✓ 6 **The Social Determinants of Health and Illness** 133
    Introduction.. 134
    Intermediate Causes 135
    The Influence of Stress on Health Status 140
    Root Causes 141
        Economic Instability..................................... 142
        Neighborhood and Physical Environment 143
        Housing Access and Quality.............................. 146
        Transportation.. 148
        Education 150
        Food Insecurity... 151
        Community and Social Context 154
        Residential Segregation.................................. 155
        Criminal Justice 158
    Summary.. 159
    Key Points.. 160
    References.. 161

✓ 7 **Paying the Piper: Health Disparities**........................... 167
    Introduction... 168
    The Stratification of Health Conditions 169
    Health Metrics Associated with Disparities 170
    The Causes of Health Disparities 173
        Poverty and Health Disparities 173
        Environmental Conditions and Health Disparities 174
        Education and Health Disparities 176
        Food Insecurity and Health Disparities................... 177
        Residential Segregation and Health Disparities 177
        Community and Social Context and Health Disparities..... 177
        Crime and Criminal Justice and Health Disparities 178
    Groups that Exhibit Disparities................................. 179
    Trends in Health Disparities 189
    Summary.. 192
    Key Points.. 194
    References.. 195

✓ 8 **Population Health and Healthcare Delivery**..................... 199
    Introduction... 199
    Population Health Principles and Healthcare Delivery............ 202
    Attributes of Population Health Management 204
    Barriers to Population Health Management 215
    The Role of Healthcare in Population Health Improvement......... 217
    The Role of the Healthcare System in Population Health 222
    A New Mindset.. 225

	Summary...	226
	Key Points...	228
	References...	228
✓ 9	**Population Health and Public Policy**.................	231
	Defining Public Policy	231
	Spheres for Policy Development..........................	234
	Macro-level Policies	235
	Public Policies.......................	237
	Organizational Policies...............	240
	Professional Policies..................	243
	Health in all Policies...................................	243
	Social Domains and Public Policy	249
	Education	249
	Housing and Community Development	250
	Transportation........................	253
	Economic Development	254
	Food Access and Security..............	255
	Criminal Justice	256
	Summary..	258
	Key Points...	258
	References...	259
✓ 10	**Traditional Approaches to Community Health Data**....	263
	Introduction...	263
	Traditional Categories of Data for Health Needs Assessment	264
	Demographic Data	264
	Epidemiological Data	266
	Health Behavior	268
	Healthcare Resources	269
	Health Services Utilization...........	276
	Non-Traditional Health Data Metrics.....................	278
	Obesity	278
	Mental Illness	278
	Disability Data	280
	Dental Health Data	282
	Sources of Data for Health Needs Assessment.............	282
	Sources of Demographic Data	282
	Sources of Epidemiological Data	283
	Sources of Healthcare Resources Data..	287
	Sources of Health Behavior Data	289
	Sources of Health Services Utilization Data...	291
	Issues with Traditional Health Data	291
	Issues with Epidemiological Data......	291
	Issues with Health Behavior Data......	293
	Issues with Health Services Utilization Data	293

Contents   xi

Summary	295
Key Points	296
References	297

11   Data Needs for the Population Health Model 299
- Introduction 299
- Nature of Relevant Data 300
  - Perspective 300
  - Individual vs. Community 300
  - Level of Data Collection 301
  - Qualitative vs. Quantitative 302
- Data Categories for Population Health Assessments 304
  - Economic Instability 304
  - Neighborhood and Physical Environment 305
  - Housing Access and Quality 306
  - Transportation 306
  - Education 308
  - Food Insecurity 309
  - Community and Social Context 310
  - Residential Segregation 311
  - Crime and Criminal Justice 312
- Sources of Data for Population Health Assessments 313
  - Sources of Data on Economic Instability 314
  - Sources of Data on the Neighborhood
    and Physical Environment 314
  - Sources of Data on Housing Access and Quality 314
  - Sources of Data on Transportation 316
  - Sources of Education Data 316
  - Sources of Data on Food Insecurity 317
  - Sources of Data on Community and Social Context 318
  - Sources of Data on Residential Segregation 318
  - Sources of Data on Crime and Criminal Justice 320
- Population Health Data Challenges 320
- Transitioning from CHNA to PHA 323
  - The Changing Context for Community Assessments 324
  - Similarities Between CHNAs and PHAs 328
  - Differences Between CHNAs and PHAs 329
- Summary 331
- Key Points 332
- References 333

12   The Role of the Community in Population Health Improvement 335
- Introduction 335
- Why Not Community? 337
- Why the Community? 338

Community Preparation	342
Steps in Community Involvement	343
Community Health Business Model	348
Policy-Setting and Population Health	351
Barriers to Community Leadership	353
Summary	355
Key Points	356
References	356

Chapter 1
Defining Population Health

Despite the growing interest in "population health" on the part of health professionals, policy analysts and government agencies, there is considerable confusion over the actual definition of the term. Different people use the term in different ways adding to the confusion. This chapter reviews the history of the population health movement, noting early proponents of this model. It then provides a definitive description of the population health concept (what it is and is not) and characterizes it in terms of its attributes.

In this chapter the reader will:

- Gain an understanding of the emerging concept of "population health"
- Be exposed to the evolving definition of "population health" and a more contemporary conceptualization of the model
- Receive a framework for viewing "population health" in a systematic manner
- Understand the different levels (micro and macro) at which the population health model can be applied
- Learn about the attributes that are thought to characterize "population health", and
- Find out what "population health" is *not*

Introduction

There is growing interest in the concept of "population health" among health professionals, policy analysts and government agencies. As an approach that assesses health from a population rather than a patient perspective, it represents an opportunity for developing a better understanding of the health status of populations—whether they are patients or not—and an innovative approach to improving a population's health status.

While "population health" has become the buzzword *du jour* in healthcare and everyone seems to have adopted this nomenclature, the term is used inconsistently and often, in the authors' opinion, erroneously. Healthcare providers claim they are using a population health approach to more efficiently manage their patients; consultants have rebranded themselves as population health experts to capitalize on this trend; and vendors claim to be able to support their clients' population health needs. Yet, it is clear when one looks beneath the surface that there is widespread misunderstanding of the concept at best and outright misuse of the term at worst. In fact, many who claim to have expertise in population health do not appear to understand the concept.

A number of factors confound the discussion of "population health." These factors contribute to a lack of clarity with regard to the term's definition and to confusion over what is meant by a population health approach to health status improvement. For example, healthcare providers generally use the term as a replacement for "patient health" and have difficulty getting past the notion of improving health one patient at a time (Raths, 2015). Managers of accountable care organizations (ACOs) see population health in terms of the status of their patient panels—especially Medicare patients—while public health officials often view the population in terms of geographically defined or racial and ethnic populations (Tompkins et al., 2013). Even federally qualified health centers that ought to be closer to this issue than most healthcare providers view providing a "medical home" for the medically underserved as their contribution to population health (Hagland, 2013). Each of these conceptualizations violates some aspect of the model, and these contradictions will become clearer as the attributes of the population health model are described below.

Defining Population Health

In formulating the population health concept one must consider the different dimensions of the definition, the levels at which the concept is applied, and the directness of the approach employed. As far back as 20 years ago, some health professionals began using the term "population health". A variety of definitions were put forth and modified over time to reflect evolving perceptions of the concept. In an attempt to clarify our understanding of the model, this chapter begins with the working definition below. A historical review of the evolution of this definition is presented in Box 1.1.

Deprez and Thomas (2017) have attempted to address the confusion surrounding the concept of population health and develop a more useful working definition. They view the definition as having two dimensions: noun and verb. As a noun, population health refers to the status of the population reflecting its health and well-being as measured by several population-based measures thought to be relevant. The emphasis is on broad measures of health, some of which might be considered the sum of individual health status and others as attributes of the group as a whole.

Box 1.1: Historical Definitions of Population Health
As with most new concepts in healthcare, several definitions abound that vary widely in both interpretation and application. The most frequently cited definition is the one formulated in 2003 by Kindig and Stoddard. This definition reads: *population health represents the health outcomes of a group of individuals, including the distribution of such outcomes within the group.* This definition has been much-discussed and many (including Kindig and Stoddard) have expressed concerns over its adequacy in the light of current thought. Interestingly, after considering the pros and cons of this definition, most parties have opted to continue its use (see for example, the Institute of Medicine [Kindig and Isham, 2014]). While this might be considered the default definition due to its widespread citation, in today's environment it seems somewhat imprecise and does not fully capture the essence of the concept as it has evolved.

Kindig (2007) subsequently attempted to expand on this definition by analyzing the meaning of the basic components. He defines '"population" as a group of individuals, in contrast to the individuals themselves, organized into many different units of analysis, depending on the research or policy purpose. Whereas many interventions (e.g., much of medical care) focus exclusively on individuals, he argues that population health policy and research concentrate on the aggregate health of population groups like those in geographic units (cities, prisons) or ones delineated based on other characteristics (ethnicity, religion, health plan membership). He rightly notes that the determinants of health have their effect at a group rather than the individual level. Kindig appreciates the modern understanding of health as a state of wellness or well-being. He further considers health in relation to all aspects of life in the environments in which we live (Kindig and Isham, 2014).

Although Kindig and Stoddard are widely cited, other definitions have been posited, some of which predated theirs. Early offerings include that of John Frank (1995), founding director of the Canadian Institute for Population Health, who stated: *Population health is a conceptual framework for thinking about why some people, and some peoples, are healthier than others [with the intent of exploring] the determinants of health at individual and population levels.* Frank makes the point that the major determinants of human health status, particularly in countries at an advanced stage of socioeconomic development, are not medical care inputs and utilization, but cultural, social and economic factors—at both the individual and population levels.

Young (1998) defined population health as: *A conceptual framework for thinking about why some people are healthier than others, as well as the policy development, research agenda, and resource allocation that flow from it.* J.M. Last (2007), the founding editor of the *Dictionary of Epidemiology* offered a simpler version that defined population health as: *the health of the population, measured by health status indicators.*

(continued)

Box 1.1 (continued)

It is worth noting that some of the early thinking on population health occurred outside the United States and, to a certain extent, remained under the radar. The work of the Canadian Institute for Population Health noted above is one example. The work of the Scottish Public Health Observatory (2014) with its emphasis on community well-being is another. Another perspective offered by Health and Welfare Canada (1994) is stated as follows: *Population health strategies address the entire range of individual and collective factors that determine health. Traditional health care focuses on risks and clinical factors related to particular diseases. Population health strategies are designed to affect whole groups of populations of people.*

In subsequent work Kindig (2015) attempted to clarify our thinking in this regard. He reviews the evolution of population health terminology and considers the new contexts in which population health is being discussed. He recognizes the shortcomings of his and other definitions and suggests that multiple definitions may be necessary. This includes a recognition of its application to individual patients on one hand and groups of people on the other. While the traditional population health definition can be reserved for geographic populations, new terms such as *population health management* or *population medicine*, he argues, are useful to describe activities limited to clinical populations and a narrower set of health outcome determinants.

Kindig feels that the second clause of their definition should receive increasing emphasis. Thus, "including the distribution of outcomes within the group" is felt to reflect the importance of addressing intragroup disparities. If the intent is to improve overall health status *and* reduce disparities, this is a critical consideration. In health status measurement, policy formulation, and research, the emphasis is typically on the aggregate health status for the population in question to the neglect of disparity reduction.

The danger in defining *population health* in terms of patient populations is that this draws attention away from the critical role that non-clinical factors play in producing health. Kindig recommends the use of more than one definition in order to address this concern or perhaps the use of some other term that more precisely describes the application of population health within a clinical setting. For this reason, Jacobson and Teutsch (2013) recommended to the National Quality Forum that "current use of the abbreviated phrase *population health* should be abandoned and replaced by the phrase *total population health*." While Kindig appreciates these concerns, he supports the decision of the Institute of Medicine to retain the shorter term population health while recognizing its limitations.

"Global" measures such as self-reported health status are examples of the former. The latter is somewhat more difficult to conceptualize and reflects attributes of the group such as poverty level, household structure, and environmental conditions that reflect the social determinants of health.

> *Population health, n.*, An assessment of the health status of a population that uses aggregate data on non-medical as well as medical factors to measure the totality of health and well-being of that population.

As a verb, population health refers to an approach to improving health status that operates at the population rather than the individual (or patient) level. The approach focuses on social pathology rather than biological pathology and involves the "treatment" of conditions within the environment and policy realms in addition to the provision of clinical services to individual patients. While an underlying assumption is that a population health approach aims to improve health status by focusing on the healthcare needs and resources of *populations* not individuals, it does not rule out specific patient-based medical treatment but views healthcare as only one component of a health improvement initiative.

> *Population health, v.*, An approach to improving community health status that focuses on populations rather individuals and addresses the root causes and structural factors rather than exclusively focusing on treating the symptoms/conditions of individuals.

Figure 1.1 presents a graphical depiction of the population health model based on the definition above. The first set of boxes indicates the factors that contribute to a community's health status. These include the attributes associated with individuals within the community and are arguably the least important of the inputs. Life circumstances refers to the conditions of everyday life that impact a member's community. These include such factors as food insecurity, housing instability and unsafe neighborhoods—factors that impinge on the everyday lives of community members. The third component is the characteristics of the groups in which community members participate. More than any other factor, this input into health status reflects the culture associated with the community and its various population subgroups. The final input—social determinants of health—has received increasing attention

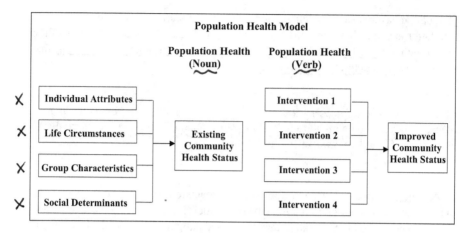

Fig. 1.1 Population Health Model

over time. As will be seen, these social determinants are playing an ever larger role in the determination of community health status. Population health at this point is represented by the health status of the population as measured by relevant community attributes. This reflects the noun aspect of the definition.

The second set of inputs (depicted here as "interventions) relate to the verb dimension of the definition. These interventions reflect efforts to address the factors (depicted in the first panel) that contribute to community health status. Little can be done to alter individual attributes, but interventions directed at life circumstances, group characteristics or cultural patterns, and, importantly, the social determinants of health reflect the dynamic dimension of the definition. In this simplified depiction, the interventions are intended to contribute to improved community health status.

Micro and Macro Dimensions of Population Health

The application of the population health model can be explored at two different levels— a micro-level view that considers population health as it relates to the delivery of care and a macro level view that considers population health from a societal perspective. At the micro-level one approach might be to identify individuals at high risk and intervene to reduce their risk. At the macro-level the approach might involve reducing the average risk level for the total population. Intervening with individuals at high risk is generally the domain of clinical medicine, although public health authorities coordinate certain clinically implemented programs in order to achieve population health objectives. Some programs such as breast cancer screening and childhood vaccinations involve individual encounters but have population-level objectives. Ultimately, some initiatives targeting individuals at the micro-level will have macro-level implication while others will not. Because of its emphasis on population-level interventions, Box 1.5 discusses the distinction between population health and public health.

At the micro-level the focus is typically on a group of individuals receiving care within a health system, or whose care is financed through a specific health plan or entity. Examples of a discrete population include employees of an organization, members of a health plan, all those within a practice patient panel, or all those enrolled within a particular ACO. The members of a discrete population can be known with some certainty. At the macro-level *regional/community populations* are inclusive population segments, defined geographically or demographically. People within a segment of a community population are unified by a common set of needs or issues, such as low-birth weight babies or older adults with complex needs. However, these individuals may receive care from a variety of systems or may be unconnected to care. Micro-level applications of population health principals are considered in more detail in Chap. 8. Box 1.2 discusses various ways of thinking about population health.

Box 1.2: Describing Population Health
In describing population health throughout this document various terms have been utilized. The concept is referred to as a population health "model", a population health "approach", or a population health "perspective". Although it would be helpful if there is one term that applies in all situations when population health is discussed, there is little consensus on population health nomenclature and on more than one occasion Kindig (1997, 2015) has tried to clarify terminology.

From this author's perspective the population health *model* refers to a context for approaching community health improvement. As a context the model attempts to integrate the various component parts of the concept into a systematic framework. A population health *approach* refers to more of a method for improving population health, and, as noted above, to the verb form of population health. Any action taken to improve community health constitute an approach.

A population health *perspective* refers to more of a mindset, a conceptual way of visually the process. In reality, implementing a population health approach requires a different worldview—a worldview that involves not individual patients but groups of consumers, not downstream treatment but upstream prevention, not clinical solutions but serious efforts to address the social determinants of health. With these thoughts in mind, these various terms will continue to be used throughout this document.

Growing numbers of observers are arguing that, in the current environment, we can not improve health status by treating one patient at a time as we have in the past. The pattern of morbidity engendered by the predominance of chronic conditions limits the ability of the healthcare system to reduce the burden of disease. An increasingly complex etiology presents challenges in the diagnosis and treatment of contemporary health problems. The growing impact of the social and physical environments and of lifestyles on the health status of the population further limits the contribution that medical care can make to reducing morbidity. It is being increasingly argued that the social, demographic and psychographic attributes of healthcare consumers play a greater role in determining population health status than does the healthcare system. These attributes of healthcare consumers are even thought to influence clinical outcomes. The population health movement is predicated in part on the conviction that our society cannot improve the health status of the population through "business as usual" but must transition into an approach that considers the social determinants of health problems and "treats" the population rather than the individual patient.

At the macro-level there is growing concern over the failure of the US healthcare system to improve the overall health status of the population. While the ability of the system to provide state-of-the-art care to individual patients is acknowledged, the system's ability to improve community health status is increasingly being questioned. The fact that the World Health Organization ranked the US system as the 37th best in the world suggests that its impact at the societal level is limited (World Health Organization, 2000). It has been estimated that medical care today contributes only 10% to observed differences in health status, and there is some evidence that Americans are actually getting sicker after a century of steady health status improvement.

One development that should be noted that ties back into the macro-level discussion involves a provision of the Patient Protection and Affordable Care Act (ACA) of 2010. Given the concern over the perceived lack of improvement in community health, the ACA mandates that not-for-profit hospitals conduct a community health needs assessment at least every three years. They must submit a report to the Department of Health and Human Services that documents the "community benefits" they are providing. This is an important consideration in that such hospitals' continued tax-exempt status will be contingent upon this documentation as well as the requisite forms required by the Internal Revenue Service. Not-for-profit hospitals must demonstrate an understanding of the health status of the communities they serve and the health problems facing residents of those communities. This is a major shift in emphasis in that their responsibilities are extended beyond their own patients to the needs of the general population. Not only must not-for-profit hospitals be knowledgeable concerning the needs of the community, they must certify that they have plans in place for addressing identified deficiencies in the provision of care to the community.

An aspect of population health that is particularly relevant to providers who confront these challenges relates to the role that non-medical factors play in the onset and progression of illness. As noted above, the population health approach is premised in part on the conviction that the social and physical environments and lifestyles—that is, non-medical aspects of health and illness—must be addressed in order to improve community health. Box 1.3 describes situations where a population health approach may be appropriate.

Box 1.3: What Do These Scenarios Have in Common?

The following scenarios might be thought of as illustrating issues increasingly common among healthcare entities:

- A hospital is penalized for unacceptably high rate of readmissions within 28 days
- A hospital realizes that its outcomes vary widely based on the demographic characteristics of its patients
- A provider loses the panel of patients allocated by a managed care plan due to failure to meet health status benchmarks
- An employee assistance provider loses money due to the high level of over-utilization of some services and under-utilization of others
- A behavioral health organization loses its contract with a state insurance plan due to its inability to effectively communicate with its plan members
- A Medicaid managed care organization loses money due to its inability to manage the utilization of its services by its enrollees
- A hospital is reprimanded by the IRS for failure to take the needs of the service area population into consideration in the preparation of it needs assessment
- A county government is faced with escalating healthcare costs due to excessive preventable admissions and inappropriate use of the emergency room at its public hospital
- An accountable care organization (ACO) fails to quality for "shared savings" under its contract with Medicare

The factor that all of these entities have in common is the need to address the issues affecting a *population*, a need that cannot be addressed using traditional methods. These challenges cannot be met by providing clinical care to individual patients. And they cannot be met unless the entity has a much more in-depth (and more nuanced) understanding of the characteristics of the affected population.

The challenges facing these organizations include cost containment, patient management, community health improvement, appropriate utilization and member retention among others. Despite these disparate challenges all are faced with the need to adopt a population health approach, an approach that allows them to view the challenge in terms of groups of people—whether they be patients, consumers, plan members, employees or others—who can be profiled in terms of their salient characteristics and be served, assessed, and managed using methods that address the groups (and subgroups) in a wholesale manner.

Attributes of Population Health

One way in which to clarify the definition of population health may be to identify the attributes thought to characterize this model. While there is still disagreement as to the exact nature of the population health model, the following attributes are thought to be salient.

1. *Recognition of the social determinants of health*. An emphasis on understanding the social determinants of health is critical to the population health model, and the importance of social pathology over biological pathology must be recognized. Social factors are powerful determinants of health status (and health services utilization). As the nature of the health problems affecting the US population has changed, the influence of social factors on health status and health behavior has become more obvious. Depending on the source it could be argued that social determinants account for 40–60% of the variation in health status among subgroups of the population. If social factors are considered the root cause of observed health problems, any solution should take these factors into consideration.
2. *Focus on populations (or subpopulations) rather than individuals*. The focus is on measuring the health status of the total population rather than simply aggregating the clinical results (e.g., reduction of A1C, blood pressure) for individual patients. Since regulators, payers and other evaluators will increasingly reward healthcare providers for their effectiveness in managing groups of patients, consumers or plan members, the attributes characterizing targeted populations will become increasingly important.
3. *Shift in focus away from patients toward consumers*. Once the healthcare industry was introduced to marketing in the 1980s, it was inevitable that "patients" would come to be seen as "consumers". The trend was already underway with baby boomers who were demanding that they be treated by the healthcare system in the manner that they were used to being treated by other entities. They wanted the benefits of quality care as patients coupled with the efficiency, convenience and value that they had come to expect as consumers in other arenas. This represented a significant conceptual leap for healthcare providers and one that foretold the future direction of the healthcare industry and, inadvertently, the emergence of a population health approach.
4. *Geography as a predictor of health status and health behavior*. There is increasing recognition of the importance of the spatial dimension in the distribution of health and ill-health. One of the most significant—and some would say disturbing—findings from decades of health services research is that the utilization of health services varies in terms of geography. Where one lives is a powerful determinant of the kind and amount of medical care received. Rates for various procedures may vary by as much as a factor of 10, reflecting local practice patterns, insurance coverage, availability of services and consumer lifestyles. Now, it has been determined that one's ZIP Code of residence is the best predictor of one's health status and, by extension, health behavior (Roeder, 2014). This would

explain the fact that certain communities exhibit persistent health problems over time regardless of who resides in the community.

5. *Health status defined at the community level*. A community-based (participatory) understanding of what the critical health issues are is a prominent feature of population health. While some argue that community health status represents the sum total of the health status of the individuals within the community, a population health approach would posit the existence of a state of health independent of the health of the individuals who make up the population (The significance of a relevant definition for health status is such that a later chapter is devoted to the topic.)

6. *The limited role of medical care* It has become increasingly clear that there is no evidence that more care translates into better health. Indeed, a premise of the population health model is that health services make a limited contribution to the overall health status of the population. As the US population consumes increasing amounts of healthcare resources per capita, our health status is not improving and may, in fact, be declining. It actually appears that the emphasis on medical care may be contributing to adverse effects, with medical errors currently the third leading cause of death.

7. *Role of the group in health behavior decisions*. As noted above, health status and the decisions made with regard to health behavior are not thought to be the result of individual volition but reflect the impact of the individual's social context, cultural milieu and life circumstances. The population health model recognizes that improvement in personal health status needs to be addressed within the context of the social or community environment in a manner that capitalizes on group influence. Even personal lifestyles (so important in determining health status) might be thought to reflect the influence of the social groups with which individuals are affiliated (See Box 1.4.).

8. *Traditional metrics used to measure health status may not be appropriate*. The ways in which health status has been historically measured depend on indicators that have relevance for health professionals. Not surprisingly these indicators represent a biomedical bias. Any assessment of health status should reflect the perspectives of the community rather than those imposed externally by health professionals. The problems identified through community input are not likely to correspond with those recognized by the healthcare establishment.

9. *Community involvement in health status improvement*. On the assumption that the healthcare system—certainly not alone—cannot improve the health of the population, the responsibility falls to the larger community. No one organization can have a significant impact on the health status of the community's population especially in light of the variety of factors that are now known to influence health. Involvement by a wide range of community organizations—supported by but not led by the healthcare system—is necessary to create the collective impact that is necessary to make a difference. This includes involvement by representatives of the education, housing, economic development, criminal justice, and transportation sectors. Involvement on the part of government agencies related to policy making is critical for the generation of the collective impact necessary to improve

community health. (Although the community is ultimately seen as the driver for population health improvement, this attribute is listed last since most of the previous attributes are prerequisites for multi-sector community collaboration.) Box 1.4 highlights the importance of group influences on decision making for healthcare consumers.

> **Box 1.4: The Myth of Individual Decision-Making**
> A common refrain whenever the plight of poor people is discussed is the contention that their condition can be attributed to bad choices that they have made in their lives. In order to accept this version of "blaming the victim", a number of assumptions must be made.
>
> Assumption 1: People act of their own volition, identifying options, weighing the relative merits and making a rational decision
> Assumption 2: There are in fact options available to members of disadvantaged populations
> Assumption 3: People know what the options are and are able to choose among the various possibilities
> Assumption 4: Knowing what the options are creates an opportunity for rational decision making
>
> A realistic assessment of these options when it comes to disadvantaged populations raises a number of issues. First, social scientists argue that we seldom make truly independent decisions without any external influence. In reality, decisions are almost always made within a social context. On a macro level it could be argued that there are always cultural constraints that influence decision making. For example, one's religious convictions may prevent them of taking certain jobs. Further, there are perceptions that have been inculcated due to our social context with regard to acceptable and unacceptable behavior. At a micro level, the role of social support as a positive force and peer pressure (as either a positive or negative force) should not be minimized. One reason that people (especially adolescents) continue to eat fast food and drink soft drinks when they know the health consequences is that acceptance by their peers demands it. Ultimately, the decisions that people make reflect the totality of their social experiences and cultural confines, reinforced by social support and peer pressure.
> The notion that people can make rational choices among the options assumes that they know what the options are. Just as social context influences decision making, it also determines the options that are available to individuals. But do those in disadvantaged populations know what the options are? How would they? If you have never known anyone who has had a job—much less a well-paying job—how would you know that is an option? If you have never known anyone who has been married how would you know that is an option? If you have never known anyone who went to college, how would you

(continued)

Box 1.4 (continued)

know that was an option? If they have never known anyone who didn't use drugs to cope, how would they know this is an option? If a teenage girl has never known any peer who has not had a child at a young age, how would she know that not having a child is an option?

It could be argued that of course people know there are options when it comes to work, marriage, education and so forth, they are just not taking advantage of them. After all, they can see these options played out on television and in the movies. American society has done a good job of, first, limiting the options for the disadvantaged and, second, preventing them from knowing what the options are. The primary mechanism for carrying this out is the pervasive and persistent residential segregation that characterizes US society. By isolating members of disadvantaged populations in areas of like individuals who themselves do not know what the options are guarantees that the worldview of these populations is limited. With regard to role models on television and in the movies, research has found that members of disadvantaged groups consider these to be fairytales perhaps open to a privileged few in society but certainly not to them.

Finally, if one knows the options, it is argued, it simply becomes a matter of making the right choice and choosing the best option. Again, our society has been very successful at limiting access to options even when they are known by members of disadvantaged groups. No one can argue that it is easy for a disadvantaged person to get a job, obtain an education or find adequate housing. Barriers are placed all along the way, limiting access to the options and insuring the likelihood of failure.

The healthcare arena provides an excellent example of how this works. Research has found that members of disadvantaged groups are actually fairly knowledgeable when it comes to health issues. After all, virtually everyone they know has a health problem of some type. And, quite often, they know what causes the health problem and how it can be addressed. There are few impoverished people who do not realize the importance of a healthy diet, but they are relegated to neighborhoods that are food deserts. They realize that they need to exercise to stay healthy, but they are restricted to areas that have limited exercise options and those that are available may be unaffordable.

If they do become ill, there is a good chance they have no healthcare options in their communities. It has become a maxim in our society that the locations of medical services and the locations of poor people are mutually exclusive. Even if there is a clinic within the community, it may not accept poor patients or there may be other barriers like transportation and hours of operation. Limiting access to health insurance for this population represents an additional barrier to access.

Despite the tendency to blame the victim for bad choices, the fact is that the options available to members of disadvantaged populations are limited and, to the extent options exist, they may not be accessible to this population.

What Population Health is <u>Not</u>

While establishing a universally accepted definition of population health is a challenge, a more immediate concern for those attempting to apply the concept in the field is specifying what population health is *not*. As with many new concepts, early proponents attempted to set the parameters of the field on their own terms. This problem appears to be particularly acute when it comes to population health since many different entities representing widely varying perspectives have gotten into the act.

There has been a tendency in the early stages of the development of the concept to conflate population health with other existing activities. This is not surprising since the proponents of these perspectives are operating from their own comfort zones. The confusion this causes can be addressed by attempting to specify the following processes that do not constitute population health:

- Population health is not "public health". Of all of the alternative iterations of population health, public health probably comes closest to the mark. It is argued that the population health movement, if not growing out of public health, was clearly inspired by the community focus of public health initiatives. It also could be argued that if any healthcare domain should have taken the lead in population health it should have been public health. Ultimately, the population health approach, while incorporating some aspects of public health, is much broader, taking into consideration a number of dimensions relative to community health that are beyond the purview of public health. In addition, the population health model can be applied by healthcare organizations in the management of their patients, an option not available within the public health context. (Box 1.5 explains why public health cannot be equated with population health.)
- Population health is not "disease management". Those who are in the trenches of providing healthcare are tempted to equate population health with disease management. Efforts toward monitoring and tracking the characteristics of patients are primarily at the individual level. In the best case, a disease management approach would identify all of those thought to be at risk for a disease and view them as a group for analytical purposes without addressing the factors that influence their health status. In the end, the disqualifying attributes of this approach are its focus on a particular disease (rather than overall health status) and on individual patients.
- Population health is not "patient management". An effort has been made by healthcare providers to broaden the approach to care management by focusing on the patient rather than patient's disease. The objective here is to manage the entire patient—not only the constellation of diseases but the non-medical factors that are under consideration—in an effort to provide more efficient care and improved outcomes. While this represents an improvement over traditional approaches that sought to reduce health problems to the lowest possible level without consideration of external factors, those in the patient management mode continue to focus on the individual patient.

Box 1.5: Why Population Health Is Not Public Health
As population health is a relatively new concept, uncertainties remain over details of how, precisely, it differs from public health. Both are concerned with patterns of health and illness in groups of people rather than in individuals; both monitor health trends, examine their determinants, propose interventions at the population level to protect and promote health, and discuss options for delivering these interventions. The distinction is subtle, but population health is seen as broader, as offering a unifying paradigm that links disciplines from the biological to the sociological. It provides a rational basis for allocating health resources that balances health protection and promotion against illness prevention and treatment.

Public health differs from clinical medicine in its application to populations rather than to individuals, and the population health model advances the application of public health beyond the basics functions of public health such as immunizations and disease control, environmental monitoring, vector control, family planning and nutrition to emphasize the significance of the root causes of health problems in US society—poverty, housing insecurity, lack of job opportunities, poor educational levels and so forth.

Despite the potential for public health to contribute to the population health movement, the distinction between public health and population health is becoming clearer over time. While many activities that fall under the heading of public health may overlap with those that are considered reflective of a population health approach, the focus of public health in general remains too narrow to fit within the parameters of population health. As noted above, most core functions of public health are not particularly supportive of a population health approach.

Even when support for a more broad-based effort is espoused, public health authorities face significant challenges in getting beyond institutional constraints. Public health, in fact, retains something of the one bug/one drug/one shot mentality that served it so well during the twentieth century. While monitoring and surveillance are important functions, they are essentially downstream activities. They determine when the horse has already left the barn or, best case, when the horse is leaving the barn. Even when addressing broader issues (e.g., environmental toxins) the response is typically more reactive than proactive.

Public health initiatives that attempt to impact the behavior of people tend to emphasize the steps that individuals can take themselves to improve their personal health status. While there is no overt attempt to blame the victim, social marketing (e.g., smoking cessation) and health education (e.g., healthy diet) are premised on the notion that members of the targeted population are involved in inappropriate behavior. In order to improve their health they must change their behavior. While these efforts represent a sort of mass marketing, their success depends on the changes in the behavior of individual actors. (To

(continued)

> **Box 1.5** (continued)
>
> be fair, the nationwide initiative to reduce smoking involved a variety of other components and, in that regard, came much closer to a population health approach.)
>
> When public health tackles a health issue, its interventions are focused on maintaining health or preventing disease. For example, the public health approach to childhood obesity might advocate education for parents and children, subsidized healthy school lunch programs, bans on soft drinks in school vending machines, tougher regulations on marketing of junk food to children, etc. A population health approach would tackle childhood obesity in a broader context. A population health approach might, for example, consider the food system itself: How do agricultural subsidies affect the price of food? Can planning policies address the problem of urban food deserts? The population health approach views issues from a broader perspective and tends to include additional considerations, such as economics, environmental sustainability, social justice, etc.
>
> The embrace of the population health model requires a conceptual shift. The view of a population as an aggregate of individuals focuses on health *in* the population. By contrast, when the population is seen in emergent terms, as an interacting whole, the focus is on the health *of* the population. In this view, a healthy community or population is one that works as a group to promote its welfare and address challenges. A healthy population supports and promotes the health of people within it, thereby contributing to individual health; examples include social equity legislation and the development of healthy public policies that characterize a society sensitive to the root causes of ill-health. (Additional discussion of the role of public health is provided in Chap. 4.)
>
> When these factors are considered *in toto* it can be argued that public health simply has not grasped the vision of population health. Under other circumstances public health professionals should be expected to be champions for the model and take the lead in its implementation. Public health would be the natural "home" for population health but through an unfortunate confluence of forces our nation's public health establishment is likely to be a spectator vis-à-vis the emerging population health movement.

- Population health is not "case management". The rationale for the case management model comes closer to the population health model than most approaches. Case management involves theoretically at least the consideration of all factors—medical and non-medical—that might affect the health and well-being of the "case". While the consideration of non-medical factors is certainly laudable, the fact that issues are being addressed one case at a time leads us back to the original rationale for the development of a population health model.

- Population health is not "population health management". Some observers (e.g., Young, 2016) have suggested that a "perversion" of the concept of population health has occurred with the emergence of population health management. They feel like the term has been co-opted by those involved in healthcare delivery. This situation is exacerbated by consultants and vendors who tout their population health approaches for managing patient care, controlling utilization or maximizing revenue. While the application of the population health approach to the delivery of care *is* addressed in this text, it is with the caveat that this is not in keeping with the original spirit of the population health approach.

There is one other aspect of population health that bears consideration. Kindig and Stoddard (2003) identify an enterprise they refer to as "population health research." There is no consensus as to the definition of population health research but those involved in in this endeavor represent an interdisciplinary perspective with researchers focusing on the health status and behavior of groups within society. These populations can be defined variously (e.g., workers at a workplace, residents of a neighborhood, people sharing a common race or social status, or the population of a nation). This research seeks to characterize, explain and/or influence the level and distributions of health within and across populations. Researchers in the field view health as the product of multiple determinants that include biologic, genetic, behavioral, social, and environmental components and their interactions with each other. As Kindig and Stoddard noted, the field addresses health outcomes, health determinants, and policies and interventions that link the two in efforts to improve population health and ameliorate health disparities. Research findings to date are included throughout this text and references are provided to on-going sources of new information on the field of population health.

Summary

Despite the growing interest in "population health" on the part of health professionals, policy analysts and government agencies, there is considerable confusion over the actual definition of the term. Different people use the term in different ways adding to the confusion. Several definitions of population health have been offered, with the most frequently cited definition formulated in 2003 by Kindig and Stoddart. This definition reads: *population health represents the health outcomes of a group of individuals, including the distribution of such outcomes within the group.* While the usefulness of this definition is debated, its emphasis on populations and their differential health outcomes represents the essence of the population health approach. Population health policy and research, it is argued, should concentrate on the aggregate health of population groups like those in geographic units (cities, prisons) or ones delineated based on other characteristics (ethnicity, religion, health plan membership). Other definitions have been offered that explicate the connection between social determinants and the health of populations. An effort to clarify the definition involves a dual conceptualization with both a noun and verb component.

In formulating the population health concept, one must consider the different dimensions of the definition, the levels at which the concept is applied, and the directness of the approach employed. Deprez and Thomas attempted to bring some clarity to the issue by making a distinction between population health as a noun and as a verb. As a noun, population health refers to the status of the population reflecting its health and well-being as measured by several population-based measures. As a verb, population health refers to an approach to improving health status that operates at the population rather than the individual (or patient) level. The approach focuses on social pathology rather than biological pathology and involves the "treatment" of conditions within the environment and policy realms in addition to the provision of clinical services to individual patients.

The application of the population health model can be explored at two different levels— a micro-level view that considers population health as it relates to the delivery of care and a macro level view that considers population health from a societal perspective. Micro-level assessments and interventions typically involve patients within a clinical setting or individual consumers involved in prevention or self-treatment activities. In this case, population health principles are adapted to interventions designed for defined populations and not the total community. Micro-level interventions target health determinants in an attempt to improve overall health, rather than to prevent specific diseases by reducing poverty or environmental threats, for example.

The primary emphasis of population health is at the macro-level and focuses on societal factors that affect groups of people rather than individuals. The growing impact of the social and physical environments and of lifestyles on the health status of the population reflects the role that social, demographic and psychographic attributes are playing in the distribution of health and illness. There has been a tendency in the early stages of the development of the concept to conflate population health with other activities that should not be confused with population health.

Although there is no formal agreement as to the attributes of the population health model, the population health approach is thought to involve: the recognition of the social determinants of health problems; a focus on populations (or subpopulations) rather than individuals; a shift in focus away from patients to consumers; the recognition of geography as a strong predictor of health services use; the measurement of health status at the community level; and recognition of the limited role that medical care in play. Importantly the collective impact engendered at the community level through multi-sector collaboration for community improvement is a hallmark of this approach.

Key Points

- Population health is increasingly being recognized as a useful approach to community health improvement.
- As an emerging concept, there is substantial confusion over what population health is and is not.

- "Population health" defined as a noun refers to a population or community's health status defined in terms appropriate for a population health approach.
- "Population health" defined as a verb refers to a methodology for improving community health that takes social determinants and other non-health factors into consideration.
- The population health approach represents a response to the realization that the US healthcare system can make a limited contribution to community health improvement.
- The attributes that define population health are:

  - Recognition of the social determinants of health
  - Focus on populations rather than individuals
  - Shift in emphasis from patients to healthcare consumers
  - Geography as a predictor of health status and health behavior
  - Health status assessed from the perspective of the community
  - A limited role for the healthcare system
  - Significance of group influences on health status and health behavior
  - A revised conceptualization of health status
  - Community involvement for generating collective impact on community health status

- Population health is *not* public health, disease management, patient management, case management or population health management.

References

- Deprez, R., & Thomas, R. (2017). Population health improvement: It's up to the community—Not the healthcare system. *Maine Policy Review Spring, 25*(2), 44–52.
- Frank, J. (1995). Why 'population health'? *Canadian Journal of Public Health, 86*, 162–164.
- Hagland, M. (2013). What federally qualified health centers can teach their provider peers about data and population health. *Health Informatics*. Downloaded from URL: http://www.healthcare-informatics.com/article/what-federally-qualified-health-centers-can-teach-their-provider-peers-about-data-and-popula.
- Health and Welfare Canada. (1994). *Strategies for population health: Investing in the health of Canadians*. Health Canada.
- Jacobson, D. M., & Teutsch, S. (2013). *An environmental scan of integrated approaches for defining and measuring total population health*. Downloaded from URL: http://www.rethinkhealth.org/resources/an-environmental-scan-of-integrated-approaches-for-defining-andmeasuring-total-population-health-by-the-clinical-care-system-the-government-public-health-systemand-stakeholder-organizations/.
- Kindig, D. A. (1997). *Purchasing population health: Paying for results*. University of Michigan Press.
- Kindig, D. A. (2007). Understanding population health terminology. *The Milbank Memorial Fund, 85*(1), 139–161.
- Kindig, D. A. (2015). *What are we talking about when we talk about population health?* Downloaded from URL: http://healthaffairs.org/blog/2015/04/06/what-are-we-talking-about-when-we-talk-about-population-health/.

Kindig, D. A., & Isham, G. (2014). Population health improvement: A community health business model that engages partners in all sectors. *Frontiers of Health Services Management, 30.4* (Summer): 3–20, 56–57.
- Kindig, D. A., & Stoddard, G. (2003). What is population health? *American Journal of Public Health, 93*, 366–389.
- Last, J. M. (2007). *A dictionary of public health*. Oxford University Press.

Raths, D. (2015). Getting beyond encounter-based care to include social determinants. *Healthcare Informatics*. Downloaded from URL: http://www.healthcare-informatics.com/blogs/david-raths/getting-beyond-encounter-based-care-include-social-determinants.
- Roeder, A. (2014). *Zip code better predictor of health than genetic code*. Downloaded from URL: http://www.hsph.harvard.edu/news/features/zip-code-better-predictor-of-health-than-genetic-code/.

Scottish Public Health Observatory. (2014). *Community well-being: Key points*. Downloaded from URL: http://www.scotpho.org.uk/life-circumstances/community-wellbeing/key-points.

Tompkins, C., Higgins, A., Perloff, J., et al. (2013). Population health management in Medicare advantage. *Health Affairs*, April 2, 2013. Downloaded from URL: http://healthaffairs.org/blog/2013/04/02/population-health-management-in-medicare-advantage/.

World Health Organization. (2000). *The world health report 2000*. World Health Organization.
- Young, T. K. (1998). *Population health: Concepts and methods*. Oxford University Press.

Young, T. K. (2016). *Personal correspondence on the use/misuse of the population health approach.*

Additional Resources

Population health blog: improvingpopulationhealth.org.

Maraccini, A. M., Galiatsatos, P., Harper, M., et al. (2017). Creating clarity: Distinguishing between community and population health. *The American Journal of Accountable Care, 5*(2). Downloaded from URL: https://www.ajmc.com/view/creating-clarity-distinguishing-between-community-and-population-health.

Riegelman, R. (2020). *Population health: A primer*. Jones and Bartlett.

Rosario, C. (2021). *The difference between population health and public health*. Downloaded from URL: https://www.adsc.com/blog/the-difference-between-population-health-public-health#:~:text=Scientists%20define%20population%20health%20with,professionals%20do%20their%20job%20properly.

Chapter 2
The Road to Population Health: A Changing Society

The emergence of population health as a strategic approach to addressing the health needs of the population can be traced to developments that have taken place over the past 25 years in US society. Without the changes that affected the characteristics of Americans toward the end of the twentieth century, we would probably not be discussing the topic of population health. While these changes have substantially transformed the American population, it is the implications of these changes for the health of the population that are particularly germane to the discussion of population health.

In this chapter, the reader will:

- Learn about developments in US society over the past quarter of a century that have modified the context for the operation of the healthcare system
- Understand how social changes have interfaced with developments within the healthcare system itself to affect the health status of the population
- Be exposed to the extent to which the new conditions of life in America have limited the effectives of our healthcare delivery system
- Understand how these developments have highlighted the need for a new paradigm in healthcare and fostered the emergence of the population health model

Introduction

The emergence of the population health movement did not occur in a vacuum but developed over a period of time within the context of a changing society. A number of developments in US society over the past three decades have helped to create an environment that is fertile for the emergence of a population health model. The convergence of a number of trends created a situation that is dynamic and unlike anything previously experienced by the US population. It is within the

© The Author(s), under exclusive license to Springer Nature
Switzerland AG 2021
R. K. Thomas, *Population Health and the Future of Healthcare*,
https://doi.org/10.1007/978-3-030-83887-4_2

context of this new social mosaic that the population health model has taken root. A variety of different trends inside and outside of healthcare contributed to the birth of the population health movement, and the major social developments in this regard are summarized in the sections that follow. (Developments within healthcare itself that reflect the changing nature of American society are considered in the next chapter.)

Changing Population Characteristics

Any healthcare system should be responsive to the characteristics of the population it serves. A population's demographic makeup is a critical determinant of the type of health services it needs and wants. As modern medicine developed in the United States in the post-WWII years, it was shaped by the health problems of the time. The population to be served was relatively young, primarily white, and increasingly middle class. Most adults were married and living in "intact" households. There was an unprecedented surge of births as America made up for lost time with regard to fertility. The "baby boom" generation constituted the largest age cohort to date, and, in contrast to past cohorts, most of these boomer babies survived infancy. Few women worked outside the home, and a majority of households included children. During the three decades following the war, immigration was at the lowest level it had been since the Great Depression, and the various minority groups truly represented statistical and cultural minorities.

The expansion of the US population, thanks to the baby boomers, was accompanied by an expansion of the healthcare system. The "golden age" of American medicine described in the next chapter witnessed an expansion of the healthcare institution in every conceivable manner. Life-saving drugs supplemented the vaccines that had been introduced in earlier years, and the battlefield experience gained during World War II introduced advanced surgical techniques to the general public. The scope of medicine expanded dramatically as new procedures and new technologies allowed clinicians to treat an ever-expanding range of problems—problems that now extended beyond the traditional ills to conditions historically thought beyond the purview of medical doctors.

For two or three decades after the war there was a comfortable fit between the healthcare system and the needs of the population it served. The healthcare system practiced what could best be described as white middle-class medicine with increasingly standardized protocols for assuring a consistent quality of care. Health insurance had become widespread, and there was a cozy relationship between health service providers and the insurance industry. The health status of the population steadily improved, and much of the credit was accorded to a healthcare system that inspired awe. Although public health measures were actually responsible for much of the improvement in health status, feats of "heroic" medicine captured the spotlight and held the general public in awe.

The primary health conditions characterizing the population in the post-war period were the acute conditions associated with a young and relatively healthy population. These conditions included respiratory diseases, gastrointestinal disorders, ear and throat infections, and, until the post-war period, the communicable diseases that had dominated the morbidity profile throughout the twentieth century. Add to these the accidents and injuries characteristic of a younger population, and a morbidity profile that is receptive to the application of "modern medicine" emerges. These needs tapered nicely with the capabilities of a system of care operating within the context of the germ theory.

"Allopathic" medicine emerged as a response to common health conditions whose biological etiology could be countered with antibiotics. The emphasis was on treatment and cure as the antidote for the predominant health conditions. Because most health problems were thought to be caused by biological pathogens, few healthcare providers emphasized prevention. The population was after all at the mercy of factors that could not be foreseen. Given the disease profile of the US post-war population the favored therapeutic modalities of drugs and surgery were considered appropriate.

While the one-size-fits-all healthcare system that evolved was effective in responding to the healthcare needs of the majority of the population, there were small but significant minority groups that did not realize the benefits of modern medicine. African Americans, in particular, were often excluded from the system's expanding capabilities—either deliberately early on or *de facto* during later years. If people did not fit the mold of white middle-class patients, they were often labeled as "bad patients" and treated accordingly. This situation was not limited to minority group members but also included poor people who were often excluded from the system or shunted off to inferior public services.

Efforts to accommodate patients that did not fit within the medical care model resulted in a dual healthcare system that included state-of-the-art treatment for white, well-insured patients and a poorly funded system of clinics and charity hospitals for the rest of the population. This development is important to note in that it planted the seeds for the significant health disparities that would become increasingly glaring over time. By the beginning of the twenty-first century these disparities had generated enough attention that they played an instrumental role in the search for a new healthcare paradigm.

A number of related trends converged to create an environment that would ultimately require a new paradigm for addressing America's healthcare needs. The societal trends described below ultimately laid the groundwork for a new approach to community health improvement.

The Changing Age Structure

The most significant demographic trend during the last quarter of the twentieth century was the aging of the US population. The importance of this phenomenon for health status, health behavior and the operation of the healthcare system cannot be overstated. By the last quarter of the twentieth century social observers were calling attention to the changing age structure of the US population. During the post-war period when women were having babies at a rate not experienced in "modern times", the United States exhibited a population pyramid similar to that of many less developed countries. By the end of the baby boom, the US population had developed a unique population structure.

As the population began to age following the baby boom the median age increased from a low of less than 28 years in 1970 to a high of over 38 years in 2019. The 1970 US population was by far the youngest the United States had been since the Great Depression and today's median age is the highest in history by far. By the end of the twentieth century, the nation's youngest age cohorts had ceased to grow. Some younger cohorts (i.e., those 25–34) had begun to experience a net loss of population as we entered the twenty-first century. Despite early predictions of a society that was growing older by the day, the trend was generally ignored and, in healthcare as elsewhere, America woke up one morning to find out that it had indeed aged significantly.

The movement of the baby boomers out of the "middle ages" made 45–65 year olds the largest age cohort in the first decade of the twenty-first century. Seniors became the fastest growing age group—abetted by the aging of the baby boomers—with the oldest-old (i.e., 85 years and above) outstripping other age groups in terms of growth rates. The proportion of the population 65 or older stood at over 16% in 2019 compared to 9% in 1960.

The baby boom cohort that dominated the last quarter of the twentieth century grew up in affluence and comfort and its members were used to having things, including their health, in working order. Boomers are now in the process of reinventing retirement just as they have influenced other social phenomena along the way. Boomers have already influenced the healthcare delivery system in significant ways, and now they are driving the demand for a wide range of services tailored to the needs of older adults.

Interestingly, health policy analysts had viewed the aging of the baby boom generation with trepidation on the assumption that, after its oldest members reached 65, there would be a surge of demand for health services—a surge for which the system was unprepared. Although the oldest of the baby boomers will be 75 by the time this book is published, the healthcare system has so far been spared the pressure on services that was anticipated. This reflects that fact that baby boomers are healthier than previous generations, allowing end-of-life services to be deferred for approximately a decade. However, as baby boomers contend with the onset of chronic disease and the natural deterioration that comes with aging increasing pressure will be put on the healthcare system.

While the population cannot expect to continue to age indefinitely, it will be a while before the median age tops out. This aging process would be even more obvious without the contribution of millions of young immigrants to the population. The changing age structure more than any other variable has laid the groundwork for the emergence of the population health movement. This process has not just created an age structure unprecedented in US society but has been the driving force in the epidemiological transition that has dramatically changed the nature of morbidity within the US population. Box 2.1 describes the epidemiological transition and its implications for America's morbidity profile.

> **Box 2.1: The Epidemiologic Transition**
> During the twentieth century, the United States and most other developed countries experienced an "epidemiologic transition". The transition involved a shift from a predominance of acute conditions to a predominance of chronic conditions for the affected populations. This phenomenon was primarily a consequence of the demographic transition occurring earlier in the century along with advances in society's ability to manage health problems. In the former case, the aging of the population resulted in a dramatic change in the types of health conditions affecting its members. In the latter, the introduction of public health measures and, to a lesser degree, advances in clinical medicine eliminated certain health conditions and inadvertently brought other conditions to the fore.
>
> While acute conditions typically result from pathogens in the environment or accidents, chronic diseases are characterized by a much more complex etiology. Acute conditions affect a cross-section of the population sometimes seemingly at random; chronic diseases are much more selective in their impact. In the twentieth century, emergent chronic diseases reflected the combined effect of heredity, environment, lifestyles and even access to healthcare. From a demographic perspective, this meant that, for the first time, demographically related disparities in health status would become common.
>
> Prior to the epidemiologic transition, the most common health conditions were respiratory conditions, gastrointestinal conditions, infectious and parasitic diseases, and injuries. Even today, in traditional societies and populations with a younger age structure, cholera, yellow fever, skin diseases, nutritional deficiencies and similar acute conditions are common. In the wake of the epidemiologic transition, populations in developed countries and those with older populations develop a morbidity profile characterized by heart disease, cancer, diabetes, arthritis, chronic respiratory diseases and similar chronic conditions. As a practical matter, most members of traditional societies did not live long enough to contract chronic conditions and, when they did, these conditions could not be managed and early death likely ensued.
>
> (continued)

> **Box 2.1** (continued)
>
> It was not until the epidemiologic transition was well underway that the focus in medical science began to shift away from acute conditions to chronic conditions. This shift has been a difficult transition for the US healthcare system due to the complexity of chronic disease etiology, its unpredictable progression, and its management challenges. More attention is now being paid to disease etiology (and, subsequently, disease prevention), disease progression and management and, importantly, the demographic disparities associated with chronic disease.
>
> For those involved in the provision of care and others concerned about the population's morbidity profile, the shift from a predominance of acute conditions to a predominance of chronic conditions has been momentous and created an environment that spawned the population health movement. Since the US healthcare system was initially designed to respond to acute conditions, the epidemiological transition ultimately resulted in a mismatch between the healthcare needs of the population and the ability of the system to address them.

The Changing Sex Ratio

An inevitable accompaniment to the aging of America has been the "feminization" of its population. Generally speaking, the older the population the greater the "excess" of females. Except at the very youngest ages, females outnumber males in every age cohort. Among seniors, females outnumber males two to one, and, at the oldest ages, there may be four times as many women as men. In 2019, the excess of females over males in the US population amounted to five million. (This figure is actually down from previous years due to the influx of millions of younger—and proportionately more male—immigrants. The immigration restrictions enacted by the Trump administration and the current pandemic have reduced immigration and affected the sex ratio. It is likely that subsequent years will see a rewidening of the male-female gap.)

As a result of this trend, the female healthcare "market" is considerably larger than the male market. Not only do women constitute a numerical majority but women are more aggressive users of health services than men. Women bear much of the burden for healthcare decision making, not only for themselves but for their families, and they are more likely to influence the health behavior of their peers than men.

Women will increase as a proportion of the total population and are particularly dominant among the patient population. Women accounted for 51% of the population in 2019 but 56% of the physician office visits. Today the typical patient in a doctor's waiting room is a 50-year-old female. If one were to extrapolate the amount of healthcare-consuming years for males and females, respectively, at age 50, we would find that the females in the US population would generate 100 million life-years more than males over the lifecycle.

The emerging female majority has had a significant impact on both health status and health behavior. The types of health problems that characterize females are clearly different from those that affect males, and we now realize that the same disease may affect men and women in different ways. At the same time, women exhibit different attributes related to health behavior. To the extent that health disparities affect the overall health status of the population, we find that females suffer disproportionately from health problems (of almost all types), are treated differently by healthcare providers, and exhibit less favorable outcomes for many types of treatment. These are issues that certainly must be addressed by the emerging population health model.

Growing Racial and Ethnic Diversity

Another demographic trend that had its origin in the last half of the twentieth century is the increasing level of racial and ethnic diversity. The racial and ethnic profile of the US population has been greatly altered since the 1980s. Increasing racial and ethnic diversity has been driven by unprecedented levels of immigration and higher fertility rates for virtually every ethnic and racial minority. America has once again become a nation of immigrants, with the number of newcomers from foreign lands during the period 1990 through 2017 exceeding historic highs. Prior to the policy changes introduced by the Trump administration, the United States welcomed around one million legal immigrants per year. In addition, long-established ethnic and racial minorities continued to grow at faster rates than native-born whites.

The cumulative effect of the trends of the past several years has been a diminishing of the relative size of the white population (especially the non-Hispanic white population) and the growing significance of the African-American, Asian and Hispanic components of the US population. Current estimates reveal an America that is becoming less "white", with percentage increases noted in the African-American, Asian-American, Hispanic and American Indian/Alaskan Native populations juxtaposed against a proportionally smaller white population. Assuming that population growth over the next two decades will return to pre-Trumpian and pre-pandemic levels, most population growth will be a function of immigration. (A telling statistic is the fact that, in 2019 racial and ethnic minorities accounted for 40% of the total population but 50% of the children under 5.)

Given that the US healthcare system has historically been geared to the needs of the mainstream white population, the trend toward greater racial and ethnic diversity cannot help but have major implications for its operation. The proliferation of distinct racial and ethnic minorities has implications for health status, health behavior, and the demands placed on the system. The significance of these trends is made all the more important by the documented level of disparities affecting racial and ethnic groups in the US. Ethnic patients will continue to grow in numbers and diversity, and the twenty-first century will come to be considered the era of the vanishing white patient. Increasingly diverse healthcare consumers will have new and often

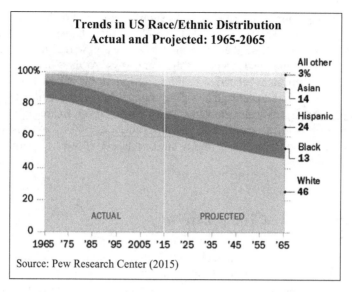

Fig. 2.1 Trends in US Race/Ethnic Distribution Actual and Projected: 1965–2065. (Source: Pew Research Center (2015))

unique requirements as well as different expectations of the healthcare system. Figure 2.1 presents actual and projected trends in the population's racial and ethnic composition.

Any effort to engage the population in desired health behavior must take into consideration its changing racial and ethnic characteristics and the demands that these changes will make on the system. From a population health perspective any efforts toward community health improvement must consider the significance of various racial and ethnic groups.

Changing Household and Family Structure

Another demographic development contributing to the changing society is the transformation of the nation's household and family structures that began in the last quarter of the twentieth century. Sometimes referred to as the "second demographic transition", this trend involves a major reshuffling of the population in terms of marital status and household structure. For decades the family has been undergoing change. First it was high divorce rates, then it was less people marrying (and those who did marry marrying at a later age); then it was less people having children (and those that did having fewer of them and at a later age). The average age at first marriage in 1960 was 22.8 years for males and 20.3 years for females. This contrasts with figures of 29.8 years and 28.0 years, respectively, for 2019 (U.S. Census Bureau, 2020a). The average number of children produced per woman was 1.93 in 2019 compared to 2.33 in 1960 (U.S. Census Bureau, 2020b).

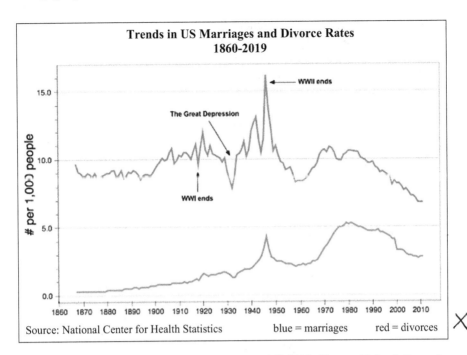

Fig. 2.2 Trends in US marriages and divorce rates 1860–2019. (Source: National Center for Health Statistics)

The transformation of US households has been dramatic. In 2019, the Census Bureau (2020b) reported that 52% of the US population age 15 and over was married, a very low figure by historical standards. Some 31% had never married, 11% were divorced, and 6% were widowed. These figures for the never married and divorced approach historic highs. The respective figures for the 1960 population are: 68% married, 22% never married, 3% divorced and 7% widowed. In two generations the US population was transformed from one of the world's most married populations to one of the world's least married. Figure 2.2 presents historical trends in marriage and divorce rates.

These changes in marital status have had major implications for US household structure. It has meant that what is popularly considered the "typical" American family (with two parents and x number of children) has become a rarity. According to the American Community Survey, only 18% of the households in 2019 fell into this "traditional" category. Today, married couple households (without children) have become the most common household but still only accounting for less than 29% of the total. This development means that family households accounted for only 64% of total households in 2019, compared to 75% in 1960. "Non-traditional" households have become the norm, and an unprecedented proportion of households are one-person households.

Health status and health behavior differ considerably among the various marital statuses. To a great extent, health services have been historically geared to the needs of traditional households involving two parents and one or more children. This has been encouraged by the extensive provision of employer-sponsored insurance that focused on the wage-earning head of household.

Further, marital status, household structure and living arrangements constitute aspects of life circumstances that influence health-related attributes. As with marital status, the changing household structure has important implications for both health status and health behavior. The demands placed on the healthcare system by two-parent families, single-parent families, and elderly people living alone are significantly different from each other and require different responses on the part of the system. The continued diversification of US household types for the foreseeable future is likely to require commensurate modifications in the healthcare delivery system.

Changing Lifestyles

A major development accompanying, and to a great extent driving, the epidemiological transition has been the changing lifestyles of the US population. While the population was aging it was also experiencing a shift in its lifestyle characteristics. Perhaps no other societal trend had as much to do with the emergence of a population health perspective as changes in the way Americans lived. "Lifestyles", simply put, refers to patterns of behavior or the way of life characterizing a population. (References are made to an individual's "lifestyle" but it is group patterns of living that are of interest to this analysis.) A lifestyle typically reflects the attitudes, values and worldview of members of a particular group as well as the behavior patterns that reflect these characteristics. A group's lifestyle provides a means of forging a sense of self for the group member and includes the cultural symbols that resonate with personal identity. While individual lifestyles are sometimes considered voluntary, members of various groups tend to have their attitudes and behaviors shaped and ultimately constrained by group norms.

It is also found that there is variation in disease incidence/prevalence based on the lifestyle characteristics of various subpopulations. Although lifestyle clusters often track demographic subpopulations, there is evidence that lifestyles may cut across demographic groups. Thus, the health circumstances of active, healthy seniors may be quite different from those of frail, incapacitated seniors although both groups have similar demographic attributes. The study of the relationship between lifestyles and health status has not been as extensive as that for demographics and health status but, with the emergence of the population health approach, there is likely to be growing interest in the role of lifestyles in affecting the health of subpopulations.

The diseases that have come to be dominant within the US population are increasingly referred to as "diseases of civilization", reflecting the notion that our "civilized" way of life is contributing to our health problems. These diseases appear to increase in frequency as countries become more industrialized and more people live to old age. Chronic conditions of this type are due to the combined effect of a lifetime of stress and wear and tear and the unhealthy lifestyles that have been simultaneously adopted overlaid on a population that is steadily aging. Box 2.2 lists health conditions considered "diseases of civilization".

> **Box 2.2: Diseases of Civilization**
> As the epidemiological transition has unfolded, it has led to a change in the types of health conditions responsible for the bulk of the morbidity—and mortality—in US society…
>
> | | |
> |---|---|
> | Alzheimer's disease | Metabolic syndrome |
> | Atherosclerosis | Crohn's disease |
> | Asthma | Nephritis and chronic renal failure |
> | Cancer | Osteoporosis |
> | Chronic liver disease and cirrhosis | Stroke |
> | Chronic obstructive pulmonary disease | Depression |
> | Type 2 diabetes | Obesity |
> | Heart disease | Sexually transmitted infections |
>
> While most of these conditions were not unknown in pre-modern societies, there occurrence was exceedingly rare if they existed at all. Diets, as sparse as they often were, lacked the types of items that today contribute to poor health status. Exercise was a regular part of everyday life. Importantly, with the short average life expectancy characterizing most premodern societies, people simply did not live long enough to contract most chronic diseases. This was especially true of those that reflected long years of wear and tear.

Today, added to these recognized diseases of civilization, epidemiologists have newly identified a subset of conditions that they refer to as "diseases of despair." The existence of this category of disease came to light with the emergence of the opioid epidemic in the United States. The increase in death rates (and concomitant decline in life expectancy) as we entered the twenty-first century led to the identification of grouping of conditions that included substance abuse (including prescription drugs), alcohol dependency, and depression, often culminating in premature death from liver disease and suicide. Given how ubiquitous diagnoses of heart disease and cancer are, it is noteworthy that these conditions could actually have an impact on the death rate.

One of the consequences of changing lifestyles has been the emergence as obesity as a disease of civilization. Over the past 50 years the US population has become increasingly obese. More than a third of the population are classified as obese and almost two-thirds as overweight or obese. Today, obesity is a concomitant diagnosis for virtually every other condition that is presented for treatment. While obesity represents a health threat in its own right, it serves as a "gateway" for the emergence of many other chronic conditions. Indeed, the increase in obesity among American children has given rise to levels of morbidity in young children unthinkable in the paste. Box 2.3 discusses the link between obesity and morbidity.

The impact of lifestyles can be clearly seen when the health status of immigrants is tracked. As new immigrants spend increasing amounts of time in the

Box 2.3: Obesity and Morbidity

Most of the world's populations throughout history have survived on restrictive diets. The challenge was being able to find enough to eat in order to survive. Thus, obesity is a "disease of civilization" and reflects the lifestyles of populations in modern society. The terms "overweight" and "obesity" refer to body weight that is greater than what is considered healthy for a certain height. People classified as "obese" have an abnormally high and unhealthy proportion of body fat. Body mass index (BMI) is the metric generally used to diagnose overweight or obesity. Obesity is considered a morbid condition in its own right and is associated with a wide range of other health conditions. The trend toward increased levels of obesity within the US population has raised concerns among health professionals over its long-term impact on morbidity. The following disorders are considered to be caused, triggered or exacerbated by obesity.

Coronary Heart Disease

As one's body mass index rises, so does the risk of coronary heart disease (CHD), a condition in which plaque builds up inside the arteries. Plaque can narrow or block the coronary arteries and cause angina or a heart attack. Obesity also can contribute to heart failure and the progressive deterioration of heart function.

High Blood Pressure

The chances of having high blood pressure is greater for people who are overweight or obese. If blood pressure rises and stays high over time, it can damage the body in a variety of ways, making it a predictor of many other health conditions.

Stroke

Being overweight or obese can lead to a buildup of plaque in the arteries. Eventually, an area of plaque can rupture, causing a blood clot to form. Blood in the brain can block the flow of blood and oxygen and cause a stroke. The risk of having a stroke rises as one's body mass index (BMI) increases.

Type 2 Diabetes

In type 2 diabetes, an acquired form of the disease, the body's cells do not use insulin properly resulting in excessive sugar in the blood. Diabetes is a leading cause of early death in its own right but also contributes to the development of CHD, stroke, kidney disease, and blindness. Most people who have type 2 diabetes are overweight.

Cancer

Obesity is associated with increased risks for several types of cancer, including cancers of the esophagus, breast (postmenopausal), endometrium

(continued)

Box 2.3 (continued)

(the lining of the uterus), colon and rectum, kidney, pancreas, thyroid, gallbladder, and, potentially, cancers affecting other sites. The percentage of cancer cases attributed to obesity varies widely for different cancer types but is as high as 40% for some cancers.

Osteoarthritis

Osteoarthritis is a common joint problem of the knees, hips, and lower back. The condition occurs if the tissue that protects the joints wears away. Extra weight can put more pressure and wear on joints, thereby triggering osteoarthritis.

Sleep Apnea

Sleep apnea is a common disorder in which a person has one or more pauses in breathing or shallow breaths during sleep. One cause of sleep apnea is excess fat stored around the neck. This can narrow the airway, making it hard to breathe.

Obesity Hypoventilation Syndrome

Obesity hypoventilation syndrome (OHS) is a breathing disorder that affects some obese people. In OHS, poor breathing results in too much carbon dioxide (hypoventilation) and too little oxygen in the blood (hypoxemia). OHS can lead to serious health problems and may even cause death.

Reproductive Problems

Obesity is associated with several reproductive disturbances due to its effect on the body's metabolism and chemical balance. Increasing evidence points to the long-term impact of early onset (childhood/adolescence) obesity as a predictor of infertility. Obesity is also a contributor to menstrual disorders.

In addition to the above, it is now realized that overweight and obesity also increase the health risks for children and teens. Type 2 diabetes, for example, once was rare in American children, but an increasing number of children are developing the disease today. Also, overweight children are more likely to become overweight or obese as adults, increasing the disease risks noted above.

Source: National Heart, Lung and Blood Institute (2013).

United States their health status declines in keeping with their adoption of American lifestyles. Further, as second- and third-generation immigrants become increasingly vested in the American way of life, they develop morbidity patterns comparable to those of the native-born population. Case Study 2.1 provides an example of the impact of lifestyles on health status.

Case Study 2.1: Lifestyles and Health

The role of lifestyles in promoting or inhibiting health has been clearly documented. While we often think of lifestyles as a reflection of personal preferences, in most case, they reflect social context and collective influences on members of the group in question. This perspective is evident when we see large segments of a population affected *en masse* by lifestyle changes.

A substantial body of research has documented that immigrants are relatively healthier than natives when they arrive in the US (Neuman, 2014). This health advantage is typically attributed to the self-selection process whereby the less healthy are discouraged from immigrating. This initial health advantage, however, deteriorates in accordance with time spent in the US and disappears during the second and third generations. Conditions that were rare in the sending country emerge and a morbidity pattern arises that is comparable to that of native-born Americans. These changes are typically attributed to the adoption of American lifestyles.

These findings are particularly striking when focusing on Hispanics. Since they are characterized by lower socio-economic status than natives, one would expect them to exhibit poorer health status. Yet, immigrants are generally assessed as healthier than native-born Americans. There is evidence, however, of a downward trajectory in health status over time and across generations despite inter-generational improvement in socioeconomic status. This phenomenon has been referred to as the "Hispanic health paradox" (George, 2013). This apparent paradox has been observed in general health status, life-expectancy, mortality due to cardiovascular diseases, cancer, and infant health outcomes. While the socio-economic status of the immigrant subpopulation improves over time and across generations, its health status deteriorates.

Some scholars emphasize the lower incidence of risk-factors among immigrants at the time of migration and of a worsening of behaviors with time spent in the US and across generations (Antecol & Bedard, 2006; Fenelon, 2012). There is evidence of a generational worsening of risky behaviors and health conditions (e.g., smoking, alcohol consumption, and, hypertension), yet second-generation Hispanics still maintain a sizeable health advantage over non-Hispanic white natives. However, the impact of changed behaviors and greater assimilation is evidenced by poorer third-generation health status. This phenomenon even shows up in birth outcomes, with the relatively low initial rate of infant mortality reverting to a level similar to the native-born population (Acevedo-Garcia, 2005).

A major consideration for this analysis on the impact of lifestyles is dietary patterns, particularly in the case of Mexican-Americans where obesity has significantly increased. The majority of the American foods that have been incorporated into the Mexican American diet are carbohydrate heavy and lacking in micronutrients. They are usually highly processed foods with added preservatives such as cookies, chips, crackers, pastries, French fries, and

(continued)

Case Study 2.1 (continued)
sugary cereals. These foods are simple carbohydrates that are flour or potato-based, as opposed to complex carbohydrates that are corn or vegetable based. In addition to the snack foods listed above, frozen and pre-made meals have also been incorporated into the Mexican-American diet. While unhealthy, processed foods that have been added to the Mexican-American diet, fresh fruit has been reduced in importance primarily due to the difficulty in obtaining them (Giuntella, 2012). While clearly more research is necessary, there is evidence that adopting an American lifestyle (particularly with regard to diet) is likely to be detrimental to the health of immigrants and, by the third generation and serves to erase any health advantage exhibited by the immigrant population.

One final point to be made concerning lifestyles relates to the discussion of the demographic correlates of morbidity. As noted above, demographic attributes are incorporated into the development of lifestyle segmentation systems. While psychographics attempt to transcend the limitations of demographic analysis, there is an inherent demographic aspect to any psychographic classification system. Indeed, it could be argued that many psychographic differences identified actually reflect underlying demographic attributes. For that reason certain lifestyles may be associated with specific demographic groups. African-American teenagers, affluent housewives with young children ("soccer moms"), college students and similar demographic groupings come to mind, with their lifestyle attributes tied very closely to their demographic roots. Further evidence of the psychographic/demographic link is provided when observed lifestyles changes as demographic status (e.g., age, marital status, income level) changes.

Changing Patient Characteristics

Today's patients have quite different characteristics than those sitting in the doctor's office during the heyday of allopathic medicine. The demographic trends that played out over the past quarter of a century dramatically reshaped the patient population. Not only did these developments create a population with traits that are mostly unprecedented, their unfolding has major consequences not only for the operation of the healthcare system but for its conceptual underpinnings.

Today's patients are several years older on the average than a generation ago, and the children who were ubiquitous 20 years earlier have become a dwindling population. The proportion of the population that is non-Hispanic white has shrunk considerably, and a majority of school-aged children are now from minority populations. While the greatest increase has been recorded for the Hispanic population, the proportion of citizens from all non-white racial and ethnic groups has increased dramatically bringing considerable diversity to the physician's waiting room. Women continue to outnumber men (by more than five million), meaning that the majority of patients are female. Importantly, the proportion of the population's adults who are married has declined dramatically since the Baby Boom generation. Not only are fewer people marrying but those who do are having fewer children. Thus, fewer patients live in intact families or are even part of a family household. The healthcare system operates to a certain extent on the assumption that people live in families (thus family insurance plans) and that patients, to the extent that providers consider such things, have support in the household to assist with healthcare needs.

This changing patient profile has been accompanied by the transformation of the "patient" into a "consumer". By the end of the twentieth century, fewer health professionals were using the term patient because of its narrow connotation. Patients came to be referred to as clients, customers, consumers, or enrollees. The major consideration, regardless of the label applied, was the fact that clients, customers, consumers, and enrollees all had different characteristics from patients. While "patient" implies a dependent, submissive status, the other terms connote a more proactive involvement in the therapeutic process.

This newly minted consumer exhibited a different attitude, was more knowledgeable about the healthcare system, more open to innovative approaches, and more intent on playing an active role in the diagnostic, therapeutic, and health maintenance processes. This has resulted in a shift from patients as passive recipients of healthcare to consumers as active players in the management of their own health. These new attitudes were fostered by baby boomers (and by extension successive groups of Generation Xers and Millennials) who have been influential in downplaying the importance of physicians and hospitals and providing the impetus for the rise of alternative therapy as a competitor to mainstream allopathic medicine. Baby boomers favor a patient-centered approach to healthcare and are more likely to recognize the nonmedical influences on health and illness.

The fact that patients now had quite different characteristics than those in the past has important implications for the operation of the healthcare system. We realize today that children are different from adults, males are different from females, whites are different from non-whites, the affluent are different from the poverty-stricken and so forth. This precludes the operation of the one-size-fits-all healthcare system of the past. This means that adult medicine (particularly older adult care) has become more important than pediatric care. Geriatric medicine has become a distinct specialty area, and there is increasing attention to long-term care, home healthcare and end-of-life care. Much of the emphasis in female healthcare has shifted from obstetrics to gynecology, and "men's health" has emerged as a specialty area. Cultural competency has become a buzzword as the diversity characterizing the American population has encroached on the healthcare system.

The increasing diversity of the population in general and the patient population in particular has had two major implications for US healthcare. First, as noted above, the patient pool has become increasingly diverse as the number of immigrants has increased over the past two decades. Further, some specialties like obstetrics and pediatrics can be expected to be dominated by minority patients for the foreseeable future. Healthcare providers have had to modify their approaches to care in order to accommodate an increasingly diverse patient pool, translating practice materials into other languages and hiring interpreters for their patients. They have found that it takes more than converting materials into a different language, since many ethnic groups have cultural patterns and social expectations quite different from the historical mainstream patient.

Second, the increased diversity of the patient pool has raised sensitivity with regard to the health disparities that exist. It has long been documented that members of racial and ethnic minority groups often suffer from inordinate health problems, lack access to care, and, when they receive care, are often treated in an inappropriate manner. Pursuing "business as usual" runs the risk not only of alienating a large segment of the patient population but of delivering ineffective care when ethnic perspectives are not taken into consideration. As discussed below, the conditions in which various racial and ethnic groups live and the way they are treated by the system have important implications for their health status. The health disparities that have emerged due to a failure of the system to accommodate a diverse patient population have contributed to the emergence of the population health model. Box 2.4 addresses the issue of distribution of disease within the population.

Box 2.4: Patterns of Disease Distribution

One of the consequences of the changing morbidity profile for the US population is the establishment of distinct patterns of distribution of health and illness. When acute conditions were predominant there were few clear patterns of disease distribution. Virtually everyone was at the same risk of exposure (and death). Communicable diseases were no respecter of age, race, sex or income, and incidence and mortality rates varied little from social group to social group.

Even a casual review of patterns of morbidity in the United States suggests that today's disease patterns are quite different from those exhibited a century ago or even a couple of decades ago. While the nature of morbidity can be expected to change over time in every society—through natural processes if nothing else—the dynamic nature of US society almost guarantees an ever-changing morbidity profile.

While the distribution of acute conditions appears random, chronic conditions affect different subgroups within the population in different ways. The knowledge that our vital processes are socially and economically structured led, in fact, to the emergence of social epidemiology as an analytical

(continued)

Box 2.4 (continued)

framework. As Wilkinson (1996) noted over 20 years ago: Medical science can address the biological pathways involved in disease…, but in so far as health is a social product and some forms of social organisation are healthier than others, advances in our understanding of health will depend on social research.

The emergence of diseases of civilization was accompanied by a clarification of patterns of disease distribution within the population. Early on, only the affluent could "afford" to acquire diseases of civilization (or initially "diseases of affluence" as some would say). Over time there was a change in the social pattern/distribution of diseases through which coronary heart disease, stomach ulceration, stroke and obesity became more common among the poorer segments of affluent societies thereby reversing their previous social distribution. Thus, while chronic conditions affect all segments of US society, their impact is greater on some segments than others.

Significant differences in mortality and morbidity rates continue to exist between income groups and social classes in most developed countries. This salient fact serves to remind us of the continuing importance of social and economic determinants of health. The persistence of poverty within the US population is a key determinant of health status. The existence of the social distribution of disease cuts across the notion of disease as an "autonomous individual affliction" and reflects that fact that the exposure to causative risk factors is a function of the society's social and cultural environment.

Patterns of disease distribution can be analyzed in terms of geographic and demographic dimensions. The geographic distribution of disease is usually top of mind as a result of our exposure to epidemiological studies that compare incidence/prevalence rates for various geographic areas. It is common to initially examine the distribution of a health condition at the state, county, ZIP Code or census tract level. This is useful information in its own right as it provides insights into the spatial aspects of disease distribution and serves as a basis for disease control. More important, however, is the clues that geographic distribution provides with regard to the social distribution of ill-health.

A significant body of research has documented the differential distribution of disease among various subgroups within the US population. An association can be demonstrated between morbidity rates and such factors as age distribution, sex ratio, racial and ethnic makeup, and even attributes such as marital status, income and education. The fact that disease patterns can be determined based on geography is more often than not a function of the demographic attributes of residents of different geographic areas. Evidence of widespread health disparities has been generated based on analyses of the differential distribution of disease among various demographically delineated subpopulations.

Conclusions concerning the distribution of disease based on demographic characteristics has to take into consideration the likelihood of the interaction

(continued)

> **Box 2.4** (continued)
> of various demographic variables. There are correlations, for example, between income and education, with these two variables often interacting with each other. If first-order analyses are conducted, erroneous conclusions may, in fact, be generated. Perhaps the best-known example of this the perceived relationship between race and health status. The generally negative health status associated with African Americans relative to non-Hispanic white Americans can be virtually eliminated when socioeconomic status is factored into the equation (Williams & Collins, 1996).
>
> It is also found that there is variation in disease incidence/prevalence based on the lifestyle characteristics of various subpopulations. Although lifestyle clusters often track demographic subpopulations, there is evidence that lifestyles may cut across demographic groups. Thus, the health circumstances of active, healthy seniors may be quite different from those of frail, incapacitated seniors although both groups have similar demographic attributes. The study of the relationship between lifestyles and health status has not been as extensive as that for demographic and health status but, with the emergence of the population health approach, there is likely to be growing interest in the role of lifestyles in affecting the health of subpopulations.

Changing Disease Etiology

The shift from a predominance of acute conditions to a predominance of chronic conditions has been accompanied by a significant change with regard to disease causation. The major killers a century ago (and throughout human history) could almost invariably be attributed to a single factor. Today's major killers, on the other hand, reflect the interaction of a variety of factors, made possible today by a long life that allows prolonged exposure to carcinogens and the development of degenerative diseases. The contemporary approach to etiology argues for a more complex view of disease causation, one that takes into consideration the interdependence of various biological and non-biological factors.

Disease etiology is considered in this chapter for two reasons: (1) the changing origin of contemporary health problems can be traced to the trends described above, and (2) the ability to implement a population health approach is contingent upon our ability to address factors that contribute to overall health status and the disparities that are observed within the US population.

The growing importance of lifestyles as a determinant of health status is symptomatic of the extent to which the etiology of disease has changed due to the epidemiological transition. Throughout much of the twentieth century it could be argued that society members were "innocent bystanders" when it came to the source of disease. After all, biological pathogens in the environment were responsible for the bulk of the health problems. Exposure to communicable disease was haphazard with disease distribution within the population essentially random.

By the turn of the century this situation no longer existed, as communicable diseases gave way to chronic conditions. Far from being at the mercy of naturally occurring organisms, members of today's population are for the most part active contributors to their own ill health. The health problems that dominate today are reflective of the things that we are doing to ourselves. The US population has transitioned from one that was very active, with many workers still in manual occupations, to one that is very sedentary, from one that walked everywhere to one that seldom walks, from one partaking in a simple diet involving fresh, unprocessed foods to one exiting primarily on processed foods. These trends, it should be noted, do not so much reflect the choices made by individuals but the forces that are brought to play on the population *en masse*. In this regard, societal influences trump individual volition.

In view of changing etiological patterns, it might be worthwhile to first consider the contributors to disease etiology that are becoming less significant. Genetic factors are perhaps the most easily identified of the various contributors to morbidity. Among the many determining factors under consideration, heredity is, in the case of each individual, the one factor which cannot be intentionally altered. Humans are born with a certain genetic makeup which, while heavily influenced by environmental factors, assigns permanent attributes to each individual.

Genetic factors are likely to play some role in high blood pressure, heart disease, and other vascular conditions. However, it is also likely that people with a family history of heart disease share common environments and risk factors that increase their susceptibility. The risk for heart disease can increase even more when heredity is combined with unhealthy lifestyle choices, such as tobacco use and poor dietary habits. Ultimately, it is believed that genetics accounts for less than 10% of the morbidity found within the US population, and this is one determinant that is not likely to be amenable to a population health approach.

While most infectious diseases have been eliminated if not eradicated in modern developed countries, the threat of biological pathogens cannot be entirely removed. Despite extraordinary advances in the management of such diseases, the ease of world travel and increased global interdependence assure the continued impact of such conditions. Public health authorities in the United States must constantly monitor disease trends in order to detect the emergence of new communicable diseases and the re-emergence of old ones. The most salient modern example of an emerging infectious disease is HIV/AIDS, which likely emerged a century ago after the virus jumped from one primate host to another and, as a result of a complex array of social and demographic factors, spread readily within the human population.

The importance of changing lifestyles for the health of the US population cannot be overstated. Diet, physical activity, obesity, alcohol consumption, and cigarette smoking have been associated with increased risk for a wide range of chronic diseases. Dietary practices alone have been found to account for 26% of deaths and 14% of disability-adjusted life-years (Murray, Abraham, Ali et al., 2013). The prevalence of conditions thought to be influenced by obesity has more than doubled during the last 40 years.

Diseases that are not transmitted genetically or via infection are typically considered environmental diseases. It may, however, be more appropriate to refer to them as environment-engendered disorders. Although the morbidity patterns of all societies everywhere have been affected by their environments (after all, biological pathogens are part of the environment), the impact of the physical and social environments has emerged in modern society as a major contributor to the nature and level of morbidity within a population.

Environmental factors (up to and including the impact of climate change) can contribute to the health of the population in a number of ways—at a micro level that affects people in their homes and communities and at a macro level that affects entire populations. The most obvious type of impact would be direct contact with an environmental toxin. This could involve contact with the skin or respiratory intake. Examples of diseases caused by physical factors in the environment include skin cancer caused by excessive exposure to ultraviolet radiation in sunlight and diseases caused by exposure to chemicals in the environment such as toxic metals.

Although direct contact certainly represents a health threat, a much greater threat involves the indirect influence of environmental factors. This would include the transmission of toxins through other often routine means. Thus, people ingest toxins through the water they drink, the food they eat, and the second-hand smoke they breath. Eating, drinking and breathing are obviously routine activities that in a polluted environment put health at risk. Cancer acquired through breathing secondary smoke is a leading example, as are diseases caused by contaminated foods.

In many disorders genetic and environmental factors work together to bring about changes in otherwise normal genes. For example, some forms of radiation or chemicals can cause cancer in people who are susceptible due to their genetic makeup. Subtle differences in genetic factors will cause people to respond differently to the same environmental exposure. This explains why some individuals have a fairly low risk of developing a disease as a result of an environmental insult, while others are much more vulnerable (National Institute of Environmental Health Sciences 2013).

Although the risks of developing chronic diseases are attributed to both genetic and environmental factors, a much higher proportion of disease risks is probably due to differences in environments. The evidence shows that environmental risk factors play at least some role in more than 80% of the diseases regularly reported by the World Health Organization. Globally, nearly one quarter of all deaths and of the total disease burden can be attributed to the environment. In children, however, environmental risk factors can account for slightly more than one-third of the disease burden. (World Health Organization, 2006).

The growing role of the environment has important implications for population health. These changing etiology patterns have significant implications for the emergence of the population health model, making an understanding of the contributors to contemporary morbidity patterns crucial. The range of impacts associated with the environment offer ample opportunity for the application of population health methods. Box 2.5 looks "upstream" to examine the *real* causes of ill-health.

Box 2.5: The Leading Determinants of Health
For at least 20 years the changing nature of the factors that contribute to the health and illness characterizing a given population have been debated. Just as the diseases that affect the US population have changed over the past century, the factors that contribute to observed morbidity patterns have also changed. McGinnis, Williams-Russo and Knickman (2002) have provided a summary (up to that date at least) of the various contributions that different factors make to the amount and nature of ill-health within the population. They envision these factors in five domains.

Genetics is certainly a factor in the health status of the population. Although genetic diseases account for a negligible proportion of deaths, gene defects account for a wide variety of health conditions and may account for up to 60% of late onset diseases such as diabetes and heart disease. Due to the large number of diseases that have some genetic component, the authors estimate that 30% of health conditions can be attributed to heredity.

A population's "social circumstances" has been increasingly cited as a determinant of health and illness. Health is influenced by education, employment, income disparities, poverty, housing, crime and social cohesion. Throughout the life cycle, the social circumstances that affect individuals contribute to their lifestyles and life chances, and exposure to various social factors is likely to affect the status of individuals many years after the fact. Poverty by itself is thought to account for 6% of mortality and presumably a similar or greater amount of morbidity. The ubiquitous nature of social circumstances caused the authors to indicate that they account for 15% of the observed differences in health status.

In considering the impact of environmental factors, the authors include biological pathogens (microbial agents) with hazards in the form of toxic agents (e.g., air/water pollution, occupational products) and structural hazards (e.g., worksite conditions, home hazards). Microbial agents have become less significant as others aspects of the environment have come to the fore. Environmental factors are thought to account for 5% of the observed differences in health status.

According to McGinnis, Williams-Russo and Knickman, behavior patterns represent the most dominant domain of influence over health status today. Referred to elsewhere as "lifestyles" the authors point out the far-reaching influence of patterns of diet, exercise and social behavior. The things that we do to ourselves—what we choose to eat, how much physical activity we participate in and what we do for recreation, for example—all affect our health status. This domain includes the positive steps we take—adequate sleep, use of automobile seatbelts, preventive checkups—and the negative influences that we avoid (or not)—alcohol, tobacco and drug abuse, risky sexual behavior. These factors taken together are thought to account for fully 40% of the observed differences in health status.

(continued)

> **Box 2.5** (continued)
> The authors note that early on various commentators noted the limited impact that medical care actually exerted on the morbidity pattern of our society. While medical care certainly benefits individual patients and available treatments and technology contribute to overall health status to some extent, these benefits are to a certain extent nullified by the negative impact of medical care on people's health. The Centers for Disease Control and Prevention (CDC) have consistently placed the impact of medical care on our population's health at around 10%.
> Braveman (Braveman & Gottlieb, 2014) returned to this topic over a decade later and, in the light of subsequent research, reinforced the initial contentions of McGinnis, Williams-Russo and Knickman, stating:
>> ...[A]dvances in knowledge that have occurred over the past 25 years leave little room for doubt that social factors are powerful determinants of health...[S]trong associations between social...factors and a multitude of health outcomes in diverse settings and populations have been well documented, and the biological plausibility of the influence of social factors on health has been established...[T]he effects of any factor are contingent upon the presence of myriad other factors—social, economic, psychological, environmental, genetic and epigenetic...[A]ppreciation of...the social factors that influence...health status itself can help clinical providers develop more effective treatment plans.

Summary

The emergence of the population health movement did not occur in a vacuum but developed over a period of time within the context of a changing society. Initially, the population to be served was relatively young, primarily white, and increasingly middle class. Most adults were married and living in "intact" households. The expansion of the US population thanks to the baby boomers was accompanied by an expansion of the healthcare system as American medicine found its footing. The scope of medicine expanded dramatically as new procedures and new technologies allowed clinicians to treat an ever-expanding range of problems—problems that now extended beyond the traditional ills to conditions historically thought beyond the purview of medical doctors.

Ever since its emergence as a major institution, the healthcare system has practiced white middle-class medicine with increasingly standardized protocols for assuring a consistent quality of care. While this one-size-fits-all healthcare system was effective at responding to the healthcare needs of the majority of the population, there were small but significant minority groups that did not benefit from modern medicine. Further, poor people were often excluded from the system as well or shunted off to inferior public services. These developments planted the seeds for the significant health disparities that would become increasingly glaring.

The most significant demographic trend during the last quarter of the twentieth century was the aging of the US population. Following the baby boom the median age increased from a low of less than 28 years in 1970 to a high of nearly 38 years, and seniors became the fastest growing age group. The aging of America was accompanied by a surge in the "feminization" of the US population. American society during this period experienced an increasing level of racial and ethnic diversity. The cumulative effect of the trends of the past several years has been a reduction in the relative size of the white population (especially the non-Hispanic white population) and the growing significance of the African-American, Asian and Hispanic components of the US population. Given that the US healthcare system has historically been geared to the needs of the mainstream white population, the trend toward greater racial and ethnic diversity cannot help but have major implications for the operation of the system particularly in view of the documented level of disparities associated with various racial and ethnic groups. The nation's household and family structures also changed dramatically during the last quarter of the twentieth century. Fewer Americans were getting married or having children, and the proportion of single (never married) Americans was at an all-time high The "typical" American family (with two parents and x number of children) had become a rarity, and "nontraditional" households became the norm.

A major development spawned by these trends is the epidemiologic transition. As the US population aged chronic conditions replaced acute conditions as the predominant health problems and the most frequent causes of death. The types of problems being presented at the doctor's office were quite different from just a generation earlier. The patterns of disease distribution that have emerged have served to highlight the disparities between various groups and have provided considerable impetus for the emergence of a population health model.

The demographic trends that played out over the past quarter of the century dramatically reshaped the patient population. Today's patients are several years older on the average than a generation ago, and the children who were ubiquitous 20 years earlier have become a dwindling population. The proportion of the population that is non-Hispanic white has shrunk considerably, and a majority of school-aged children are now from minority populations. Women continue to outnumber men, and the proportion of the population's adults who are married has declined dramatically since the Baby Boom generation. The increasing diversity of the population is having a significant impact on our health care system, and some specialties like obstetrics and pediatrics can be expected to be dominated by minority patients for the foreseeable future.

Ultimately, these developments have contributed to the emergence of the population health model. The surge in chronic conditions has served to exacerbate the health disparities observed within the population. The current characteristics of the US population and its health status profile present a challenge for a healthcare system that is still operating under a twentieth century model.

Key Points

- Changes in the characteristics of the US population laid the groundwork for the emergence of the population health model
- These changes include:
  - The aging of the population
  - Increasing "feminization" of the population
  - Increasing racial and ethnic diversity
  - Changes in household structure and marital status
- These developments contributed to the epidemiological transition whereby chronic diseases replaced acute diseases
- "Diseases of civilization" became common as lifestyles played an increasing part
- Biologic pathogens became increasingly irrelevant
- The characteristics of patients were changed as a result of these developments, with females, non-whites and the elderly becoming increasingly important
- The nature of patients also changed as they adopted the attributes of consumers

References

Acevedo-Garcia, D. (2005). The differential effect of foreign-born status on low birth weight by race/ethnicity and education. *Pediatrics, 115*(1), e20–e30.

Antecol, H., & Bedard, K. (2006). Unhealthy assimilation: Why do immigrants converge to American health status levels? *Demography, 43*(2), 337–360.

Braveman, P., & Gottlieb, L. (2014). The social determinants of health: It's time to consider the causes of the causes. *Public Health Reports, 129*(S2), 19–130.

George, M. P. (2013). The Mexican American health paradox: The collective influence of sociocultural factors on Hispanic health outcomes. *Discussions, 9*(2), 1–3.

Giuntella, O. (2012). *Why does the health of immigrants deteriorate?* Downloaded from URL: https://www.dartmouth.edu/~neudc2012/docs/paper_232.pdf.

McGinnis, J. M., Williams-Russo, P., & Knickman, J. R. (2002). The case for more active policy attention to health promotion. *Health Affairs, 21*(2), 78–93.

Murray, C. J. L., Abraham, J., Ali, M. K., et al. (2013). The state of US Health, 1990–2010: Burden of diseases, injuries, and risk factors. *Journal of the American Medical Association, 310*(6), 591–606.

National Heart, Lung and Blood Institute. (2013). *What are the health risks of overweight and obesity?* Downloaded from URL: http://www.nhlbi.nih.gov/health/health-topics/topics/obe/risks.html.

National Institute of Environmental Health Sciences. (2013). *Gene-environment interaction.* Downloaded from URL: http://www.niehs.nih.gov/health/topics/science/gene-env/.

Neuman, S. (2014). Are immigrants healthier than native residents? *IZA World of Labor*. Downloaded from URL: http://wol.iza.org/articles/are-immigrants-healthier-than-native-residents.pdf.

Pew Research Center. (2015). *Modern immigration wave brings 59 Million to US, driving population growth and change through 2065.* Downloaded from URL: https://www.pewresearch.org/fact-tank/2016/03/31/10-demographic-trends-that-are-shaping-the-us-and-the-world/.

U.S. Census Bureau. (2020a). *Historical marital status tables*. Downloaded from URL: https://www.census.gov/data/tables/time-series/demo/families/marital.html.
U.S. Census Bureau. (2020b). *Historical families tables*. Downloaded from URL: https://www.census.gov/data/tables/time-series/demo/families/families.html.
Williams, D. R., & Collins, C. (1996). U.S. socioeconomic and racial differences in health: Patterns and explanations. In P. Brown (Ed.), *Perspectives in medical sociology* (2nd ed.). Waveland Press.
Wilkinson, R. G. (1996). *Unhealthy societies: The afflictions of inequality*. Routledge.
World Health Organization. (2006). *Preventing disease through healthy environments: Towards an estimate of the environmental burden of disease*. Downloaded from URL: http://www.who.int/quantifying_ehimpacts/publications/preventingdisease/en/.

Additional Resources

DeSalvo, K. B., Wang, Y. C., Harris, A., et al. (2017). *Public health 3.0: A call to action for public health to meet the challenges of the 21st century*. National Academies of Medicine.
Health Knowledge. (2016). *Public health textbook*. Downloaded from URL: http://www.healthknowledge.org.uk/public-health-textbook.
Pew Research Center. (2019). *6 Demographic trends shaping the US and the world in 2019*. Downloaded from URL: https://www.pewresearch.org/fact-tank/2019/04/11/6-demographic-trends-shaping-the-u-s-and-the-world-in-2019/.
Population Reference Bureau (www.prb.org).
White, N. E. (2016). *A comparative analysis of the Mexican vs Mexican-American diet and rates of obesity through two case studies*. Unpublished honors thesis (University of Wyoming). Downloaded from URL: http://repository.uwyo.edu/honors_theses_15-16/53/.
World Health Organization (www.who.int).

Chapter 3
The Road to Population Health: A Changing Healthcare System

As the US population was evolving into its contemporary demographic profile, its healthcare system was undergoing a major transformation of its own. Driven in part by the convergence of the social trends discussed in the previous chapter, the healthcare system experienced a series of events that created a continuously evolving situation calling for constant adaptation to a changing environment. Over a period of 20 years the system went through a number of changes before arriving to a point amenable to the introduction of a population health approach.

In this chapter the reader will:

- Come to understand the evolution of the US healthcare system and the factors that contributed to its modern iteration
- Be exposed to the attributes of modern Western medicine that led to its twentieth century success while laying the groundwork for its demise
- Understand the increasing deficiencies of the US healthcare system in the face of contemporary health problems
- Review the shift from an emphasis on "medical care" to an emphasis on "healthcare"
- Be exposed to the reasons for the limitations of the healthcare paradigm
- Learn the factors that have contributed to the decline in efficacy of the medical model

Introduction

The goal of the healthcare system in every society is to provide for the health and well-being of its population. As health systems are established or evolve their primary intent is to develop a means to advance the population's health status. Societies differ in how they interpret this goal and in the means they employ to pursue it. This effort can take a wide range of forms, however, from rear-guard efforts to stave off death on one end of the spectrum to proactively enhancing the health status of the population on the other. For that reason, the healthcare systems in different societies may differ in a variety of aspects as they establish society-specific approaches to similar goals.

The process of establishing a healthcare system is complicated by the fact that a society may explicitly or implicitly establish multiple goals for the system. While addressing the health and well-being needs of the population may be an important consideration, it is not necessarily the only—or even the primary—goal of every healthcare system. In some societies the stated purpose of the system may be quite different from, and even at odds with, health improvement goals. To wit, the stated goal of the "social medicine" officially sanctioned by the nineteenth century Prussian empire was to assure a steady flow of healthy soldiers; the sprawling system of the Soviet Union was designed to maintain social control of the population by the central government; and even today, the stated purpose of the National Health Service in Great Britain is to efficiently allocate scarce societal resources.

Ostensibly, the goal of the US healthcare system is to manage illness and advance the health status of the population. It could be argued, however, that the system at some point became diverted from its primary goal as competition on the part of various vested interests influenced the course of American medicine. Some, in fact, would argue that the needs of the patient became subordinated to the needs of the system—especially in view of the for-profit component of the industry. Ultimately, it will be argued, the perversion of the primary goal of the US healthcare system established the foundation for the emergence of the population health model. Box 3.1 discusses the multiple functions of the US healthcare system.

The Emergence of Modern Medicine

When modern healthcare systems were developing, the United States shared many traits with other similar countries. The period leading up to WWII saw the emergence of allopathic medicine, steeped in the germ theory. This model focused on the acute conditions that affected the population at that time. In this regard, the US system resembled the other systems that were emerging in their modern forms. After the war, however, the economies (and with them the healthcare systems) of most comparable countries were devastated. While the US system was expanding and actually benefited significantly from the lessons learned during the war, European countries, along with Russia, China and Japan were faced with essentially building healthcare systems from the ground up.

One of the consequences of this situation was the establishment of the twentieth century as the "American century" in medicine. Prior to WWII, European medicine represented the world standard, and any American clinician who sought to

Box 3.1: The Multiple Functions of the US Healthcare System

The primary objective of any healthcare system is to provide for the health and well-being of the population it serves. However, this is not the only function of the healthcare system and, in a society as complex as the United States, this institution serves a number of other purposes as well. The US healthcare system addresses the healthcare needs of the population through curing sickness when it occurs and, secondarily, preventing its onset when possible. Implicit in this function is the staving off of death and the prolongation of life.

These clearly overt functions of the system are not its only functions, however, and other functions exist. One overt function of the healthcare system is the promotion of public health and safety. Thus, assuring that society members have safe drinking water and clean air to breath, along with the myriad other functions carried out by public health agencies and government organizations such as the Environmental Protection Agency, is an important but often overlooked function of the healthcare system. Indeed, without the successful operation of this function, treatment and cure on the part of the medical practitioner would face an uphill battle in its efforts to maintain the health status of the population.

The US healthcare system performs many other functions that indirectly contribute to the goals of the system. Healthcare organizations—often the same ones involved in patient care—provide training for health professionals and participate in research toward the furtherance of our understanding of the nature of health and illness. At the same time, these organizations typically perform humanitarian and community service functions, through the provision of free or discounted care, community education programs, and the sponsorship of community events. Further, many healthcare organizations serve as conduits for the transmission of religious tenets.

The healthcare system also performs an important economic function in US society. As a three trillion dollar a year industry, healthcare contributes to the creation of wealth and provides jobs for over 10 percent of the workforce while accounting for nearly 20% of the gross domestic product. For-profit healthcare organizations are expected to return a profit to their owners. In many small communities, the local hospital may be the largest employer in the area.

These are all generally recognized functions of the healthcare system in the United States and, to a lesser degree, in other developed countries. There are also some not so overt functions of healthcare systems that are found in varying forms in most societies. One of these functions is resource management. In centrally planned healthcare systems (e.g., the British National Health Service), the major goal of the system may be the efficient management of government resources. Promoting health is an important, albeit secondary, function.

(continued)

Box 3.1 (continued)

The healthcare system also provides an answer for the "why" of sickness and death. Whether the explanatory system is based on supernaturalism as in traditional systems or the rationality of the medical model, the system helps explain why people get sick and why they die. It doesn't change the reality of sickness and death, but human beings seem to require at least some explanation for the events that befall them.

The healthcare system also contributes to the overall operation and stability of the society in which it resides. The system often serves as a method of social control. Sickness represents a form of deviance in the eyes of society, and some means of controlling deviance and restoring functionality must be established. By identifying the biologically abnormal, the representatives of the system can isolate them and provide them the care that will restore them to normality and, at the same time, protect the rest of society from the potentially harmful effects of deviants within its midst.

One other function of the healthcare system identified by anthropologists is the integrative role it performs. The operation of the system in the face of sickness serves to bring the community together in a common effort and reaffirms the belief system of the society. By rallying around the sick person and participating in shared rituals, the community is brought together and its cultural traditions reinforced. The degree to which the healthcare system embodies the values of society helps explain why many Americans have a visceral reaction to any criticism of the system.

The United States in the twentieth century went further than any other society in establishing healthcare as a dominant institution. The system involves a wide range of activities that not only contribute to the health and welfare of the Americans but also perform a number of other functions in contemporary US society. While many of these functions are laudable, it could be argued that the multiple goals of the system have served to divert it from what should be its primary goal: advancing the health status of the population.

distinguish himself would study in Scotland or Germany. During that period medicine was still at a primitive stage everywhere but considered more advanced prior to the war in the established academic centers of Europe than in the United States.

Within two decades after the war the United States had established itself as the leading light in medicine. Throughout the rest of the century, most of the advances in treatment, innovations in technology, and refinements in medical education were generated by the US system. Clinicians from Europe and around the world were drawn to the United States to study the world's most advanced system of care.

The impetus for the ascendancy of "Western" medicine was the adoption of the germ theory as a basis for its disease theory system. This led to the establishment of what came to be labeled the "medical model" approach to health and illness. This perspective emphasized the existence of clearly identifiable clinical symptoms, reflecting the conviction that illness represents the presence of biological pathology. Thus, illness is seen as a state involving the presence of distinct symptoms while health is seen as the negative, residual state reflecting an absence of symptoms. Both medical education and the organization of care reinforce the medical model perspective.

The medical model also assumed that illness could be reduced to disordered bodily (biochemical or neurophysiological) functions. This physical reductionism excluded any social, psychological, and behavior dimensions of illness (Engle, 1977). The result of this reductionism, together with medicine's mind-body dualism, was the locating of pathology within the individual body. Such conceptions prevented the medical model from considering external factors such as the effect of the individual's social or emotional life on his physical health.

A related assumption of this model was the belief that each disease is caused by a specific identifiable agent. This notion emerged from the nineteenth century work of Pasteur and Koch, who demonstrated that the introduction of specific virulent microorganisms (germs) into the body produced specific agents with a causal link to specific diseases. This doctrine of specific etiology was later extended beyond infectious diseases.

Proponents of the medical model deliberately discarded most vestiges of previous systems for managing health and wellness. "Bedside manner", an important resource for traditional healers and one of the few tools available to the early twentieth century physician, was demeaned in favor of efficient, impersonal patient management. The contribution that the patient and his social support group could make to the therapeutic process—another important resource for the traditional healer— was also discounted to the point that patients were not told their test results and family members were banned from the bedside. The natural remedies that had stood the test of time (and later became the basis for hundreds of drugs) were denounced as "home remedies" if not outright quackery.

While the healthcare system grew and expanded its scope, other entities were emerging that would have significant implications for the system and for the nation's future health. Although health insurance existed prior to WWII, it was only after the war that insurance coverage became widespread. Early insurance plans were typically established by not-for-profit associations or community welfare organizations. After the war the burgeoning middle class enthusiastically embraced the concept of insurance coverage. As demand grew, for-profit companies entered the field. Although these new entrants expanded the available options for consumers, they introduced the profit motive into the industry and subordinated charitable concerns to the "bottom line". Box 3.2 presents the various stages in the evolution of US healthcare.

Entering the 1970s the healthcare system appeared to be continuing along a track of expansion and growth. New treatment modalities continued to be introduced, and there appeared to be no limit to the application of technology. Even more new health

> **Box 3.2: Stages in the Evolution of the US Healthcare System**
> 1950s Emergence of "modern" medicine
> 1960s The "golden age" of American medicine
> 1970s Chinks in the armor
> 1980s The "great transformation"
> 1990s A shifting paradigm
> 2000s New millennial healthcare
> 2010s Emergence of the population health model

conditions were identified, and increasing numbers of citizens were brought under medical management. This expansion of scope was abetted through private insurance and government-subsidized insurance plans. The hospital became entrenched as the focal point of the system, and the physician continued to control more than 80% of the expenditures for health services.

To this point in time, all of the players in the system had shared in its success. Hospitals were viewed positively by the community and were able to concentrate financial resources for the advancement of medicine. Even not-for-profit hospitals were able to generate significant surpluses for use in expanding their capabilities and influence. Physicians were seen as "gods" during this period and were compensated accordingly. There was a cozy relationship between healthcare providers and insurers as everyone cooperated to share the wealth. Patients for the most part felt well cared for and, with expanding health insurance, were able to benefit from the system's growing capabilities.

The developments within the healthcare system in the 1960s and 1970s primarily served to consolidate and expand the influence of the healthcare system. There was little reason to assume that the system would not continue on its current trajectory. Ideas on the etiology of disease, the types of conditions treated, and the available level of technology spawned a system that focused on individual morbidity and attempted to achieve the system's stated goals one patient at a time.

To this point the only dissension concerning the healthcare system was heard on the part of those few advocates for segments of the population that were not sharing in this "golden age". The "discovery" of poverty was accompanied by the identification of groups that were excluded from the healthcare system. Issues of access and equity reached a point where they could no longer be ignored as large segments of the population appeared to be excluded from mainstream medicine. Further, the effectiveness of the system in dealing with the overall health status of the population was brought into question for the first time. The health status indicators of the day suggested that the US population was lagging behind other comparable countries in improving health status.

A major concern during this period was the rapidly increasing cost of care. Clearly, the United States had the world's most expensive healthcare system. The costs were high and they were increasing much faster than those in other sectors of the economy. While it was once assumed that resources for the provision of healthcare were infinite, it became clear that there was a limit to what could be spent to provide health services.

This "golden age" of medicine in the United States contained the seeds of its own downfall. The last decades of the twentieth century witnessed developments that would have significant implications for the health of the US population going forward and laid the groundwork for the emergence of the population health model. In some ways it could be argued that the system became a victim of its own success and ended up overselling its capabilities. Along the way it spawned circumstances that would detract from the achievement of the system's goals.

The 1980s will no doubt be seen by historians as a watershed for US healthcare. The numerous issues that had been emerging over the previous two decades came to a head as the 1980s began. By the end of the decade, American healthcare had become almost unrecognizable to veteran health professionals. Virtually every aspect of the system had undergone transformation, and a new paradigm began to emerge as the basis for the disease theory system.

The escalating–and seemingly uncontrollable–costs associated with healthcare prompted the Medicare administration to introduce the prospective payment system. Other insurers soon followed suit with a variety of cost containment methods. Employers, who were footing much of the bill for increasing healthcare costs, began to take a more active role in the management of the health of their employees.

This transformation of the 1980s resulted in considerable shifts in both power and risk within the system. The power that resided in hospital administrators and physicians was blamed for much of the cost and inefficiency in the system. Third-party payors, employers and consumers began to attempt to share in this power. Large groups of purchasers emerged that were able to negotiate for lower costs in exchange for their "wholesale" business. Insurers, who had historically borne most of the risk involved in the financing of health services, began shifting some of this risk to providers and consumers. As something of a precursor to the population health movement, much of the discussion began to surround the management of groups of patients for the first time.

As for-profit insurers became dominant (and even not-for-profits took on similar characteristics) the aims of the system became perverted. Health insurers were less and less concerned about the needs of their plan members and increasingly concerned about the needs of their shareholders. The involvement of insurers ran up the cost of care and diverted resources away from patient care to administrative costs. The focus on profits over people led to a wide range of abuses that, due to the political influence of a now-powerful insurance industry, went unaddressed. This situation ultimately influenced the enactment of the 2010 Patient Protection and Affordable Care Act (ACA) which sought to address the worst of the abuses. However, to a great extent the damage had been done by this point. Health insurers were firmly entrenched as "middlemen" between patients and the healthcare system. For better or worse, the ACA assured that this would continue.

Another major development was the emergence of the pharmaceutical industry during this period. Originally established as a community resource and supported by the federal government, a private pharmaceutical industry emerged in the second half of the twentieth century to become a major player on the healthcare scene. Previous success in the creation of vaccines and life-saving drugs gave the pharmaceutical industry unwarranted credibility. Drug therapy became the fastest growing component of healthcare delivery, and pharmaceutical companies came to be among the most profitable of American industries.

As pharmaceutical companies expanded their clinical impact, they increased their political influence, becoming among the most powerful lobbying groups in government. "Big pharma" was able to gain concessions from the federal government and exerted an inordinate influence over the Food and Drug Administration, the organization charged with regulating it. Perhaps the influence of the industry is best epitomized in the form of Medicare D, the pharmaceutical component of the Medicare program for seniors. The law specified that the federal government that was paying for drugs under the program could not negotiate with pharmaceutical companies for better prices. That is, drug companies were able to charge whatever they wanted to Medicare patients and, ultimately, the federal government.

Other organizations not involved in the provision of care further influenced the course of healthcare. The American Medical Association (AMA) had emerged as a strident voice for the interests of doctors. Their constituency clearly was not patients, and at various points in time the AMA has been the largest contributor to political campaigns and the most aggressive lobbyist at the federal level. The position of organized medicine has been clearly stated when the US Public Health Service (USPHS) was established in 1899. The USPHS was not to be allowed to provide clinical services to patients or the medical establishment would oppose its organization. Similarly, the American Hospital Association became a major lobbyist in Washington and, although not as self-serving as the AMA appeared to be, still made it clear that it was working for the benefit of hospitals and not patients.

Americans increasingly turned to the healthcare institution in the late twentieth century despite its obvious deficiencies for a wide range of social, psychological and even spiritual issues. Physicians came to be regarded as experts on virtually any human problem. This expansion of scope is evidenced by the fact that even today less than half of the people in a primary care practitioner's waiting room suffer from a clear-cut medical problem. They are there because of emotional disorders, sexual dysfunction, social adjustment issues, nutritional problems, or some other non-clinical threat to their well-being. Despite the fact that physicians are generally not trained to deal with these conditions, the healthcare system is seen as an appropriate place to seek solutions to these and other non-medical maladies. (Box 3.3 reviews topics that doctors should be taught about in medical school but seldom are).

> **Box 3.3: What Every Doctor Should Know… But Doesn't Learn in Medical School**
> Since the mid-twentieth century Americans have come to rely upon the skills of physicians to cure them when they are sick and to prolong their lives to the extent possible. Physicians are increasingly called upon to address issues in realms outside standard medical practice. This approach to personal health has worked well—at least in the past. Today it is being suggested that there is a mismatch between the training doctors receive and the tasks they are asked to perform.

(continued)

Box 3.3 (continued)

Research on patients visiting physician offices has found that a large portion of those presenting for care do not actually have physical health problems. While non-medical conditions may manifest themselves through physical symptoms, in a large proportion of the cases a non-medical condition has prompted the office visit. Increasingly patients are presenting with emotional or mental disturbances, nutritional, weight or metabolic problems, sexual disorders, addictive behaviors, and other conditions that do not lend themselves to a medical solution. While physicians make every effort to address these issues with tools they have at their disposal, the medical school curriculum offers limited training in these areas and does not accord them the attention that their prevalence merits.

Despite revisions in medical school curricula in recent years, doctors-in-training still receive limited information on a wide range of topics. Most patients today have issues related to diet, yet physicians receive little training in nutrition, weight management and even eating disorders. Their advice on healthy lifestyles, in fact, is likely to be limited to "eat less and exercise more." Although there is typically a clinical rotation in psychiatry, there is limited exposure to psychological and emotional issues, behavioral health issues and addictive behaviors. Limited attention is paid to domestic violence and child abuse and the whole notion of family health (physical and mental) is honored more in concept than in practice. There is little exposure to sexuality and sexual dysfunction, and women's health issues in particular are given short shrift except for those specializing in obstetrics. Although chronic disease management is being increasingly emphasized, there is little emphasis on geriatric care despite the elderly population accounting for most chronic conditions. Despite the increased recognition given to oral health as a factor in physical health, this topic is mostly absent from the medical school curriculum The importance of spirituality to health has been neglected for decades and is only now being revisited in medical school.

Beyond these deficiencies related to the delivery of care, other factors that limit physicians' appreciation of population health issues is their lack of exposure to the social determinants of ill-health or to the influence of the physical and social environment on their patients' health. They even receive limited exposure to public health. Given the content of medical education it is not difficult to understand the lack of appreciation on the part of physicians of the significance of population health.

The result: American medicine has become less and less capable of addressing the health problems of contemporary America, leading to the now indisputable conclusion that Americans are getting sicker. Because of the mismatch between physician skills and the needs of the patient population, continued deterioration of our nation's health could be expected short of a total rethinking of our approach to improving population health.

Emerging Deficiencies

Although the medical model had its flaws, its effectiveness in addressing health problems during the twentieth century helped it maintain it positive standing. One of the undisputed trends over the past century was the steady improvement in the health status of the US population. Using the year 1900 as a convenient starting point, it is possible, based on a variety of indicators, to trace the continuous decline in mortality, the increase in life expectancy, the reduction or elimination of many of the major killers at the beginning of the twentieth century. This was accompanied by overall improvement in health status based on both objective and subjective measures. Over the course of the century, it is agreed, Americans became bigger, stronger and generally healthier.

In retrospect it is clear that medical science received too much credit for the health advances of the twentieth century. While millions of lives were undoubtedly saved by the healthcare system from the scourges of the day, the general improvement in the overall health status of the population is now attributed to a rising standard of living, better nutrition, and the introduction of preventive measures. To the extent that the healthcare system did have an impact, it was primarily through the machinations of the expanding public health system. Clean water, safe foods, and the reduction of environmental threats played a greater role in improved health status than direct patient care. Even many of the much-touted vaccines that eliminated common communicable diseases were introduced *after* most diseases had begun to decline as health threats (McKinlay & McKinlay, 1977).

Despite admitted advances, a growing amount of upsetting evidence indicting the US system of care emerged. One of the most scathing critiques of modern American medicine in provided by Bailey (2014) in *The End of Healing*. Presented in novel format, Bailey examines all aspects of our system of care. Driven by a concern that our healthcare system was actually bad for our health, he finds fault with virtually every component. He begins with the delivery of care, the component of most salience here, and sees a system that has been perverted from its primary goal (that is, advancing health) to serve the needs of clinicians and institutions. He argues that even laudable efforts to advance therapeutic techniques are often driven by self-interest and greed, with the needs of individual patients (and ultimately the entire population) subjugated to the needs and interests of researchers, ambitious specialists and administrators more concerned with acquiring power and resources than serving the needs of patients. These factors led Bailey to suggest that the increasing intensity of care has had a negative impact on the health of the US population. Box 3.4 discusses the relationship between more care and better health.

Bailey finds fault with the insurance industry, arguing that, while lining its own pockets, it works to the detriment of patients. Although some of the worst abuses of the health insurance industry were addressed through the 2010 Affordable Care Act, there is ample evidence that insurers continue to pursue their own interests rather than those of the insured.

Box 3.4: Does More Care Mean Better Health?
For most of the modern medical era in the United States the conventional wisdom has stated that more care equates to better health. The assumption has been that the more health services that the population consumes the better its health status. This approach has been applied at the individual patient level where over-treatment is preferred to under-treatment. The potential harm from therapeutic "overkill" has been considered preferable to the perceived danger of limiting diagnosis and treatment.

The relationship between the provision of care and the health status of the population has become an issue of increasing importance to health professionals. There are growing doubts about the benefits of incremental "doses" of care and some accusations that over-diagnosis and over-treatment are health threats in their own right. This question is relevant as policies are set and decisions made with regard to the funding of health services and is particularly salient if one is considering healthcare reform. This question also has relevance for the population health model in that its implementation would involve decisions on the allocation of resources to other sectors of society rather than to health services.

The US healthcare system has exhibited a steady increase in the expenditure of resources on healthcare. Many different measures of resource allocation support this contention, with one of the most straightforward being per capita expenditures. Per capita expenditures for health services almost doubled between 1990 and 2000 and then almost double again between 2000 and 2010. While there is evidence of a slowing in the increase in healthcare costs, a 46% increase in expenditures was recorded between 2010 and 2019.

The question for us here is whether or not this increased spending has led to improved health. Unfortunately, while it is easy enough to calculate healthcare expenditures, it is much more difficult to determine the impact of these expenditures. While it is possible to measure the use of formal health services, that does not tell us whether the consumption of services led to improved health status. While we can determine that more expenditures have been incurred, it is difficult to determine the impact of incremental expenditures.

Improvement in health status cannot be as easily measured in that there is no available metric for this purpose. There is no agreement on how to measure the population's health status and, even if there were, access to the necessary data would be problematic. An examination of the experience with Medicaid in the United States found that enrollment in the Medicaid program led to increased access to services and greater utilization of services for enrollees. Compared with uninsured adults, Medicaid-covered adults were 25% more likely to report they were in good to excellent health (versus fair to poor health), 40% less likely to report health declines in the last 6 months, and 10% more likely to screen negative for depression. In addition, access to Medicaid improved adults' mental health markedly.

(continued)

Box 3.4 (continued)

Medicaid's impact on physical health, however, could not be conclusively verified. While having Medicaid coverage led to a 30% reduction in the rate of positive screens for depression, gains in physical health were more limited. The Medicaid program did increase the detection of diabetes and use of diabetes medication, but it did not have a statistically significant effect on the ability to control diabetes, high blood pressure, or high cholesterol. It is contended that multiple factors may mitigate the impact of coverage on clinical outcomes, including unmeasured barriers to access, missed diagnoses, inappropriate medication, patient noncompliance, and ineffectiveness of treatments (Paradise & Garfield, 2013).

A study conducted in Canada (Cooper, 2016) found that publicly insured low-income patients used healthcare services more than did their counterparts who had higher levels of income and education. However, their clinical outcomes appeared to worsen over time, leading patients to record ever more primary care visits. Overall, patients' use of health services had little cumulative explanatory impact on the associations between mortality and socioeconomic status. Another study suggests that Canada's Medicare program has improved access to health services for poorer Canadians thereby flattening the slope of the relationship between wealth and health. However, other findings suggest that universal access alone cannot eliminate health disparities (Alter et al., 2011).

The one consistent measure of health status available over time—self-reported health status—may offer some insight into the relationship between healthcare expenditures and health status. If we compare trends in expenditures with trends in self-reported health status, this should give us an indication of what if any impact more care has on health. As noted above, per capita expenditures for healthcare have been steadily and dramatically increasing for a quarter of a century.

If we examine trends in self-reported health status it is difficult to claim improvement commensurate with the growth in expenditures. In fact, over the past decade and a half there appears to be no improvement and perhaps even some decline in self-reported health status for the population overall. According to the Behavioral Risk Factor Surveillance System (BRFSS), the proportion of the population reporting only poor or fair health increased from 8.9% in 2000 to 10.1% in 2010 and more drastically to 18.8% in 2019. While one should not conclude too much about declining health status from these figures, it certainly appears that the population's perceived health status declined while healthcare expenditures were skyrocketing.

There is a growing contention that the health status of the US population is actually *declining*. Today there is convincing evidence that the longstanding trend toward improved health status has stagnated and, on some measures, has been reversed (Thomas, 2016) despite the continued escalation of healthcare expenditures.

Even "watchdog" organizations and research institutes within the federal government have been co-opted by private interests. The FDA (responsible for oversight of drugs and medical devices) is underfunded to the point that it has to rely on data from the parties that the agency is monitoring in order to carry out its functions. Even the National Institutes of Health are not immune to outside influences, with research funding decisions often made at the behest of vested interests rather than based on the objective health-related needs of the population.

Bailey was driven to produce this critique because of the system's propensity to kill its patients. Medical errors arising from the operation of the system contribute to at least 400,000 unnecessary deaths a year. Medical errors in addition to excessive diagnostic testing, often unnecessary invasive treatment, and pharmaceutical-related deaths reflect a healthcare environment that is fraught with danger. Even after the enactment of the Affordable Care Act tens of millions of Americans still lack health insurance with 40,000 of them dying each year as a result. When the indirect impact of the operation of the healthcare system is examined it is clear that the healthcare system itself is a leading cause of death.

There are a number of implications for the healthcare system—and ultimately the health of the population—related to these developments. The manner in which care is delivered coupled with the mechanism for financing it has created an inefficient and ineffective systems. The impact of the cost of care remains glaring as healthcare spending accounts for an increasing share of America's gross domestic product. Today, healthcare spending accounts for nearly 20% of the GDP, twice or more than that of other comparable countries. This massive spending, however, is not particularly productive in that the structure of the system results in 35% or more of the healthcare dollar going to something other than patient care. While systems with universal coverage are spending 10% or less on non-medical expenses, the United States is spending more than one-third of its healthcare dollar on overhead and administrative costs.

These developments have served to distract the system from its ultimate goal. The impact of care has been diluted while competing interests have shifted the emphasis away from patient care. Importantly, these factors have led to the extreme misallocation of resources. Resources are focused on specialty care rather than primary care, on extensive diagnostic techniques, and on the most expensive but often least effective treatments. Even the distribution of clinical personnel and facilities reflects this misallocation, as the maldistribution of resources leaves many segments of the population with limited access to care. (Box 3.5 discusses the possibility that modern Western medicine may have outlasted its usefulness.)

Box 3.5: Western Medicine: An Idea Whose Time Has Come…and Gone?

The emergence of modern Western medicine based on the germ theory ushered in a revolution in the treatment of health problems. For the first time there was scientific support for a system of care, and evidence-based medicine emerged in respect to the causes of disease and death in human societies. An allopathic approach to treatment was tailor made for the diseases that threatened human populations at that time. This "medical model" found fertile ground in post-WWII America as the United States was emerging as a world power.

Modern medicine represented a departure from traditional forms of care and, indeed, its practitioners sought to distance themselves from most aspects of traditional medical systems. "Traditional medicine", for lack of a better term, has been used to address the health needs of human populations for millennia. Most such systems emphasized a oneness with the universe and all other objects in nature and sought a balance between the individual and his social group. The notion of equilibrium pervades the lore of primitive societies, and the first function of diagnosis was to determine the extent to which an imbalance contributed to the health condition. Consequently, the examination by the practitioner deemphasized physical symptoms and concentrated on social psychological factors. The social history thus took on more importance than the medical history.

The approach to primitive healthcare was holistic in that the individual was not only seen as a total entity (as opposed to a collection of tissue, organs, etc.), but was viewed as inextricably tied into a social network. Diagnosis could only be made with reference to the patient's social milieu, and treatment almost always involved other members of society. It was believed that treatment should only occur within the individual's familiar surroundings, and isolation of the patient was rare. Recovery, in fact, required the marshalling of all available social and emotional support, with family and friends usually participating in the therapy.

As the healthcare system in the United States experienced unprecedented expansion during the 1960s it was quick to discard any vestiges of "folk medicine". The hospital emerged as the center of the system, and the physician–much maligned in earlier decades–came to occupy the pivotal role in the treatment of disease. Physician salaries and the prestige associated with their positions grew astronomically.

The medical model operated on the assumption that there was a single identifiable cause for every disease, a logical assumption given the nature of disease in early twentieth century America. It was contended that an approach that counteracted this cause (allopathy) was the only appropriate response. This perspective led to an effort to isolate clinical pathology—not only from other co-morbidities but from the external environment. In support of this

(continued)

Box 3.5 (continued)

emphasis on reductionism the body was segmented into organ systems, organ systems into individual organs, organs into tissue, tissue into cells and, more recently, cells into cell components and even DNA.

Modern medicine became the antithesis of holism as it reduced the body to its component parts and isolated pathology not only from the whole person but from non-medical factors. The influence of the social environment, cultural context and life circumstances were ignored on the assumption that the more a problem could be isolated the more effective the treatment. Unlike the traditional healer, modern clinicians did not consider the external factors that might affect the onset, progression and/or outcome of the health condition.

During the course of the twentieth century, remarkable progress was made in eliminating the diseases that accounted for high rates of both morbidity and mortality. The communicable and infectious diseases ("notifiable diseases" in CDC parlance) that were the scourge of the population at the beginning of the twentieth century were reduced in significance if not eliminated entirely by the end of the century. The major killers of 1900—like tuberculosis, diphtheria, and diarrhea—were supplanted by heart disease, cancer and stroke during the course of the century.

But, after a century-long run, the form of medicine practiced in the United States and most industrialized countries appears to have lost its efficacy. Deficiencies in the US healthcare system were noted as early as the 1960s when it was realized that mainstream healthcare was not available to large portions of the population. During the 1970s and 1980s the list of grievances expanded to include in addition to inaccessibility, inequitable care for different groups, questionable quality of care, and vast differences in practice patterns from one community to the next among other concerns. The cost of the system to the nation was spiraling out of control, and the inefficiencies of such a massive system meant that resources were frequently misallocated or otherwise wasted. The increasing cost of the system far outweighed any incremental benefits.

The epidemiological transition lead to a growing mismatch between the health problems of the population and the treatment modalities offered in response. The system was clearly geared toward the treatment and cure of acute conditions and not the management of chronic problems. Doctors were trained to save lives not to "nurse" patients with chronic conditions and no hope of recovery. Medical education, the organization of medical practice, and reimbursement incentives were all geared to the treatment of acute conditions, conditions that were increasingly rare by the end of the twentieth century.

Given what we know now, it could be argued that Western medicine as practiced in the United States is an aberration in the evolution of healthcare.

(continued)

> **Box 3.5** (continued)
> It appears that there was a century-long window of opportunity where the health conditions of the day lent themselves to the therapeutic approaches fostered by the medical model. An approach that worked reasonably well for acute conditions had limited effectiveness, however, with chronic conditions. A century was spent creating the foundation for this form of treatment, only to realize that it was being made obsolete by developments in both society and healthcare.

Late-Century Paradigm Shift

Since the beginning of the twentieth century, the dominant paradigm in Western medical science has been the medical model of disease. Built on the germ theory formulated late in the nineteenth century, the medical model provided an appropriate framework within which to respond to the acute health conditions prevalent throughout that century. By the 1970s, however, enough anomalies had been identified to bring the prevailing paradigm into question. Despite the ever-increasing sophistication of medical technology, the importance of the non-medical aspects of care was increasingly being recognized.

Although change occurs unevenly throughout a system as complex as American healthcare, some observers contend that by the late 1990s a true paradigm shift was occurring. Simply put, this involved a shift from an emphasis on "medical care" to an emphasis on "healthcare". *Medical care* is narrowly defined in terms of the formal services provided by the healthcare system and refers primarily to those functions of the healthcare system that are under the influence of medical doctors. This concept focuses on the clinical or treatment aspects of care, and excludes the non-medical factors contributing to health and illness. *Healthcare* refers to any function that might be directly or indirectly related to preserving, maintaining, and/or enhancing health status. This concept includes not only formal activities (such as visiting a health professional) but also such informal activities as preventive care, exercise, proper diet, and other health maintenance activities. The growing awareness of the connection between health status and lifestyle and the realization that medical care is limited in its ability to control the disorders of modern society have prompted movement away from a strictly medical model of health and illness to more of a biopsychosocial model (Engel, 1977).

Clearly, the epidemiologic transition—by which acute conditions were displaced by chronic disorders—has played a major role. As acute conditions waned in importance and chronic and degenerative conditions came to the forefront, the medical model began to lose some of its salience. Once the cause of most health conditions ceased to be environmental microorganisms and became aspects of lifestyle, a new model of health and illness was required. The chronic conditions that had come to account for most health problems did not respond well to the treatment-and-cure approach of the medical model.

Independent of this trend, patients were increasingly expressing dissatisfaction with the operation of the healthcare system. The traditional approach to care was not a comfortable fit with the attitudes baby boomers were bringing to the doctor's office. This population—more than any other group in US society—has led the movement toward advances in healthcare delivery. This cohort emphasizes convenience, value, responsiveness, patient participation, and other attributes not traditionally incorporated into the medical model. Further, the runaway costs of the system have led observers to question the wisdom of pursuing the one-size-fits-all approach to solving health problems that is traditional in medical care.

Despite this changing orientation, an imbalance remained in the system with regard to the allocation of resources to its various components. Treatment still commanded the lion's share of the healthcare dollar, and most research still focused on developing cures rather than preventive measures. The hospital remained the focal point of the system, and the physician continued to be its primary gatekeeper. Nevertheless, each of these underpinnings of medical care was substantially weakened during the 1980s, with a definitive shift toward a healthcare-oriented paradigm evident during the 1990s.

The transition from the medical care model to the healthcare model has affected every aspect of care—from the standard definitions of health and illness to the manner in which healthcare is delivered. *Health status* is now defined as a continuous process rather than as a static condition. Causes of ill health are now sought in the environment, and the patient's social context is now often "under the microscope". The importance of the non-medical component of therapy has come to be recognized to the point that fathers are now allowed to participate in childbirth and families are encouraged to participate in the treatment of cancer patients.

Well into the twenty-first century this paradigm shift is still on-going. Not surprisingly, there are many barriers to the complete acceptance of the healthcare model. Not the least of which is pushback from the medical establishment that has a vested interest in the traditional medical model approach. While it is anticipated that there will be continued movement toward a more holistic approach to clinical care, the possibility exists that the population health model may overtake its plodding implementation.

The Impact of Medical Science on Population Health

The *raison d'etre* for medical science is the management of morbidity and the reduction of mortality. It could be argued that the level and nature of morbidity in contemporary US society is a function of the contribution that medical science has made in the control and/or eradication of various diseases. The fact that we do not suffer today, it could argued, from polio, measles or other communicable diseases is a reflection of the application of medical science. While this appears a plausible explanation for the observed level of health, this conventional wisdom, as shown below, is not universally accepted.

Unquestionably, there are a number of ways in which the actions of medical practitioners contribute to the morbidity patterns that exist within the US population today. As noted above, the development of therapies, drugs and, in particular, immunizations to combat the communicable diseases that plagued the population until well into the twentieth century played a significant role in eliminating the epidemic diseases that accounted for most of the morbidity (and mortality) at the beginning of that century. These developments in medical science had the dual effect, however, of eliminating certain diseases and laying the groundwork for the emergence of others. By eliminating the diseases that were common in childhood along with other acute conditions, and, thus, extending the life expectancy for large portions of the population, medical science contributed to the shift toward the chronic conditions that emerged in the last half of the century. Four generations ago, relatively few people died from cancer or degenerative diseases since few people lived long enough to contract them. Thus, medical science did not so much eliminate disease from the population but engendered a trade-off of acute conditions for chronic conditions.

Another way in which medical science has contributed to morbidity patterns reflects its past application of drug therapy. Through the widespread use of antibiotics, for example, medical science has, on the one hand, relieved considerable suffering and saved lives but, on the other, has contributed to the mutation of micro-organisms resulting in the emergence of new—and often antibiotic-resistant—strains of pathogens. Again, it could be argued, that this amounted not so much to the eradication of disease but to a swapping of one disease for another.

It should also be noted that the success of medical science has led to the emergence of additional health problems. A case in point would be medicine's ability to save the lives—and maintain the viability—of individuals who would not have survived in previous eras. Through emergency and trauma care many lives are saved, and individuals are able to return to society. Similarly, modern technology can keep severely premature babies alive who would have died in the past. The downside of the intervention of medical science is the existence of a large number of disabled individuals within the population. This means that the number and proportion of disabled Americans are greater today than at any time in the past. This fact is not solely the consequence of the application of medical science, of course, but our society's ability to save lives and maintain viability has clearly been a contributor.

An additional argument for the role of medical science in contemporary morbidity patterns is the negative impact of the healthcare system itself on the health of the population. Health problems that are caused by the healthcare system—iatrogenic conditions—have become increasingly common. A leading example would be the proportion of hospital patients who contract some condition while hospitalized other than the one for which they were admitted. Or the fact that accidental falls in hospitals are a major health consideration. Then there are the situations of missed diagnoses, inappropriate or inadequate treatment, or outright negligence on the part of healthcare providers. The high rate at which patients require emergency care and hospital admission as a result of the actions of the healthcare system has been clearly documented by the Centers for Disease Control and Prevention (Bernstein et al., 2003).

In addition to suffering from the side-effects of many therapies, particularly drug therapy, a large proportion of the population has become dependent on prescription drugs. While the therapeutic benefit of most drugs is not in dispute, the negative impact of "polypharmacy" is also indisputable, with addiction to prescription drugs becoming an increasingly common disorder. Indeed, by 2015 overdoses attributed to prescription drugs exceeded overdose deaths from all illegal drugs. Box 3.6 discusses the impact of the US healthcare system on the health status of the population.

> **Box 3.6: The Contribution of the Healthcare System to Ill Health**
> The ostensible goal of any healthcare system is the promotion of personal and community health. The assumption is that the operation of the system will have a positive impact on the health of both individuals and society at large. That assumption is arguably valid when applied to the system that dominated US healthcare during the twentieth century. This system was generally credited—rightly or wrongly—with a reduction in mortality, an increase in longevity and the steadily improving health status of the population. However, it is now being argued by some that the US healthcare system as currently operating may not be contributing to health improvement but, in fact, may have a negative impact on American's health status.
>
> Few knowledgeable people today support the contention that the United States has the best healthcare system in the world. However, even some who agree that there are deficiencies in the system still contend that, for those who can obtain care, the advanced techniques offered by modern medicine provide unprecedented life-saving capabilities. Yet even this contention is being called into question. Those benefits, it is argued, only accrue to those who are well-insured, actually have access to top quality care, and do not suffer from health disparities.
>
> For some time now, it has been argued that medical errors are a serious problem within the US healthcare system, with some citing as many as 400,000 deaths per year. Although this number has been disputed, there is no doubt that medical errors—particularly in hospitals—account for tens of thousands of deaths annually. Even if this figure overstates the number, medical errors are only one contribution to mortality—and ill-health in general--that can be attributed to the healthcare system. Many die as a result of medically appropriate treatment and many others die from hospital acquired infections.
>
> These deaths represent direct ways in which the healthcare system contributes to ill-health. Everyday there are situations when providers refuse to treat

(continued)

> **Box 3.6** (continued)
>
> a patient because they are <u>uninsured</u> or are insured by a <u>plan the provider doesn't accept</u>. When patients present to a hospital emergency department with a serious problem, <u>delays in treatment</u> may have <u>life-threatening consequences</u>. Moreover, although hospitals cannot refuse to treat emergency cases, they can transfer patients to another facility once they are stabilized. The wait involved in making the transfer to what may be an inferior facility can also contribute to the body count.
>
> Hospitals and doctors are notorious for locating their facilities in select communities where patients have the ability to pay for health services although the level of morbidity is low. This leaves a large portion of the community with limited access to care due to their distance from sources of medical treatment. Even routine problems can become life threatening if they are not addressed. Sadly, the <u>sickest groups in US society</u> have the <u>least access to care</u>.
>
> One other consideration is the role that insurance plays in creating ill-health within the population. Even after the passage of the 2010 Affordable Care Act, tens of millions of Americans do not have health insurance coverage and tens of millions more could be considered underinsured. This usually means that these Americans have no access to care and at best have to settle for substandard care if they can obtain any care at all. As a result, an estimated 40,000 Americans die each year as a result of not having health insurance.
>
> There are a number of other factors that indirectly contribute to the deaths attributed to the healthcare system—too many to discuss in the limited space here. If the system's contribution to ill-health is added to healthcare-caused deaths, the negative impact of the healthcare system on the population's health is indeed substantial.

Ultimately, a case can be made that, while medical science has had a significant impact on personal health, it has had much less impact on "population health" which, of course, is the focus of this book. The improvement in the health status of the population observed during the twentieth century can be primarily attributed to improved standards of living, better housing, better nutrition, and better public sanitation. To the extent that medical science played a role, it was primarily by means of the application of public health principles through which the health status of the population as a whole was improved, rather than through the application of medical science to individual members of society. Conventional wisdom suggests that as little as 10% of the variation in morbidity in contemporary society can be attributed to medical science.

Deficiencies in the "Healthcare" Model

The paradigm shift that emerged during the last years of the twentieth century from medical care to healthcare was hailed by many as a major development with the potential to improve the effectiveness of the healthcare delivery system. An approach that emphasized "healthcare" more broadly defined was seen as having the potential to address many of the issues plaguing the US healthcare system. The new paradigm recognizes the significance of changes in the nature of the health problems affecting the US population and encourages a holistic approach for improving the effectiveness of care, while emphasizing prevention and positive lifestyles to supplement clinical care.

While the population health approach is clearly emerging within the context of this paradigm shift, there are important distinctions that should be noted. The major distinction is that, with the healthcare model, the emphasis remains on the individual patient. While recognizing that today's patients have different characteristics from yesterday's and, thus, should be treated differently, it still focuses on the individual patient. This continued emphasis on the individual patient makes the population health approach an uncomfortable partner within this shifting paradigm given the emphasis placed on populations not individuals (Box 3.7 reviews the data that suggests Americans are actually getting sicker).

> **Box 3.7: Americans Are Getting Sicker**
> Americans have benefited from a 100-year run of improving health status. During the twentieth century we saw dramatic decreases in mortality (particularly maternal and infant mortality) accompanied by significant increases in life expectancy (from less than 50 years in 1900 to around 80 years today). The introduction of public health measures, advances in medicine and, importantly, increasing standards of living combined to create a population that was becoming healthier decade by decade.
>
> But, today, there is a nagging sense among social epidemiologists and other healthcare experts that all of this is changing—that Americans are, in fact, getting sicker. While few observers have been willing to state unequivocally that the health status of our population is declining, there is ample evidence that something has gone awry when it comes to the health of Americans.
>
> In the absence of a single indicator of health status, a variety of disparate types of data must be consulted, and the fragmented evidence that is available paints an increasingly pessimistic picture of the health status of Americans. When certain subgroups are examined, the results are even more sobering. When trends in chronic disease are reviewed, for example, an increase in disease prevalence has been observed across the board but with some groups affected more than others.

(continued)

Box 3.7 (continued)

Some of the trends observed were not totally unexpected. Declines in the death rate cannot continue indefinitely nor can life expectancy continue to increase at the same rate as in the past. However, the leveling off of these trends is uniquely American, with the rates for comparable countries continuing to improve. Even worse is the fact that rates for some subgroups within the population have actually reversed direction with some experiencing increasing mortality and declining life expectancy—trends virtually unprecedented in modern industrial societies. Further, there has been a dismaying increase in maternal mortality in the U.S., also unprecedented among developed nations.

Since mortality is a less salient measure of population health today than in the past, social epidemiologists now focus more on morbidity rates—that is the level of sickness and disability within the population. Today, however, the United States is experiencing a resurgence in the incidence of many diseases once thought relegated to the "dustpan of history". While the numbers are not large to this point, it is nevertheless concerning to see an uptick in cases of measles, whooping cough, tuberculosis and malaria. None of these acute conditions represent a significant threat to the general population but the fact that they are an issue at all is a reason for concern.

Although the incidence of acute conditions is an issue, it is chronic diseases that are the scourge of today's population. These "diseases of civilization" represent the predominant health threats and account for 80% of the nation's deaths. The increase in the prevalence of chronic conditions has not been a surprise to epidemiologists and represents to a great extent a natural process accompanying the aging of the US population.

Of course, aging is not the only explanation for the surge in chronic disease. Much of the increase can be attributed to changes in the lifestyles of the US population. We have been transformed from an active population with relatively healthy eating habits to a sedentary population raised on fast food. The obesity rate for the population has exploded with a third or more of the population found to be obese. While a morbid condition in its own right, obesity represents a contributor to a wide range of chronic conditions. Abetted by unhealthy activities such as smoking, drinking and drug use, not to mention stressful life circumstances, chronic disease now affects more than 50% of the population.

The increase in the prevalence of chronic disease first noted in the last couple of decades in the twentieth century was not totally unanticipated but the speed at which the prevalence rate has increased is surprising Investigators who found that the level of chronic disease is increasing at a rate not warranted by the aging of the population. When age cohorts were examined across generations it was found, for example, that although contemporary seniors were living longer on the average than seniors a generation ago, today's oldsters exhibited higher rates of chronic disease and disability. Longer life, it seems, was not being accompanied by a higher quality of life.

(continued)

> **Box 3.7** (continued)
>
> To a certain extent it is possible to rationalize the increase in prevalence of chronic disease among adults in the US population. What is hard to rationalize, however, is the surge in chronic disease among young adults, teenagers and children. Heart disease and diabetes have become increasingly common among younger populations and allergies and asthma are at epidemic proportions. Even more so than for adults, these conditions reflect the high rate of obesity among American children. Obesity lays the groundwork for a lifetime of chronic diseases and the impact of the current high rate is already becoming evident in the morbidity levels observed for America's children.
>
> At the end of the day, the question of whether Americans are getting sicker or not does not lend itself to a definitive answer. The evidence for continued improved health status is weak as even the positive metrics exhibit evidence of stagnation and unfavorable comparisons to comparable countries. While the evidence of declining health status is inconclusive, there are certainly enough examples to cause concern among epidemiologists.

While the emergence of this new paradigm was considered a positive sign by many observers (if not yet fully embraced by healthcare providers), the celebration was relatively short lived. It was realized as the body of research expanded that the US population was possibly getting sicker. After a century of improving health status, the unthinkable appeared to be occurring: the health status of the US population was declining. As far back as the 1980s and 1990s some observers argued that there were signs that the trend toward continuously improving health was being compromised. There was scattered evidence at first and, as is the case with any paradigm shift, these isolated cases of declining health status were seen as anomalies that were not reflective of the overall trend. Indeed, the scattered evidence of a downturn in health was typically related to trends in selected chronic conditions. For example, the increasing prevalence of diabetes was often cited. However, since these "anomalies" related primarily to chronic conditions, the argument could be made that, since the US population was aging, one should expect an increase in the prevalence of chronic conditions.

Subsequent research has found—although not conclusively—that the US population is, in fact, getting sicker. More evidence of an increase in the prevalence of chronic diseases has been produced and, alarmingly, accompanied by evidence that these conditions are becoming prevalent at younger and younger ages. Even certain communicable diseases, long thought eliminated if not eradicated, have re-emerged. Although the numbers are small, any increase in conditions like whooping cough, measles, and tuberculosis is reason for concern. Now, something even more unthinkable has been uncovered: the mortality rate for some segments of the population has actually increased and life expectancy has decreased. And, perhaps even more disturbing is the documented increase in the rate of maternal mortality.

These developments are incurring in the face of unprecedented healthcare expenditures. Further, counties spending half as much per capita or less than the U.S., are not exhibiting signs of declining health status. In fact, the United States is bucking the trend for other comparable countries on almost every health indicator. Clearly, there is no correspondence between high healthcare expenditures and high health status.

A major reason that the new paradigm is not effective at improving population health is that it continues to treat health conditions as the problems. It has become increasingly clear that most health problems represent *symptoms* of some deeper issue rather than the problems themselves. It is increasingly recognized that the public does not define health problems the same way that health professionals do. When clearly sick populations are surveyed with regard to their health status, they often conceptualize health and illness differently from those performing the survey. The public may point to a different set of health problems from those conventionally identified by health professionals. Further, members of the public may classify non-medical problems as medical problems—citing poverty, lack of housing, lack of access to healthy food and open space as "health problems". In fact, when asked what problems they face they may not even list "health problems" in the top ten since there are many other problems that take priority.

The "inconvenient truth" that emerges from these realizations is that our healthcare system—really, any healthcare system—is not up to the task of improving population health in today's environment. This can be demonstrated in any number of ways. The emphasis remains on treatment and cure rather than prevention, maintenance and enhancement. The focus on acute conditions still lingers despite the predominance of chronic conditions. When one considers the reasons that people present themselves for treatment we find a mismatch between the skills characterizing the practitioner and the problems presented by patients. Less than half of patients in primary care settings are thought to present with a physical health problem, with large portions exhibiting emotional, psychological or addiction issues or dietary or nutritional issues or some other non-medical problem.

At the same time, it has become increasingly clear that our society's health problems are being driven by factors that are outside the purview of the healthcare system. In reality, these forces—which are all apparent to health professionals by now—impact groups of people as much as individuals. Poverty doesn't affect individuals one at a time nor does a toxic environment. The extreme health disparities that have been observed are not a reflection of individual morbidity but of unfavorable health status at the group level.

The unescapable conclusion is that the approach taken by the US healthcare system that emphasizes treating one patient at a time is not an effective model in the face of today's health problems. While the shift from an emphasis on medical care to healthcare involved an improvement in the management of patients, that was also its Achilles heel: It still focused on individual patients albeit in a different manner. The real shift that needs to occur is a focus on populations not individuals.

Whether or not one agrees with this conclusion, the handwriting is already on the wall. Under provisions of the Affordable Care Act not-for-profit hospitals must demonstrate strategies and tactics that address the needs of the entire service area population and not just their patients. The current emphasis on better access to care, improved quality of care and cost-effectiveness requires healthcare providers to acquire an in-depth understanding of not only their existing patients but of all healthcare consumers within their service areas. Reimbursement models that emphasize pay for performance further reinforce the notion that providers will be rewarded based on their impact on groups of patients or consumers and not individual success stories. Providers with capitated patient populations will similarly be rewarded based on the health status of the entire panel rather than any individual outcomes. Box 3.8 argues that, conflict theory may be more applicable to the healthcare arena than previously believed.

> **Box 3.8: A Conflict Theory View of Healthcare**
> Conflict theory is a sociological theory that views social and economic institutions as tools of the struggle between groups in society wherein these tools are used to maintain inequality and the dominance of the ruling class. In recent years few observers have been willing to apply conflict theory analyses to the US healthcare system. However, in many ways the system could be considered the "poster child" for a conflict-based system. Society's inequities along social class, race and ethnicity, and gender lines are reflected in our health and in the operation of the healthcare system. People from disadvantaged social backgrounds are more likely to become ill, less likely to receive adequate care, and more likely to have unfavorable outcomes. The fact that these disparities are distributed along demographic dimensions makes the healthcare situation in the United States amenable to analysis from both conflict theory and population health perspectives.
>
> The conflict perspective is a theoretical approach in sociology that views social interaction as a struggle for the resources of society between conflicting groups. This conflict may be political, legal, economic, or even familial. (The best-known conflict perspective is Marxism, which focuses on the expected clash between social and economic groups.) As noted by C. Wright Mills a power elite in the United States controls the operation of society, and much of our thinking related to conflict theory and healthcare was promulgated by Waitzkin (1978). Marxist studies of medical care emphasize political power and economic dominance in capitalist society.
>
> The healthcare system mirrors the society's class structure through control over health institutions, stratification of health workers, and limited occupational mobility into health professions. Monopoly capital is manifest in the growth of medical centers, financial penetration by large corporations, and the "medical-industrial complex." Health policy recommendations reflect different interest groups' political and economic goals. The state's intervention in healthcare generally protects the capitalist economic system and the private sector. Medical ideology helps maintain class structure and patterns of domination

(continued)

Box 3.8 (continued)

The theory cites the efforts by representatives of the healthcare system—primarily physicians and hospital administrators but also proponents of pharmaceutical, insurance and other vested interests—to control the practice of medicine and to define various social problems as medical ones. While physicians and hospital administrators may believe they are the most qualified professionals to diagnose problems and to manage the care of people who have these problem, it is clear that their financial interests rest on characterizing social problems as medical problems and in monopolizing the treatment of these problems. Once these problems become "medicalized," their social roots become conveniently forgotten.

As Weitz (2013) noted: Critics argue that the conflict approach's assessment of health and medicine is overly harsh and its criticism of physicians' motivation far too cynical. Although physicians are certainly motivated, as many people are, by economic considerations, their efforts to extend their scope into previously nonmedical areas also stem from honest beliefs that people's health and lives will improve if these efforts succeed. While there is some validity to this criticism of the conflict approach, the evidence for inequality in health and medicine and for the negative aspects of the medical establishment's motivation for extending its reach remains compelling.

One consequence of control by the elite is to obscure the "causes of the causes"—the underlying factors that create the observed patterns of health and illness in society—and shift the blame for illness onto the affected individuals. If it is possible to "blame the victims" the real focus of blame could be avoided. People are blamed for smoking and poor diets without questioning the forces in society that encourage these behaviors or, in the case of diets, even make unhealthy diets unavoidable. The ideology it sells includes an overemphasis on individual lifestyle choices. The power elite is able to distract attention from its behind-the-scenes machinations by emphasizing the role of personal volition.

This brings us to the aspect of this topic that relates to population health. This perspective recognizes that a corporatist class exists for whom such concepts as the maximization of profit, shareholder value, the extraction of natural resources and market solutions for various social, political and health issues are the driving motivations. This corporate class continues to own, manage and control the means of production, distribution and exchange, and the production of ruling ideas. This corporate class wants and needs a healthy workforce only as long as the costs are not threatening to profits. Hence the health needs of the poverty-stricken are not a priority unless their labor is needed. The healthcare needs of unproductive members of society: children, students, the elderly, the sick, learning disabled and mentally ill are a costly burden to be born by individuals and families. The elites allow enough access to healthcare to keep the working classes alive (but strapped by debt from medical expenses), but not enough to keep them healthy.

Summary

As the US population was evolving into its contemporary profile, the US healthcare system was undergoing a transformation of its own. The period leading up to WWII saw the emergence of allopathic medicine, steeped in the germ theory, and focused on the acute conditions that affected the population at the time. The twentieth century came to be known as the "American century" as most advances in treatment, innovations in technology, and refinements in medical education were generated by the US system. Its foundation was the "medical model" which reflected the conviction that illness represents the presence of biological pathogens.

Developments within the healthcare system in the 1960s and 1970s primarily served to consolidate and expand the influence of the healthcare system. New treatment modalities continued to be introduced, and there appeared to be no limit to the application of technology. Hospitals were viewed positively by the community and were able to concentrate financial resources for the advancement of medicine. Insurance companies became major players, and the pharmaceutical industry began to assert its dominance. A major concern during this period, however, was the rapidly increasing cost of care, and major efforts were undertaken to control costs. The 1980s will no doubt be seen by historians as a watershed for US healthcare, as the healthcare system experienced a major transformation.

Although the medical model had its flaws, one of the undisputed trends over the past century was the steady improvement in the health status of the US population. It has been pointed out, however, that medical science received too much credit for these health advances. The general improvement in the overall health status of the population is now attributed to a rising standard of living, better nutrition, and the introduction of preventive measures. The shortcomings of both the traditional medical care approach and the emerging healthcare approach were recognized when research found that, after a century of improving health status the US population was probably getting sicker.

During the late 1990s a paradigm shift was observed that involved movement from an emphasis on "medical care" to an emphasis on "healthcare". As acute conditions waned in importance and chronic and degenerative conditions came to the forefront, the medical model began to lose some of its salience. An increasingly holistic healthcare model emerged that took into consideration the patient's social and cultural circumstances. This paradigm shift is still underway despite pushback from a medical establishment that has a vested interest in the traditional medical model approach.

Although the paradigm shift that began emerging during the last years of the twentieth century was hailed by many as a major development with the potential to improve the effectiveness of the healthcare delivery system, its emphasis remains on the individual patient, making this approach an uncomfortable partner for population health.

A major reason that the new paradigm has not been effective in improving population health is that it continues to treat health conditions as the problems. It has become increasingly clear that most health problems represent *symptoms* of some deeper issue rather than the problems themselves. It has also become clear that our society's health problems are being driven by factors that are outside the purview of the healthcare system. The extreme health disparities that have been observed are not a reflection of individual morbidity but of unfavorable health status at the group level. The inescapable conclusion is that the approach taken by the US healthcare system that emphasizes treating one patient at a time is not an effective model in the face of today's health problems, a conclusion that points to the importance of the population health approach.

Key Points

- During the last quarter of the twentieth century the US healthcare system underwent a number of significant changes
- The medical model of care that had been so successful for much of the twentieth century had lost its salience in the face of changes in the nature of patients and in predominant health problems
- Baby boomer patients wanted to be thought of as "customers" and came to expect a high level of service from the system
- With the epidemiologic transition chronic diseases came to predominate while the healthcare system remained focused on acute conditions
- While the system continued to be effective with regard to "heroic" procedures, it failed to contribute to overall population health
- In many ways the healthcare system was having a negative effect on population health
- In response to deficiencies in the system a new paradigm emerged that involved a shift in emphasis from "medical care" to "healthcare"
- The healthcare model was characterized by a broader view of health and illness and emphasized a biopsychosocial approach to supplement the medical model
- While the new paradigm was welcomed by those seeking to improve the effectiveness of the healthcare system, it did little to support community health improvement
- The paradigm continued to focus on one patient at a time—albeit in a more effective manner—while failing to address the barriers to population health improvement
- These developments helped lay the groundwork for the emergence of the population health movement

References

Alter, D. A., Stukel, T., Chong, A., et al. (2011, February). Lesson from Canada's universal care: Socially disadvantaged patients use more health services, still have poorer health. *Health Affairs, 30*(2), 274–228.

Bailey, J. (2014). *The end of healing*. The Healthy City Press.

Bernstein, A. B., Hing, E., Moss, A. J., Allen, K. F., Siller, A. B., & Tiggle, R. B. (2003). *Health care in America: Trends in utilization*. National Center for Health Statistics.

Cooper, R. (2016). *Poverty and the myths of welfare reform*. John Hopkins University Press.

Engle, G. L. (1977). The need for a new medical model: A challenge for biomedicine. *Science, 196*, 129–135. [left out SDoH causes]

McKinlay, J. B., & McKinlay, S. M. (1977). "The questionable contribution of medical measures to the decline of mortality in the United States in the twentieth century," the Milbank Memorial Fund quarterly. *Health and Society, 55*(3), 405–428.

Paradise, J., & Garfield, R. (2013). *What is Medicaid's impact on access to care, health outcomes, and quality of care? Setting the record straight on the evidence*. Downloaded from URL: http://kff.org/report-section/what-is-medicaids-impact-on-access-to-care-health-outcomes-and-quality-of-care-setting-the-record-straight-on-the-evidence-issue-brief/.

Thomas, R. K. (2016). *In sickness and in health: Disease and disability in contemporary America*. Springer.

Waitzkin, H. (1978). A Marxist view of medical care. *Annals of Internal Medicine, 89*(2), 264–278.

Weitz, R. (2013). *The sociology of health, illness, and health care: A critical approach* (6th ed.). Wadsworth.

Wilkerson, I. (2020). *Caste*. Penguin Random House.

Additional Resources

Braveman, P., & Gottlieb, L. (2014). The social determinants of health: It's time to consider the causes of the causes. *Public Health Report, 129*(Supplement 2), 19–31.

Gorski, D. (2019). Are medical errors really the third most common cause of death in the U.S.? (2019 edition). *Science Based Medicine*. Downloaded from URL: https://sciencebasedmedicine.org/are-medical-errors-really-the-third-most-common-cause-of-death-in-the-u-s-2019-edition/.

Chapter 4
The Roots of Population Health

> A number of disciplines have contributed to the evolution of population health, with public health foremost among these. In some ways, <u>population health</u> may be thought of as "<u>public health on steroids</u>" in that the movement <u>adopts</u> many of the precepts of public health and modifies them for application to a new healthcare environment. This chapter describes the contribution made to the evolution of population health by public health professionals and by demography, social epidemiology and social sciences such as medical sociology.
>
> In this chapter, the reader will:
>
> - Learn about the disciplines that have contributed to the emergence of the population health model
> - Understand the role that public health plays in US healthcare and its limitations in terms of contributing to population health
> - Be exposed to the principles drawn from various disciplines to the field of population health
> - Learn about the contributions demography, social epidemiology and medical sociology have made to the field

Introduction

The emergence of population health as a model for community health improvement has been driven by changes in the characteristics of the US population and developments within healthcare. As with many innovative trends, there is no one factor that can claim responsibility. At the same time that changes were playing out in the larger society, developments were taking place within several disciplinary areas that would have implications of one type or another for the emergence of population health.

Advancing population health involves describing the health status of a population, explaining the causes of diseases, predicting health risks in individuals and communities, and offering solutions to prevent and control health problems. To achieve these aims, population health requires collaboration between the core science of epidemiology, several social sciences that are concerned with population attributes, the humanities, and laboratory-based biomedical sciences (Young, 1998). The roles of these various contributors are discussed as appropriate in the sections that follow.

The Contribution of Public Health

History of Public Health

The most obvious "parent" of population health is public health, the component of the US healthcare system that has been most directly focused on the health of populations. Generally excluded from an active role in the provision of clinical services, public health departments have focused on activities that serve the public good rather than the individual good. This is not to say that some public health activities have not targeted individuals (think vaccinations), but that initiatives related to safe food and water, waste management, vector control and environmental safety—activities with a "wholesale" impact on community health—have been the primary concern of public health authorities.

Although the establishment of health services in the United States was not originally addressed in the US Constitution, the need to address matters of public health was recognized early in the nation's history. The 10th amendment to the Constitution called for the establishment of a public health authority endowed with emergency powers. The federal role in public health can trace its origins back to 1798 and the Marine Hospital Fund that established a system of hospitals providing care for merchant sailors arriving in US ports. In 1870, the administration of the system was brought under the auspices of the Marine Hospital Service led by Supervising Surgeon (later called Surgeon General), and medical officers were sent around the country to combat outbreaks of smallpox, yellow fever and cholera. In 1889, the Commissioned Corps was recognized as the official uniformed arm of the Marine Hospital Service.

In 1912, the organization's name was changed to the Public Health Service (PHS), and its focus was expanded to include human diseases, sanitation, water supplies, and sewage disposal. The Public Health Service was subsequently folded into the Department of Health, Education and Welfare in 1953, and, when the Department of Health and Human Services was formed in 1980, the PHS came under its jurisdiction. State and local health departments were established over the course several decades and were eventually brought under the auspices of the PHS.

The Organization of Public Health

Three levels or tiers exist in the US public health system: federal, state, and local. The Department of Health and Human Services (DHHS) is the principal national organization charged with protecting the health of Americans. As a federal Department, the DHHS serves as a source of policy, guidance, and funding but does not directly administer programs. DHHS works with state and local (i.e., county or city) governments to ensure that health information and services reach the public. This support involves financial resources, technical assistance, education, and policy making. The fact that almost one-fourth of the federal budget is spent on DHHS programs indicates the significance of healthcare in the federal budget.

The Centers for Disease Control and Prevention (CDC) is a major component of the DHHS and represents its front-line public health agency. Its main goal is to protect public health and safety through the control and prevention of disease, injury, and disability. The CDC focuses national attention on developing and applying disease control and prevention. It has historically focused on infectious disease, food-borne pathogens, environmental health, occupational, health promotion, and injury prevention, as well as educational activities designed to improve the health of Americans. (See Box 4.1 for a list of key federal agencies related to public health.)

Box 4.1: Relevant Programs: Department of Health and Human Services

Centers of Disease Control and Prevention (CDC) is the nation's first responder in health emergencies and supports people in living healthier and longer lives.

Food and Drug Administration (FDA) ensures that food, drugs, medical devices, and cosmetics that come to market are safe and effective.

Health Resources and Services Administration (HRSA) provides support for healthcare providers as they deliver health services in US communities.

Indian Health Service (IHS) funds health services and local facilities that serve American Indian and Alaska Native populations.

Substance Abuse and Mental Health Services Administration (SAMHSA) supports communities in providing treatment and preventive services to improve behavioral health outcomes.

Administration for Community Living coordinates the efforts of the Administration on Aging, the Administration on Intellectual and Developmental Disabilities, and the Department of Health and Human Services Office on Disability to address the needs of older Americans and people with disabilities across the lifespan.

Box 4.2: Core Public Health Functions

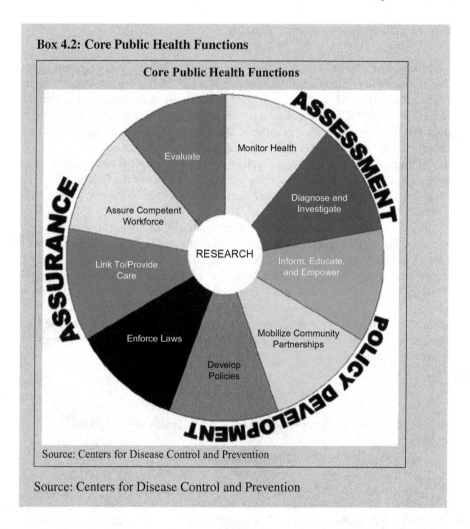

Source: Centers for Disease Control and Prevention

State health agencies are under the direction of the Health Officer (or Medical Officer) whose work is guided by the state's Board of Health. The structure of state health departments and boards vary by state. The scope of state-level public health activities also varies widely, with the responsibilities of the state health department arising from basic legal requirements to the inclusion of a wide range of state-specific activities (e.g., insurance monitoring, professional credentialing, provision of mental health services, management of hospitals). See Box 4.2 for a depiction of core public health functions.

Local agencies may be established at the county, city, or neighborhood level depending on the state system and the size of the population served. There are approximately

2800 local health departments operating in the United States today. Public health agencies may be as simple as a single health officer or as complex as a multi-state, multi-center complex of services provided by thousands of individuals. Tribal agencies operate at a level that is most similar to the state level public health agencies. Counties that do not have an extant public health agency typically have a health professional to serve as the local health officer. Larger metropolitan areas may have a city health department in addition to its county health departmen(s)t. In rural or frontier areas where the populations are sparse, the department may consist of a single person. In other areas, the city and county departments may be combined into a single entity. The local government decides how it will delegate the authority and the scope of that authority.

Most programs are administered at this level, local citizens are involved on the Boards to provide the community perspective, and vital statistics and disease surveillance reports are collected at the local level prior to being transmitted to state health officials. It is at the local level that citizens are most likely to interact with public health due to the local agency's responsibility for birth and death certificates, provision of vaccinations, and the control of sexually transmitted infections, among other functions that bring the local agency face to face with the public.

The Functions of Public Health

Public health, according to the Institute of Medicine (1988) is "what we as a society do collectively to assure the conditions in which people can be healthy." The earliest approach, termed "public hygiene", focused on environmental sanitation. Then, between 1920 and 1940, in a society concerned with diseases transmitted by immigration and increasing travel, the term and focus shifted to "health protection". As diseases of lifestyle became more common in the 1950s and 1960s, the emphasis shifted towards behavior and "health education" was born. Subsequent recognition that education alone was insufficient broadened the field to "health promotion". The social context was formally recognized when university departments of "community health" or "community medicine" began to appear.

The health promotion movement also changed the perspective on the role of individual people, who moved from being recipients of health education to active participants who should take active responsibility for their health, mainly through improving lifestyles. National programs promoted exercise, nutrition, and smoking cessation. These often implied environmental change (e.g., building sports facilities, walking paths, pedestrian malls). In the 1980s the healthy cities movement focused attention on the built environment.

Critiques of health education efforts argued that many people, especially those who were poorer, had a limited capacity to improve their lifestyles because they were deeply constrained by their socioeconomic and cultural milieux. There was concern that the health education movement could be viewed as "blaming the victim" and that, by focusing on lifestyle changes, underlying health determinants would be ignored. In a preview of population health, behaviors came to be seen as *symptoms* of underlying social determinants rather than the main causes of poor health. Box 4.3 addresses concerns over "blaming the victim" in the context of health education programs.

> **Box 4.3: Blaming the Victim: The Case of Obesity**
> Observers of the impact of various social programs have increasingly raised concerns about the appearance of "blaming the victim". The situation with regard to obesity epitomizes the issues surrounding efforts to understand and improve health behavior. Concerns over the possibility of blaming the victim, in fact, reflect the tension between the traditional medical model approach to healthcare and the population health approach.
>
> US obesity rates have escalated rapidly over the last 25 years, and today two-thirds of US adults are overweight and one-third are obese. The increase in obesity is so widespread that being overweight has become the "new normal." Obesity is now the second leading contributor to death in the United States—implicated in one of two heart disease deaths and one of three cancer deaths (Trust for America's Health, 2014). Unless the obesity epidemic is successfully addressed, life expectancy for the US population will decline, with this generation of children having shorter life expectancies than their parents (Olshansky et al., 2005).
>
> Unlike most other health problems there is a stigma associated with obesity in American society. Obese individuals may face discrimination in employment, education, interpersonal relationships, healthcare and the media (Heuer et al., 2011). Overweight children and adults are stereotyped as lazy, unmotivated and lacking in self-discipline (Puhl & Heuer, 2009). Importantly, overweight people are often blamed for their condition, with obesity indicating a lack of personal responsibility.
>
> The problem is further inflamed by the recent proclamation by the American Medical Association that "obesity is a disease" (Stoner & Cornwall, 2014). Such a designation ignores obesity's root causes and calls for a medical model solution. Conveniently, new prescription weight loss drugs have recently been released, and obesity vaccines are under development.
>
> The victim-blaming perspective emphasizes the importance of the individual's behavior when it comes to the obesity epidemic. Yet it is clear that obesity is not an idiosyncratic attribute associated with individuals but is a group phenomenon. Like most risk factors, obesity is found more often in socially disadvantaged groups. Based on 2011–14 average, the proportion of adults that was obese was 36.4%. However, this figure for African-Americans was 48.8% and for Hispanics 42.6%. Similar figures are generated for children (2–19 years). African-American and Mexican-American women are more likely to be obese than are non-Hispanic white women (Chang & Lauderdale, 2005).). Obesity is more common among lower-income

(continued)

Box 4.3 (continued)
individuals and those with less education. Some 39.2% of those living below the poverty level and 42.6% of those between 100% and 199% of the poverty level were obese, compared with less than 30% of those with incomes 400% or more of the poverty level (National Center for Health Statistics, 2015).

Despite the disparities in the distribution of obesity within the US population, conventional medical wisdom urges patients to eat less and exercise more. If individuals continue to be obese despite this "counseling", it is attributed to a personal failing. But by blaming the individual, the real culprit behind the obesity epidemic—an obesogenic environment—escapes the spotlight. This epidemic, rather than being a consequence of a lack of motivation and self-discipline among US adults and children, is a function of our food culture. The fast food industry—a central player in our obesogenic environment—specifically targets minority populations. To exacerbate the situation the fast food industry distributes misinformation that promotes obesity as a personal choice.

Policies and interventions to reduce obesity should be informed by our understanding of its underlying causes. The two predominant models that have historically been used to explain the occurrence of obesity—and of ill-health more generally—are the medical model and the public health model. These models are based on different assumptions, derive from different intellectual traditions, and have vastly different implications for policy and intervention (Adler & Steward, 2009).

The medical model focuses on curing disease and focuses on the individual patient and his or her characteristics. The main purpose of interventions regarding overweight and obesity, along with other behavioral risk factors, is providing information that allows individuals to make more informed behavioral choices. This model views individuals as responsible agents, capable of acting on their own behalf. Well-informed and properly motivated obese individuals should be able to control their weight.

In reality, few people obtain much support in controlling their weight from their healthcare providers since they have virtually no training in health maintenance. Information on weight management is more frequently obtained from diet books, interpersonal contacts, and weight management groups (e.g., Weight Watchers). A recent statement from the American Heart Association regarding our current approach to obesity notes the "limited ability to deliver enough treatment to enough people" (Kumanyika et al., 2008) and argues for more broadly based prevention strategies at the population level, recognizing the fact that this is an epidemic that cannot be cured one person at a time.

In contrast, the public health perspective does not assign responsibility for the obesity epidemic primarily to individuals who eat too much and move too little but to the obesogenic environment. Social and economic conditions have been linked to the prevalence of obesity and its recent increase. Environmental

(continued)

Box 4.3 (continued)

influences have increasingly made unhealthy choices the default option. By opting for what is available in their communities, disadvantaged residents adopt an unhealthy lifestyle out of necessity.

The public health model also looks at environmental conditions that contribute to the obesity epidemic through their effects on food consumption. The pervasive and powerful marketing of energy-dense foods has come under increasing scrutiny. The supersizing of cheap sources of energy-dense foods and the proliferation of fast-food outlets pit healthy food choices against convenience and getting "the most bang for your buck." The food industry's marketing of foods that exploit evolutionarily programmed human preferences for sugar and fat affects food preferences and their associated caloric intake.

Although some public health efforts have focused on structural factors (e.g., eliminating soft drinks from school cafeterias), regulatory efforts (e.g., food product labeling), and/or policy formulation, most of the effort has been geared toward changing individual behavior. Taking a cue from the medical model, public health public service announcements emphasize individual responsibility and assume that providing information will encourage behavioral change. Yet, it has been found that educational interventions alone are relatively ineffective (Jeffery & French, 1999).

A population health approach would expand on the traditional public health approach by addressing the social determinants of obesity and associated morbid conditions. It is clear that personal actions alone cannot stem the obesity tide and in many ways are self-defeating. An approach that focuses on the life circumstances that influence the behavior of group members should be emphasized. Further, it should call for greater control over the influence of the food industry in the political process—an accomplishment that is easier said than done. Such an approach should address the "food deserts" that exist in many communities, restricting the ingredients included in processed foods (and appropriately labeling them), and assuring the availability of greenspaces for disadvantaged populations.

An important function of public health agencies at all levels is the provision of health education to the public. Educational initiatives can take a variety of forms with much of it falling under the rubric of "social marketing." This is one public health activity that perhaps foreshadowed some of the techniques that should be applied in a population health model. The intent of social marketing is to employ standard marketing techniques developed in the private sector to disseminate information on health issues and encourage members of the general public to pursue positive health behaviors. Most of these initiatives involve mass marketing techniques although some may target specific populations (e.g., demographic groups, at-risk populations). Techniques utilized include public service announcements, community events, health fairs and other activities targeting a wide swath of the population.

Some social marketing initiatives may be viewed as "crusades" to change policies and practices. These approaches may include legislative and regulatory means to remove obstacles to healthy eating and activity habits and/or to create incentives to support them. Examples are nutrition standards for school lunch programs; bans on sugar-sweetened beverages in schools' vending machines; requirements for physical education in schools; requirements for developers of residential subdivisions to include bicycle paths, sidewalks, and parks; and zoning regulations for fast-food outlets. Box 4.4 describes a successful social marketing initiative.

Box 4.4: Social Marketing and the Reduction of Smoking: The CDC "Tips" Campaign

The Centers for Disease Control and Prevention (CDC) has been a major advocate for health education and has initiated a number of programs to promote healthy living. One of its long-term "crusades" promotes smoking cessation. A number of initiatives have been launched and its "Tips from Former Smokers" campaign has been successful beyond expectations. Since the initiation of the program an estimated 1.6 million smokers attempted to quit smoking. This national ad campaign carried out in 2012 resulted in more than 200,000 Americans quitting smoking immediately following the 3-month campaign. These results exceed the campaign's original goals of 500,000 quit attempts and 50,000 successful quits.

For this project thousands of adult smokers and nonsmokers were surveyed before and after the campaign. Findings showed that, by quitting, former smokers added more than a third of a million years of life to the US population. The Tips campaign, which aired from March 19 to June 10 was the first time a federal agency had developed and placed paid advertisements for a national tobacco education campaign. Ads featured emotionally powerful stories of former smokers living with smoking-related diseases and disabilities. The campaign encouraged people to call a toll-free number to access quit support across the country, or visit a quit-assistance website.

The evaluation of the campaign found that millions of nonsmokers reported talking to friends and family about the dangers of smoking and referring smokers to quit services. Almost 80 percent of smokers and almost 75 percent of non-smokers recalled seeing at least one of the ads during the 3-month campaign. Calls to the quitline more than doubled during the campaign and visits to the website were more than five times higher than for the same 12-week period in 2011, according to a 2012 report. It was estimated that through this initiative it was possible to save a year of life for less than $200, making this an extremely cost-effective prevention effort.

(continued)

> **Box 4.4** (continued)
>
> The Tips campaign was launched to counter the more than $8 billion in marketing annually by the tobacco industry to make cigarettes more attractive and more available. Investments in educational campaigns such as Tips have been found to save lives and reduce healthcare costs. The Affordable Care Act's Prevention and Public Health Fund paid for the $54 million Tips 2012 campaign.
>
> Source: Centers for Disease Control and Prevention (2016).

The Current State of Public Health

It is surprisingly difficult to profile the public health field due to the wide range of occupations, types of organizations, and variations in function of public health entities, but it is clear that, as the coronavirus has highlighted, public health resources are unevenly distributed across the nation. There are some areas that would be considered public health rich in that certain states, counties or municipalities have invested heavily in public health infrastructure, personnel and programs. On the other hand, there are many jurisdictions that are public health poor and lack even the most basic public health resources.

Although it is difficult to obtain accurate data on the number of health professionals one thing is clear: The absolute number of public health professionals and the professional-to-population ratio have declined significantly in recent years. There are an estimated 280,000 public health workers today spread over the United States in a wide range of different occupations. This figure is down from the 450,000 public health workers enumerated in 2000. This decline has been underway for some time with the professional-to-population ratio declining from 220/100,000 in 1980 to 158/100,000 in 2000. The current figure represents a ratio of only 85 per 100,000.

Virtually all funding for public health is derived from one level of government or another. Government budget allocations and grants are supplemented in some cases by fees charged to the public. These fees, however, represent an insignificant source of revenue. Funds for public health services at the federal level are allocated by Congress and, thus, subject to the whims of political decision makers. Despite the fact that healthcare accounts for a growing proportion of the federal budget, the amount allocated to public health has experienced the opposite trend. Trends in federal expenditures for public health ebb and flow based upon emerging needs, such as increases in emergency preparedness funding following the 2001 terrorist attacks or pandemic flu funding following a disease outbreak. Federal expenditures for public health, in fact, make up a very small proportion of federal health-related funding. Annual federal public health expenditures in 2014 accounted for only 2.5% of national healthcare expenditures. This factors out to less than $240 per capita in that year compared to $10,000 per capita spent on private health services.

Each state allocates a significant proportion of its budget for public health. Although not all state health spending is on public health, this is always a major line item, with health services accounting for either the first or second largest budget allocation in most states. Because of the variation in the activities that fall under public health at the various states, it is difficult to compare spending on a state-by-state basis. Public health funding represents discretionary spending in most states and is therefore at high risk for significant cuts during economic downturns.

Local health departments derive funding from a variety of sources, and these sources vary from state to state. The largest source of funding is local (county and/or city) government budgets (accounting for a fourth of funds). This is followed by state allocations, with federal funding combined with federal government pass-throughs accounting for most of the rest. The only other major source of funding is Medicaid, a source of funding typically only available to those agencies that provide primary care services. Dependence on state funding has contributed to the decreasing level of resources available to local health departments.

The Current Focus of Public Health

The driving force for US public health initiatives is the Centers for Disease Control and Prevention (CDC), the front-line public health agency in the United States. Its main goal is to protect public health and safety through the control and prevention of disease, injury, and disability.

Although recognizing the need to improve population health overall, most of the agency's initiatives reflect traditional public health activities. Its current emphases include combating antibiotic resistance, reducing prescription drug overdose reduction, promoting global health security, and assuring laboratory safety and quality. Further, the CDC seeks to reduce the impact of the two leading killers—cardiovascular disease and cancer—emphasizing the implementation of comprehensive tobacco control and heart health campaigns.

A new initiative by the CDC (2014) attempts to contribute to improved health status through an emphasis on prevention. The overarching goal of the National Prevention Strategy is to increase the number of Americans who are healthy at every stage of life. The strategy provides evidence-based recommendations for improving the nation's health through four broad strategies:

- Building healthy and safe community environments that encourage employees to increase physical activity and reduce pollution
- Expanding quality preventive services in both clinical and community settings by expanding the linkages between clinical and community prevention initiatives to support preventive efforts among underserved groups and improve access to preventive services.
- Empowering people to make healthy choices by providing access to actionable and easy-to-understand information and resources and culturally competent methods that support more traditional written and oral communication.

- Eliminating the health disparities that divide the US population into the healthy and unhealthy, the well cared for and the poorly cared for.

These are clearly goals that should contribute to the advancement of the population health model and to community health improvement. However, in the implementation of the actions that supposedly support these goals, the CDC typically falls back on traditional public health initiatives. The efforts to reduce the burden of leading causes of preventable death and major illness focus on:

- Tobacco-free living
- Preventing drug abuse and excessive alcohol use
- Healthy eating
- Active living
- Injury- and violence-free living
- Reproductive and sexual health
- Mental and emotional wellbeing

While these are laudable actions and, in their way, contribute to improved personal health status, their contribution to overall health status improvement is questionable.

Another initiative in which the CDC has taken steps that could be linked to population health is its Climate and Health program. This program has helped states prepare for health impacts of climate change such as increased air pollution, extreme weather, and the faster spread of food and waterborne diseases. The CDC's Building Resilience Against Climate Effects (BRACE) framework is designed to help health officials prepare for climate change. Box 4.6 describes an effort by the CDC that foreshadows a population health approach.

In response to the emerging population health model, federal health professionals are working to refine the national health agenda around social determinants through the Public Health 3.0. initiative. This initiative is led by the US Department of Health and Human Services (HHS) Office of the Assistant Secretary for Health (OASH) and builds on the work of Healthy People 2020. It encourages collaborations across communities and sectors. Public Health 3.0 represents a major upgrade in public health practice that emphasizes cross-sectoral environmental, policy, and systems-level actions that directly affect the social determinants of health and advance health equity. It challenges business leaders, community leaders, state lawmakers, and Federal policymakers to incorporate health into all areas of governance.

Public Health 3.0 is premised upon the fact that society has a responsibility to create conditions that allow all members of our communities to make healthy choices. Yet public health initiatives often exist in silos, resulting in missed opportunities to leverage the critical knowledge of communities to improve health at the local level.

Public Health 3.0 calls for the expansion of the scope of public health to address *all* aspects of life that promote health and well-being, including:

- Economic development
- Education

- Transportation
- Food
- Environment
- Housing
- Safe neighborhoods

Foreshadowing the population health model, partners from these sectors are being encouraged to work collaboratively to improve health outcomes and advance health equity. By involving stakeholders and working to foster creativity and innovation across sectors, public health authorities hope to improve the health status of the nation's increasingly diverse communities. Box 4.5 describes a federal program that reflects the growing interest in population health.

> **Box 4.5: The Community Transformation Grant Program**
>
> One initiative of the CDC that could be viewed as a step toward population health is its Community Transformation Grant program (CTG). This major initiative supported by the Prevention and Public Health Fund under the Affordable Care Act is designed to address the leading causes of chronic diseases, improve the overall health of Americans, and reduce healthcare costs over the long term. This initiative is intended to encourage people to take personal responsibility for their health outside of the doctor's office and, importantly, allow communities to address their greatest health needs. This program was prompted by a concern that unhealthy Americans generate costs for communities, taxpayers, and businesses in healthcare expenditures, lost productivity, and lower academic achievement. While individuals must take personal responsibility for their health, they must have the support of their communities so that they do not face obstacles to healthy living.
>
> Community transformation grants allow communities to design specific interventions that meet the most pressing needs of their populations through proven, effective community-based interventions that focus on the leading causes of chronic disease. Communities receiving grants are expected to meet strict performance measures, including reducing death and disability due to tobacco use, the rate of obesity through nutrition and physical activity interventions, and death and disability due to heart disease and stroke. Community transformation programs are required to base their efforts on proven, evidence-based approaches and must meet measurable, achievable outcomes to continue receiving federal dollars. Importantly, these initiatives are developed and administered by community members working together at the local level, not by Washington bureaucrats who may not understand the specific community needs.
>
> Although not initially designed based on a population health model, community transformation grants arguably have the potential for promoting a population health approach in that the local community is directed to focus on the social determinants of health and illness.
>
> Unfortunately, funding for the Community Transformation Grant Program was eliminated in 2014.

Public Health Professional Organizations

Efforts by public health departments to achieve their goals are supported by certain key professional associations. The American Public Health Association (APHA) is the professional organization that represents most public health professionals. The APHA is in many ways the most visible of the entities involved with public health since it represents the individual professionals who interface with the public. It generates considerable publicity with regard to its policy stances and priority issues. The APHA aggressively lobbies governments at all levels and is outspoken in terms of its advocacy for public health causes.

Like the CDC, the APHA is highly vested in traditional issues related to public health. Among its stated areas of emphasis are: communicable disease, chronic disease, reproductive and sexual health, vaccines, injury and violence prevention, tobacco, and prescription drug overdose. Most of these issues are traditional areas of interest to public health authorities, although chronic disease and prescription drug overdose issues are more recent concerns. The APHA has added gun violence to its areas of interest, a topic not historically addressed by public health officials. Arguably, none of these areas of emphasis has significant implications for population health but instead focus on individual health improvement.

The APHA, however, is targeting some other issues with more salience for the population health movement. These include: school graduation rates and school-based health, environmental health and climate change, and transportation issues. Broader areas of concern that relate even closer to the population health model include health equity, health in all policies, healthcare reform, and healthy community design.

While giving tacit support to the population health model, the APHA functions as a professional association and not a vehicle for program administration. The organization can and does provide information, education, resources and tools for use by its members in pursuit of various goals. And, as noted above, it supports a robust advocacy effort with regard to regulations, laws and policies related to public health. Ultimately, however, the association has limited ability to act on these issues or to directly influence the health of the population. The best it can do is to encourage its members to support these causes while providing supporting resources.

One activity of the APHA that borders on population health is a new program geared toward the health of the public. Its Generation Public Health campaign attempts to include everyone and everything that impacts health—from housing, education and income to community design, transportation and the environment. Generation Public Health builds on a key concept: every aspect of business, government, education, and communication involves health at some level. Its emphasis is on partnering with organizations in diverse sectors of society to encourage effective, evidence-based programs that improve health. A "health in all policies" approach recognizes this interconnectedness and the synergies that can be achieved when all segments of society work together for collective impact.

The overarching priorities with regard to APHA advocacy are expanding public health capacity, assuring the right to health for all citizens, and promoting health equity. Current causes for which political support is being sought include: child nutrition, climate change and the environment, reducing gun violence, and preserving provisions of the Affordable Care Act. However, in keeping with the organization's historical stance, most initiatives are of necessity limited in scope and would not be thought to contribute to overall community health improvement.

The APHA is certainly aware of the emerging population health model but has failed to engage in any meaningful way. While this should be a natural domain for the public health establishment, few professionals are in a position to promote the new model. In fact, as recently as the 2015 APHA annual conference the program literally included *no* mention of "population health", despite its theme of "health in all policies."

Another public health professional organization, the Association of State and Territorial Health Officers (ASTHO), reflects the same themes that characterize the CDC's priorities. Its membership is composed primarily of public health administrators rather than the broad range of representation found in the APHA. The priority issues that it identified for 2015 (ASTHO, 2015) include: infectious disease outbreaks, electronic cigarettes, prescription drug abuse, motor vehicle injuries, and marijuana possession. A major ASTHO priority has been the reduction of the non-medical use of and unintentional overdose deaths involving controlled prescription drugs.

The major advocate for local health departments is the National Association of County and City Health Officials (NACCHO). Since the 1960s NACCHO has sought to improve the public's health while adhering to a set of core values: equity, excellence, participation, respect, integrity, leadership, science and innovation. Today, NACCHO represents over 2800 local health departments across the nation. As the nation's strongest advocate for local health departments, NACCHO provides educational tools and resources to its members.

NACCHO's Chronic Disease Prevention Learning Communities program engages local health departments to enhance their capacity to implement, evaluate, and sustain evidence- and practice-based chronic disease prevention activities in their communities. The Big Cities Community of Practice (BC-CoP) is a forum for the leaders of America's largest metropolitan health departments to exchange strategies and jointly address initiatives that promote and protect the health and safety of the 51 million people they serve. NACCHO's environmental health portfolio focuses on the interrelationships between people and their environments and includes a number of projects that address the most pressing environmental health issues facing the world today, including climate change, food safety and security, vector-borne disease transmission, and hydraulic fracturing.

The organization's environmental health programs come closer to population health than most of its other activities. These programs address the disproportionate environmental risks borne by low-income communities and communities of color affected by poor housing stock, poor nutrition, lack of access to healthcare, unemployment, underemployment, and employment in the most hazardous jobs.

The Defunding of Public Health and Its Consequences

Public health faces significant challenges due to tightening budgets and unpredictable funding streams, with health departments suffering significant cuts reflecting national economic setbacks. While some of the most dramatic decreases came from diminished state revenue and reductions in tobacco Master Settlement Agreement allocations, federal funding, including categorical funding and block grants, has also decreased. This decline in available funds has resulted in program reductions, service cutbacks, and staff layoffs.

These developments reflect a steady decline over the past several years in national support for public health. Public health funding has historically represented only a fraction of what the federal government spends on health annually. Core discretionary budgets for the Centers for Disease Control and Prevention and the Health Resources Services Administration have suffered significant cuts although there has been some— if inadequate—restoration of funding in recent years. Since the bulk of federal public health dollars—for CDC, as much as 70 percent—flows directly to state and local health departments and other external partners, these cuts trickle down to state and local agencies. Funding specifically for public health has been cut from $740 million in 2010 to $675 million in 2019 (Wilson et al. 2020).

Funding at the state level has faced even greater cuts. According to an analysis by the Trust for America's Health (2015). From FY 2008 to FY 2013, the median per capita state spending decreased from $33.71 to $27.49. This represents a cut of more than $1.3 billion in state funding for public health (adjusted for inflation) over the 5-year period.

In addition to decreases in revenue, some states are facing increases in various costs and expenditures. State health departments may have to make up shortfalls when expenditures increase but revenue remains flat. Some states face the obligations of growing costs associated with state-level healthcare reform. These costs, coupled with the growing cost of pensions and education, are crowding out funding for public health. These added pressures make it increasingly difficult to get the public health budget back to its pre-recession level.

As a result, a number of states have enacted funding cuts across the board for public health, leaving health departments to determine how those cuts will impact their state's public health system. Some states have made this decision by prioritizing public health programs. Often, program-specific cuts made at the federal level are passed on to state health departments and, subsequently, onto local health departments.

Funding cuts at the federal and state levels obviously have an impact at the local level. Numerous analyses have found significant cuts to programs, workforce and budgets at the nation's local health departments. Local health departments lost over

43,000 jobs due to layoffs and attrition between 2008 and 2012 alone (National Association of County and City Health Officials, 2013).

The impact of budget cuts and staff reductions on the operation of America's public health machinery has been significant. Losing one-fifth of the public health workforce at the state and local level has necessitated the elimination of critical services, including immunizations, maternal and child health, food and water safety, public hospitals and clinics, and programs that prevent diseases such as diabetes, cancer, and HIV/AIDS. At the same time, the US population is facing a resurgence of a number of communicable diseases long thought eliminated or eradicated. Outbreaks of measles, whooping cough, malaria and tuberculosis are occurring across the nation.

No one factor accounts for the re-emergence of communicable diseases, but it is clear that cutbacks in testing and surveillance are considerations. While funding shortfalls have resulted in reduced surveillance, public health has perhaps been a victim of its own success. A level of complacency has been suggested as a result of past success at reducing the burden of communicable disease, leading to less monitoring urgency. In addition, fewer and fewer public health officials have had exposure to communicable diseases and are less likely to detect them within the population. The anti-vaccination movement has not helped, of course, in efforts to control some diseases.

The consequences of de-emphasizing public health have been put on full display in the wake of the coronavirus pandemic that emerged early in 2020. While there is plenty of blame for an inadequate response to this disastrous development, it became clear very early that the public health infrastructure was ill-suited to respond to such an emergency. It was obvious that many if not most public health agencies did not have the capabilities to respond in an effective manner. Most were already understaffed, and the pandemic prompted the addition of myriad more responsibilities on public health departments. The inability to systematically test for COVID-19, carry out contact tracing and institute quarantine measures, and, once a vaccine became available, efficiently manage vaccine distribution were all areas of concern.

In the light of the above developments it could be argued that our national commitment to public health has waned. While changing levels of commitment are hard to quantify there has been an undisputed reduction in funding for public health functions. The Affordable Care Act held promise for the infusion of significant new funding for public health but, due to Congressional resistance and sequestration, less than half of the budgeted funding has materialized. It is now forecast that by 2023 public health spending will account for only 2.4% of total health dollars, a decline of 25% over a period of 20 years (Himmilstein & Woolhandler, 2016).

Public Health Does Not Equate to Population Health

As population health is a relatively new concept, uncertainties remain over details of how, precisely, it differs from public health. Both are concerned with patterns of health and illness in groups of people rather than in individuals; both monitor health trends, examine their determinants, propose interventions at the population level and weigh options for delivering these interventions. The distinction is subtle, but population health is seen as broader, as offering a unifying paradigm that links disciplines from the biological to the sociological. It provides a rational basis for allocating health resources that balances health protection and promotion against illness prevention and treatment.

Public health differs from clinical medicine in its application to populations rather than to individuals, and the population health model advances the application of public health beyond the basic functions of public health to emphasize the significance of the root causes of health problems in US society—poverty, housing insecurity, lack of job opportunities, poor educational levels and so forth.

Despite the potential for public health to contribute to the population health movement, the distinction between public health and population health is becoming clearer over time. While many activities that fall under the heading of public health may overlap with those that are considered reflective of a population health approach, the focus of public health in general remains too narrow to fit within the parameters of population health.

Even when support for a more broad-based effort is espoused, public health authorities face significant challenges in getting beyond institutional constraints. Public health, in fact, retains something of the one bug/one drug/one shot mentality that served it so well during the twentieth century. While monitoring and surveillance are important functions, they are essentially downstream activities. They determine when the horse has already left the barn or, best case, when the horse is leaving the barn. Even when addressing broader issues (e.g., environmental toxins) the response is typically more reactive than proactive.

Public health initiatives that attempt to impact the behavior of people tend to emphasize the steps that individuals can take themselves to improve their personal health status. While there is no overt attempt to blame the victim, social marketing (e.g., smoking cessation) and health education (e.g., healthy diet) are premised on the notion that members of the targeted population exhibit inappropriate behavior. In order to improve their health status, they must change their behavior. While these efforts represent a sort of mass marketing, their success depends on the changes in the behavior of individual actors.

When public health tackles a health issue, its interventions are focused on maintaining health or preventing disease. For example, the public health approach to childhood obesity might advocate education for parents and children, subsidized healthy school lunch programs, bans on soft drinks in school vending machines, tougher regulations on marketing of junk food to children, etc. While these activities move public health in the direction of population health, they fall short of what would be considered population health under our definition. A population health approach might, for example, consider the food system itself: How do agricultural subsidies affect the price of food? Are there policy solutions to the problem of urban food deserts? The population health approach views issues from a broader perspective and tends to include additional considerations, such as economics, environmental sustainability, social justice, etc.

Although, in general we think of a population in geographic terms, for instance the population of a country, city, neighborhood, a population can also be defined by any factor a group of people might have in common, such as age, socio-economic status, language, or lifestyle. Further, a population can be seen simply as an aggregate of people, or it can be seen as something more than the sum of its members, as a collective organism, as people acting as a group.

The embrace of the population health model requires a conceptual shift. The view of a population as an aggregate of individuals focuses on health *in* the population. By contrast, when the population is seen in emergent terms, as an interacting whole, population health can analyse the health *of* the population. In this view, a healthy community or population is one that works as a group to promote its welfare and address challenges. For example, a healthy population would rally to a natural disaster to establish an effective collective response. Hence, in this view, a healthy population supports and promotes the health of people within it, thereby contributing to individual health.

Discussions of this type have expanded the health promotion approach into a hybrid sometimes termed population health promotion. Many public health units now take a dynamic view and develop programs that foster the ability of community groups to work together for the improvement of their own health. A key driver to the effective implementation of a population health model is the involvement of the community, and this issue is discussed in detail in a later chapter.

Why Public Health Cannot Champion Population Health

There are a number of factors that limit the ability of the public health field to champion population health. Many of them are obvious from the previous section. Despite some overlap, public health and population health represent two different conceptual frameworks. While public health might be considered a player in the implementation of a population health approach, public health cannot be a leader for the following reasons:

- The scope of public health is narrower than that of population health. Population health takes into consideration a number of dimensions relative to community health that are beyond the purview of public health.
- Public health does not have the political or financial clout to effect community health improvement through a population health approach. Within healthcare

itself, public health is the stepchild and, despite the best efforts of the APHA and other advocates, it does not have the influence of other vested interests.
- Public health has virtually no control over the populations in the communities where it would attempt to improve community health status. Many other entities in health such as managed care organizations, insurance plans, and even provider patient pools can, unlike public health, exert considerable leverage over their target populations.
- Although the population health model minimizes the role of the healthcare system in improving community health, healthcare providers do have a role to play. In fact, they are increasingly being incentivized to take a population approach to the management of their patient panels. Public health is for all practical purposes excluded from this process
- Public health authorities are limited in their ability to carry out many of the actions that support a population health approach, even if they so desired. As government agencies they face substantial constraints in the scope of their activities and limited latitude in changing their focus. At the local level in particular there are three levels of bureaucracy that constrain their activities.
- Public health will continue for the foreseeable future to suffer from funding shortfalls at all levels of government. Over the past several years most public health agencies have faced retrenchment in terms of their scope of services. Efforts toward health education and promotion, health needs assessment, community health planning and other activities invariably suffer when public health authorities must reduce their involvement due to a lack of funds and personnel.
- Public health personnel have limited understanding of population health, and this factor constrains their ability to serve as implementers of a population health approach. Despite the growing interest in population health among a wide range of health professionals, few in any sector of healthcare clearly understand the model, and the public health sector is thought to lag behind even these.
- Public health agencies are limited to actions within their specified jurisdictions. Many public health problems extend beyond local borders, for example toxic waste spills, infectious diseases, wars, and natural disasters. These problems may require the involvement of counties, states, the nation, or even other countries to fully understand the scope of the problem and respond to it.

Public health should be the natural "home" for population health but through an unfortunate confluence of forces our nation's public health establishment is unlikely to take the lead with regard to the emerging population health movement. Box 4.6 discussions the manner in which a population's environment might affect its health.

> **Box 4.6: Where you Live Should Not Determine how Healthy You Are**
> Where you live, learn, work and play make a big difference in how healthy you are. According to the Robert Wood Johnson Foundation, a range of factors, like education, employment, income, family and social support, community safety, and the physical environment, impact a population's health. These factors have led the Foundation to promote a "culture of health." In many communities, healthy choices are easy choices for their residents. In these communities, there are plenty of gyms, safe places to jog and community recreation centers with high-quality swimming pools and sports fields. Children play and exercise in well-maintained parks and have access to affordable nutritious foods.
>
> But in many other American communities, there are obstacles to healthy living. Parks and playgrounds are littered, broken or unsafe. School meals are low in nutritional value, school vending machines sell junk food, and students are not provided regular physical education classes. There are few places to get out and exercise, and some communities do not even have sidewalks for walking. Access to fruit and vegetables is limited because there are no supermarkets. Dilapidated housing, crumbling schools, abandoned factories, and freeway noise and fumes cause illness and injury. These unfavorable conditions contribute to higher levels of obesity and chronic disease, including diabetes, heart disease and cancer, and lead to higher healthcare costs.
>
> Public health departments should help improve the health of communities. They are responsible for finding ways to address the systemic reasons why some communities are healthier than others and for developing policies and programs to remove obstacles that make healthy choices impossible. Yet, there is increasing concern about the ability of public health to fulfill this function. Clearly, this is a matter that requires a population health approach on the grounds that unless a healthy environment can be created, clinical medicine has limited ability to contribute to community health improvement.

The Contribution of Demography

Demography is the study of human populations and seeks to analyze human groups and profile them in terms of their salient characteristics and the dynamic processes that influence these characteristics. The characteristics of interest to demographers are those that are relevant within a social and cultural context. Thus, demographers study biosocial traits such as age, sex and race and sociocultural traits such as marital status, education, income, occupation and even religion.

Although other sciences also study human beings, demographers focus on the attributes of populations rather than individuals (recognizing, of course, that population attributes are often but not always the aggregate of individual attributes). Thus, the emphasis of demographers is on the attributes of aggregates—a community, a state or a nation. This approach, of course, is a prerequisite for adopting a population health model.

Much of demographic analysis involves examining the relationship between demographic attributes and other population characteristics. One conclusion generated by looking at the population through "demographic eyes" is that virtually no demographic and social attribute is randomly distributed. All social phenomena (including demographics) display patterns. When demographers look at a population they do not see an amorphous mass of individuals but as clusters of characteristics and patterns reflecting the distribution of various demographic traits. Identifying patterns of distribution is a primary focus of demographers, and their work in establishing the association between demographic traits like income and education with health attributes has been instrumental in raising awareness of the social determinants of health and illness. A subdiscipline of "health demography" has developed around this field of study.

Because of the tendency for demographic attributes to cluster within populations, demographers often segment populations into meaningful subgroups along some relevant demographic dimension. There may be significant variation within any group in terms of its attributes, and an analysis of subgroup variation helps explain the characteristics of any population. This work has heightened sensitivity to health disparities that have been identified between various groups within the US population. Much of the health-related efforts of federal health agencies is focused on addressing persistent disparities in health status among various groups.

The role of demographics in creating a context for the emergence of the population health movement is indisputable. The aging of the US population prompted the epidemiologic transition that increased the significance of chronic disease at the expense of acute conditions. At the same time, the relationship between changing demographic attributes and changing lifestyles is a significant consideration when it comes to population health. The changing disease etiology (from an emphasis on biological pathogens and genetics) to an emphasis on environmental factors and lifestyles is also a factor. Ultimately, in order to understand the potential for the population health model the ramifications of demographic change must be recognized.

Of particular importance in this regard is the increasing stratification of morbidity along demographic dimensions. When acute conditions dominated there was little correlation between demographic characteristics and health status. Everyone was essentially at the same risk for disease. With the emergence of chronic conditions (and the social context that spawned them) clear-cut patterns of morbidity emerged reflecting a correlation between demographic attributes and various health conditions. Differences in health status were increasingly observed based on demography and geography. To a great extent demography became destiny as the ZIP Code became the best predictor of health status.

The study of the distribution of health and illness within the population—and the demographic correlates of these patterns—has contributed to an understanding of the social determinants of health so central to the population health model. To the extent that social determinants are influencing the health status of the US population, most of the determinants would be considered demographic attributes. Thus, poverty, housing instability, food insecurity, unemployment and other contributors to poor health are clearly demographic attributes.

Given that demographic trends have created an environment fertile for the emergence of a population health model and that most of the social determinants are demographic in nature, it only follows that efforts to implement a population health approach should address demographic attributes. Thus, early efforts to improve health status using a population health approach have emphasized job training, reduction of food deserts, improved access to adequate housing, and crime reduction as ameliorative efforts.

The Contribution of Social Epidemiology

Social epidemiology is a branch of epidemiology that focuses particularly on the effects of social-structural factors on the distribution of health and illness within a population. Social epidemiology seeks to identify societal characteristics that affect observed patterns of disease and health distribution and to understand the mechanisms that contribute to these patterns. The central question of social epidemiology to be answered is: what effect do social factors have on individual and population health—and this, of course, has become the central premise of population health.

This field in many ways represents the interface between public health and population health in that it has expanded on basic public health precepts to increase our understanding of the linkage between community health and a wide range of other factors. A primary contribution of social epidemiology has been the shift in focus away from the historical etiological sources of disease to the factors that are responsible for the bulk of today's health problems. This includes the fact that health and illness are not randomly distributed within a population but follow observable patterns. These assertions have become the bedrock on which much of population health rests.

In many ways social epidemiology represents a convergence of demography and public health. It recognizes the association between social attributes and patterns of morbidity and mortality. While public health laid the groundwork for looking beyond biological contributors to ill-health, social epidemiology has raised our consciousness with regard to the social determinants of health and illness. Because of the work of social epidemiologists, the relationship between social class and health has long been a major subject for research.

Social epidemiology provides a foundation for acquiring an understanding of the origin and distribution of disease within a population and a means for determining the appropriate response. Social epidemiologists have generated insights into the distribution of health and illness within the population along with an appreciation for the social determinants of health. In a sense, social epidemiologists have extended the knowledge generated by demographers who have demonstrated the association between demographic attributes and health status without necessarily positing an explanation. This field has taken the matter a step further by exploring causation and seeking to understand the mechanisms through which social circumstances are transformed into health problems.

The Contribution of Medical Sociology

Various social sciences have made considerable contributions to the emerging field of population health, mostly independent of the public health field. *Medical anthropologists* have led the way in the examination of subcultural differences in perceptions of and responses to health conditions and have sensitized the field to the influence of ethnic and subcultural factors on health status and health behavior. Anthropologists have also led us to understand that symptoms may be interpreted quite differently by various subgroups in society. *Medical geographers* have offered insights into the spatial distribution of health-related phenomena and provided the foundation for examining geographical variations in health conditions and health services utilization, further underscoring the significance of patterns of disease distribution. *Health economists* have sensitized us to the role that financing plays in influencing both health status and health behavior. The potential contribution of reimbursement management to the improvement of community health is becoming increasingly obvious.

Of the various social sciences, *medical sociology* has had the most to contribute to the emergence of the population health model. By its very nature medical sociology had an interest in the social factors that influence health and illness within a population well before the "social determinants of health" became a buzzword. Sociologists are sensitive to the influence of social attributes on health and for 50 years have emphasized that health status and health behavior reflect group attributes rather than individual idiosyncrasies. Medical sociology has also effectively incorporated many of the concepts and methods from the social sciences noted above and, for that matter, from public health.

As sociology emerged as a discipline in the late nineteenth century, it founders ignored the healthcare institution in their analysis of society. Unlike frequently studied institutions like the family, the political system and religion, healthcare was neglected because it had yet to emerge as a full-blown social institution. For this reason, medical sociology as an accepted field did not emerge until after World War II, nor did it achieve any significant development until the 1960s. Consequently, medical sociology matured in an intellectual climate far different from the nineteenth- and early twentieth-century environment that spawned early social thought.

Medical sociology was established as a specialized field within sociology in the United States during the 1940s and 1950s. The emergence of this subdiscipline was given impetus by virtue of the interest in social medicine that had surfaced in the 1920s and 30s and the emergence of the field of social epidemiology in the 1940s and 50s. These two movements bolstered the belief that social science had something to contribute to medical research. As a result, the first applications of this new subdiscipline within sociology were in the medical schools. However, because of the apparent success of the medical model in dealing with sickness and its domination of medical thought for a century, the significance of non-clinical factors for the health and illness equation were essentially ignored. In fact, it was only in the last third of the twentieth century that the contribution of the sociological perspective to the study of health and healthcare came to be appreciated.

Recognition of the complex relationships between social factors and the level of health characteristic of various groups has made the sociology of health and illness an important substantive area within the general field of sociology. Just as sociology is concerned with the social causes and consequences of human behavior, the sociology of health is concerned with the social causes and consequences of health and illness. The sociology of health brings sociological perspectives, theories, and methods to the study of health and healthcare.

The work of the sociologist in medicine is intended to be directly applicable to patient care or to the solving of a public health problem. These analyses are made available to health practitioners, health planners and policy setters to assist them in addressing health problems and problems in the delivery of care. Thus, sociology in medicine can be characterized as "applied research and analysis primarily motivated by a medical problem" rather than a sociological problem (Cockerham, 2001).

The shift to the perception of health and illness as social issues bolstered the contribution of medical sociology to the emerging population health movement. In fact, Link (2008) has suggested the need for an epidemiological sociology that would address issues relevant to population health. He argues that the transformation of disease causation from cruel fate, accident, and bad luck to circumstances that are under some degree of human control facilitates a "social shaping" of disease and death. This reflects the notion that, now that we as human beings are really the source of our health problems, the solutions must be sought within the social sphere.

Support for this approach is garnered from evidence of dramatic differences in health status among different populations and the uneven distribution of improvements in health status in the face of interventions. Link (1998) urged a well-supported "epidemiological sociology" that uses a wide range of sociological concepts and theories to elucidate the social shaping of disease and death. Absent a robust societal investment in epidemiological sociology, population health will reside below its optimal level, and the maldistribution of health-enhancing innovations will continue to create health disparities.

Clearly medical sociology can play a pivotal role in the development and application of a population health model. In a sense, it represents the convergence of public health, demography and social epidemiology into a comprehensive framework for examining the health status of a population and the factors that contribute to its observed status. As the emphasis in population health edges further toward the social determinants of ill-health, the role of the medical sociologist can be expected to expand.

Summary

The population health movement has its roots in a number of disciplines, and public health represents the most direct antecedent. Population health might be thought of as "public health on steroids" since many of its methods are rooted in that field. Public health in the United States has a long history dating back to the beginning of the republic. Over the decades the field has adapted to a constantly changing healthcare environment while maintaining its core responsibilities.

In the United States there is a three-tiered public health system that includes public health activities at the federal, state and local levels. At the federal level the US Public Health Service within the Department of Health and Human Services is the primary agency. Working in conjunction with other federal agencies such as the Centers for Disease Control and Prevention, the PHS serves as the leading advocate for population health. Each state and territory has a public health agency as does each county and county equivalent. State health departments are supported through state budgets with generous contributions from the federal government. Federal public health agencies, however, have limited influence on the activities of state health departments (apart from the programs they directly fund), and the structure and function of state health departments varies from state to state.

Local health departments are the point of contact for most citizens since city and county health departments provide services that directly interface with residents. These include acquiring vital statistics data (e.g., births, deaths, marriages and divorces) and supporting local disease surveillance activities. They are also responsible for local environmental safety, vector control and food inspection. Some funding for local health departments is generated locally but they depend heavily on state funding (much of which is passed down from the federal level). As with state health departments, local health department perform a variety of different functions beyond their core responsibilities.

Although public health can be credited with much of the improvement in health status during the twentieth century, the field has experienced a decline in funding in recent years. Federal funding has steadily decreased, and this means that the deficits are passed down to state and local health departments. Per capita funding for public health has steadily decreased resulting in a steadily declining work force.

While public health should be the natural home for population health it has failed to take up the challenge for a variety of reasons. Addressing population health requires a broader scope than historically evinced by public health with the latter wedded to his traditional areas of emphasis. As funding has declined health departments have been forced to retrench with regard to the services provided, typically falling back on their traditional functions without being able to expand into new areas. The lack of interface between public health and the private healthcare sector isolates them from the "space" in which most of healthcare takes place. Population health is not public health and public health is not in a position to take a leading role in its promotion.

Population health also has its roots in demography, social epidemiology, and the social sciences, particularly medical sociology. The field of "health demography" has been instrumental in raising sensitivity to the changing nature of health problems. The emergence of an environment that is fertile for a population health approach reflects the demographic trends of past decades that have involved an aging population and an epidemiological transition. Changing population characteristics were transformed to new and different health problems with a major consequence of these developments being the increasing association between demographic characteristics and disease distribution. Changing lifestyles accompanied the aging of the population, and the growing role of the environment and social determinants in health and illness further emphasized the importance of demography for the emerging paradigm.

Social epidemiology has also helped lay the groundwork for the population health model. Social epidemiologists early on identified the relationship between certain population characteristics and patterns of morbidity and mortality. The fact that health problems were increasingly becoming concentrated within particular population segments reflected emerging patterns of disease, and the growing disparities noted among various subpopulations raised sensitivity to the role of non-biological factors in the nation's morbidity configuration. Emerging evidence that the US population is becoming sicker can be attributed to the work of social epidemiologists.

A variety of social sciences have helped establish the framework for the development of a population health approach, with anthropology, geography and economics among others making contributions. The primary contribution has been made by medical sociology through its efforts to analyze the social aspects of health and illness. The population health model questions historical notions of health and illness, and medical sociologists have been instrumental in highlighting the biopsychosocial dimension.

Key Points

- Public health has historically been considered the primary guardian of the nation's health
- Federal involvement in public health dates back to the early days of the republic
- In the nineteenth century the US Public Health Service emerged with responsibility for public health at the national level
- Over time the role of the PHS expanded and the agency was ultimately incorporated into the Department of Health and Human Services
- Public health functions at the federal, state and local (city/county) levels, with each level having its respective responsibilities.

- Through the Centers for Disease Control and Prevention and other agencies the federal government attempts to protect the people's health at the national level, with responsibility for disease surveillance and vital statistics registration
- Each state and territory maintains a health department and, while certain core functions are universal, the activities of these departments vary from state to state
- Local health departments are the primary point of interaction between the public and public health, performing functions that directly affect the local population.
- Federal public health operations depend on funding from Congress and are susceptible to changing political whims
- At the state level, health is one of the largest items in state budgets with state funding supplemented with federal public health dollars
- Local health departments are funded through a variety of avenues—city and county budgets, state funding and federal funding (typically passed through the state)
- Financial support for public health has steadily eroded in recent years with a decline in budgets at all levels
- Declining financial resources have led to staffing cuts and the curtailment in some cases of all but legally mandated services
- This declining support has implications for population health in that public health should be driving the population health movement
- Unfortunately, population health does not equate to public health and the public health field has not taken the lead with this emerging paradigm
- While there is a role for public health in the implementation of population health it is not likely to be a lead role
- The field of demography has contributed significantly to our understanding of the factors that affect the health of the population, and demographic trends, in fact, have created an environment that is ripe for the emergence of this new paradigm
- Social epidemiology has established a body of evidence concerning the distribution of morbidity and mortality within the US population
- Research by epidemiologists has led us to understand the relationship between population characteristics and health status and to develop a perspective on health disparities
- Various social sciences have helped lay the groundwork for our understanding of the changing nature of health and illness
- Medical sociology in particular has contributed to our appreciation of the social aspects of health and illness.
- Raising sensitivity to the biopsychosocial nature of health conditions has established a context for applying population health methods

References

Adler, N. E., & Steward, J. (2009). Reducing obesity: Motivating action while not blaming the victim. *Milbank Quarterly, 87*(1), 49–70.

Centers for Disease Control and Prevention. (2014). *National prevention strategy: America's plan for better health and wellness*. Downloaded from: https://www.google.com/#q=a+better+plan+for+health+and+wellness

References

Centers for Disease Control and Prevention. (2016). Downloaded from: https://www.cdc.gov/media/releases/2013/p0909-tips-campaign-results.html.

Chang, V. W., & Lauderdale, D. S. (2005). Income disparities in body mass index and obesity in the United States, 1971–2002. *Archives of Internal Medicine, 165*, 2122–2126.

Cockerham, W. C. (2001). *Medical Sociology*. Prentice Hall.

Heuer, C. A., McClure, K. J., & Puhl, R. M. (2011). Obesity Stigma in online news: A visual content analysis. *Journal of Health Communication*. Downloaded from URL: http://www.tandfonline.com/doi/full/10.1080/10810730.2011.561915.

Himmilstein, D. U., & Woolhandler, S. (2016). Public health's falling share of U.S. health spending. *American Journal of Public Health, 106*(1), 56–57.

Institute of Medicine. (1988). *The future of public health*. Institute of Medicine.

Jeffery, R. W., & French, S. A. (1999). Preventing weight gain in adults: The pound of prevention study. *American Journal of Public Health, 89*, 747–751.

Kumanyika, S. K., Obarzanek, E., Stettler, N., et al. (2008). Population-based prevention of obesity: The need for comprehensive promotion of healthful eating, physical activity, and energy balance: A scientific statement from the American Heart Association Council on epidemiology and prevention, interdisciplinary Committee for Prevention. *Circulation, 118*(4), 428–464.

Link, B. G. (1998). Epidemiological sociology and the social shaping of population health. *Journal of Health and Social Behavior, 49*(4), 367–384.

Link, B.G. (2008). Epidemiological Sociology and the Social Shaping of Population Health, *Journal of Health and Social Behavior 49*(4):367–384.

National Association of County and City Health Officials. (2013). *Local Health Department job losses and program cuts: Findings from the 2013 profile study*. Downloaded from: https://www.naccho.org/uploads/downloadable-resources/Survey-Findings-Brief-8-13-13.pdf

National Center for Health Statistics. (2015). *Health: United States 2015*. National Center for Health Statistics.

Olshansky, S. J., Passaro, D. J., Hershow, R. C., et al. (2005). A potential decline in life expectancy in the United States in the 21st century. *New England Journal of Medicine, 352*, 1138–1145.

Puhl, R. M., & Heuer, C. A. (2009). The stigma of obesity: A review and update. *Obesity, 17*(5), 941–964.

Stoner, L., & Cornwall, J. (2014). Did the American Medical Association make the correct decision classifying obesity as a disease? *Australian Medical Journal, 7*(11), 462–464.

Trust for America's Health. (2014). *The state of obesity: 2014*. Trust for America's Health.

Trust for America's Health. (2015). *Investing in America's health: A state-by-state look at public health funding and key health facts*. Downloaded from URL: https://www.tfah.org/report-details/investing-in-americas-health-a-state-by-state-look-at-public-health-funding-key-health-facts-1/

Wilson, R. T., Troisi, C. L., & Gary-Webb, T. L. (2020). A Deficit of More Than 250,000 Public Health Workers is No Way to Fight COVID-19. *Stat*. Downloaded from URL: https://www.statnews.com/2020/04/05/deficit-public-health-workers-no-way-to-fight-covid-19/

Young, T. (1998). *Population health: Concepts and methods*. Oxford University Press.

Additional Resources

Arias, E., Escobedo, L. A., Kennedy, J., Fu, C., & Cisewski, J. (2018). U.S. Small-area Life Expectancy Estimates Project: Methodology and Results Summary. *Vital Health Statistics, 2*(181), 1–31.

Association of State and Territorial Health Officers. (2015). Downloaded from: http://www.astho.org/StatePublicHealth/Public-Health-Issues-to-Watch-in-2015/3-3-15/

Institute of Medicine. (2012). *For the Public's health: Investing in a healthier future*. The National Academies Press.

Chapter 5
Health Status and How to Measure It

The ultimate goal of the population health model is the improvement of the health status for defined populations. While the model has some application to the health status of individuals, the primary focus is on the health of the community. This chapter examines the concept of health status and reviews the ways in which it can be defined and measured as a prerequisite for introducing the population health approach. A key issue is the ability to define health status within the context of the population health model.

In this chapter, the reader will:

- Learn the importance of defining health and health status in contemporary terms
- Discover why the traditional conceptualization of health status is incompatible with a population health approach
- Be introduced to the health status metrics that are more appropriate for the population health model
- Be exposed to some contemporary attempts at health status measurement
- Learn the difference between a traditional community health needs assessment and a population health assessment

Introduction

The ultimate goal of the population health approach is community health improvement. In order to accomplish this, a clear and widely accepted definition of health status is required. This requirement presents a challenge at the outset. First, there is no consensus on how to define "health" much less "health status". Health professionals use both terms regularly without much thought to the specific definitions. Second, if agreement can be reached on the definition of health status, the metrics to be used to measure it must be specified. This is problematic as well in that experts disagree about what indicators are relevant since the metrics should reflect the definition that is ultimately formulated. Third, even if the metrics to be used can be specified, there are challenges in acquiring the necessary data for generating the calculations. Finally, the ability to interpret the data is required, representing another potential challenge. Each of these issues is discussed in detail below.

Conceptual Issues

Health professionals regularly use the term "health status" without much thought to its meaning. The term as conventionally applied refers to the level of health and well-being associated with an individual or a population. Within the population health context, it refers primarily but not exclusively to the health status of groups or populations rather than individuals. However, in order to conceptualize health status a clear notion of what constitutes "health" is required. In the sections that follow both "health" and "health status" are conceptualized in a manner relevant for the population health model.

Defining "Health"

The first step in defining health status is to agree on what we mean when we refer to "health". Unfortunately, there is no single definition of health, and how the term is defined depends on the context and the perspective of those defining it. Health may be variously defined in reference to: the presence or absence of biological pathology; the ability of an individual to function in society; the individual's mental perception of his health; and so forth. It may be defined in narrow terms as in the medical model definition (the absence of disease) or in more holistic terms such as that promulgated by the World Health Organization—that is, a state of complete physical, mental and spiritual health and not just the absence of disease. Clearly, the population health approach calls for a broad definition of health, realizing, of course, the challenges in operationalizing such a definition.

While deriving a generally accepted definition of health is a challenge in its own right, the definition of health may change over time. In fact, "health" as we know it today did not even exist as a concept in our society three generations ago. The dynamic nature of the definition can be observed as US healthcare experienced a paradigm shift from medical care to healthcare (discussed in a previous chapter) in which the notion of health was radically modified. Further, there may be a considerable difference between professional conceptualizations of health and lay perceptions. A challenge for proponents of a population health approach is reconciling professional definitions of health with those held by the general public. (Box 5.1 discusses lay perceptions of health and illness.)

In order to measure health status, it is necessary to make assumptions about what constitutes health. The use of some measures of health status may, in fact, be misleading to the extent that an inappropriate definition of health is utilized. For our purposes we feel a population health approach requires the broadest possible definition of health and, for most purposes will defer to the definition developed in the document *Greenprint 2015/2040* (Shelby County [TN] Government, 2015):

> *Health is a dynamic process for achieving a state of physical, mental, emotional, intellectual, spiritual and social well-being throughout the lifespan. Implicit in this definition are assumptions related to supporting conditions, e.g., adequate personal safety, housing stability, food security, and adequate access to healthcare and social services.*

Box 5.1: Lay Perceptions of Health and Illness

It has been well documented that lay perceptions of health and illness frequently vary—often significantly—from those held by health professionals (encyclopedia.com, 2021). Long before any outside help (medical or otherwise) is sought, individuals interpret their own health conditions. Underlying all such evaluations is a set of ideas about health and illness. These notions of health and illness are not those of science or medicine, although they may be borrowed, accurately or inaccurately, from those formal systems of knowledge. They are the perceptions held by ordinary people whose experiences, cultural background, and social networks shape and continually modify their notions of health and illness. Access to health-related websites fostered by social media have further encouraged lay definitions of health and illness.

Researchers have found that laymen's perceptions of health and illness vary widely from group to group (Conrad & Barker, 2010). Members of some social groups think of health as simply the absence of illness. Others describe health in terms of equilibrium in daily life or the capacity to work. While both working-class and middle-class persons share the notion that health means the absence of illness, working-class people tended to emphasize what was essential for their everyday lives–the ability to carry out their tasks, especially job and family duties. Middle-class persons are more likely to mention broader, positive conceptions of health that included such factors as energy, positive attitudes, and the ability to cope well and to be in control of one's life.

(continued)

Box 5.1 (continued)

The sense of being in control is particularly important to the middle class. It meshes with their sense of having a degree of control in their work and daily lives. This value may be remote or inconceivable to working-class persons who have control over far fewer areas of their lives. American middle-class values have actually expanded the notion of health to something that must be actively achieved.

Americans raised in different ethnic subcultures typically incorporate their group's ideas about health and illness, including perceptions of the nature of health, the causes of illness, and appropriate responses in the face of symptoms. Religious subcultures likewise influence not only their members' responses to illness but also their very definitions of health and illness. From a fundamentalist Christian perspective "health" and "wholeness" are words that reflect "salvation". A healthy person would be one that is whole in spirit, soul, mind, and body.

Just as lay notions of health are shaped by individuals' social and cultural backgrounds, so are the ways people understand their illnesses. People seek to comprehend what is wrong within a context that makes sense to them. Individual belief systems about illness are typically drawn from larger cultural belief systems, which give shape to the illness experience, help the individual to interpret what is happening, and offer a number of choices about how to respond.

Lay images of various diseases reveal why certain responses "make sense". The image allows ill persons to distance themselves from their problems. The concept of disease as an "it" also meshes with notions that the problem had its source in some external agent that invaded the body. Thus, the causal categories used by laypersons to explain illness onset may not be correct in bioscientific terms but are generally rational and based upon the kinds of empirical evidence available to them.

When members of disadvantaged populations are asked about their health status, they are likely to assess it not in medical terms but in terms of:

- How safe they feel
- How secure they feel
- How stress-free they feel
- How "well fed" they feel
- How well they can work, care-give, provide social support

Ultimately, individuals develop notions of health and illness that are consistent with the worldviews of their respective cultural milieux. People rely on their social group to provide an understanding of illness, its causation, and acceptable reactions, not only because individuals may not have access to a "professional" framework for analyzing the situation but also because, even if they did, the professional perspective may not answer questions that are important to the affected individual but outside the scope of the clinician.

Source: Freund and McGuire (1999)

Defining Health Status

Developing a definition of health status assumes that we can conceptualize health in an acceptable way and subsequently operationalize it in order to quantify health status. This has emerged as one of the major challenges in the implementation of a population health approach and raises some of the same questions as with the definition of health: *Whose* definition of health status is the appropriate one? Should health status be considered a phenomenon viewed from the top down by policy makers concerned with the "big picture"? Should it be viewed from the perspective of clinicians who are dealing directly with the health issues of individuals? Should it be viewed from the perspective of the general public who may not share the same vision of health conditions as health professionals? There is no simple answer and these questions will continue to be raised throughout this text.

Discussing the nature of health status raises the issue of how appropriate our vision of health status is. An argument could be made, in fact, that we are really talking about "illness status" rather than "health status", that we are measuring the inverse of what we are actually trying to measure. The typical approach is more focused on why some people are sick rather than why some people are healthy. Perhaps the real question should be: Given the widespread exposure to health threats, why doesn't everyone become ill? This issue was raised early on by the medical sociologist Aaron Antonovsky (1979) who introduced the term "salutogenesis." This term describes an approach to assessing health status that focuses on factors that support health and well-being, rather than on factors that cause disease (pathogenesis).

Antonovsky felt that health status was influenced by a variety of factors that were unrelated to physical or biological considerations, including the presence of a sense of "cohesion." He argued that this attribute influenced the extent to which members of various groups were susceptible to disease, were able to cope with health problems when they arose, and were likely to experience favorable outcomes. While it could be argued that this sense of coherence is an individual trait (and, indeed, Antonovsky developed a questionnaire for use by individuals), it could also be argued that these attributes of individuals arise from and are influenced by their social contexts.

Another more recent perspective has been offered by Gunderson and Pray (2009) in *The Leading Causes of Life*. In this book they emphasize the importance of identifying and capitalizing on the health-inducing assets that populations and communities have access to rather than their liabilities. Although approaching the issue from a faith-based perspective, this approach has relevance for population health to the extent that it focuses on "connection, coherence, agency, hope, and blessing". It offers insights into how *populations* cope with health challenges in the absence of the types of resources that most Americans take for granted. Box 5.2 addresses the issue of the appropriateness of our view of health status.

Like the definition of health itself, health status can be defined in a variety of ways from a variety of perspectives. This raises the question of whether it is

Box 5.2: Health Status: Are We Measuring the Right Thing?
Various parties utilize the term "health status" without giving the concept too much thought. Historically, primitive measures of health status were used by health professionals and policy makers because of their simplicity and the availability of relevant data, with mortality data as the default indicator. This metric may be supplemented with data on infant mortality or mortality for various causes of death. While the latter two options offer a refinement over the overall mortality rate, these indicators are increasingly thought to be limited in their usefulness. A spinoff from the mortality rate is life expectancy as a measure of health status. While better related to *health status* rather than *sickness status*, mortality and life expectancy indicators are top-level measures that exist a long way from the people "on the ground".

Another measure that is closer to the source is self-reported health status whereby individuals indicate their health status as "poor", "fair", "good", "very good" or "excellent". This is a widely used indicator and has been determined to provide a meaningful view of the population's health status (Snead, 2007). It should be realized that such measures, to the extent that they are valid, reflect the aggregate responses of individuals and, in this regard, may not be reflective of group health status. The long history of collecting data on self-reported health status is useful for tracking trends over time.

As well respected as the work done on self-reported health status by the National Center for Health Statistics is, there are issues with self-reports that have implications for a population health approach. One concern that can be laid to rest on the front end is the danger of using subjective assessments of an objective situation. Past research (Dorian et al., 2014) found that, when actual patient records are available, self-reported assessments correspond fairly well with objectively measured health status. Further, there is a reasonably good correlation between self-reported health status and mortality—that is, those who report poor health are at greater risk of dying (Lorem et al., 2020).

The problem from a population health perspective is that different segments of the population view health in different ways, thereby creating variations in self-reported health status. Responses are influenced by age, sex and ethnicity, and by cultural background, educational level and access to health services, among other factors. How we recognize, define, name, and categorize disease states and attribute them to a cause or set of causes influence our perception of health status.

Attempts have been made to improve our assessments of health status by examining morbidity patterns which, in today's world, mean the prevalence of chronic disease. While this represents an improvement over global measures like mortality and life expectancy, these data are not as readily available. They

(continued)

Box 5.2 (continued)

must be acquired from patient records or community surveys, both of which have their drawbacks. Even if readily available, such data may not provide the insights into health status that we expect. We would still be looking at health status from the perspective of the health professional who understandably would focus on the prevalence of easily classified disease states.

The community health indicators movement has produced several examples of health status indices that pull together data on a variety of attributes thought to reflect and/or contribute to the health of the population. These approaches pay heed in various degrees to the social determinants of health and attempt to combine disparate types of data in a meaningful model. While these efforts constitute an improvement in our attempts to understand and quantify health status, they still approach the issue from the health professional's perspective.

In attempting to measure health status, the perceptions of those who are affected by the social determinants of health are typically not taken into consideration. The Affordable Care Act of 2010 recognized this and emphasized the importance of obtaining input from the general public with regard to their perspective on health status.

How, then, would lay people characterize health status. First, it would probably never be based on mortality rates. Although death is a more frequent visitor to those with poor health status, mortality rates are clearly not top of mind. The deaths that do occur are not nearly as impactful as the constant pressure of chronic disease and disability. While chronic disease is particularly rampant in disadvantaged communities, members of the affected populations are likely to view them differently from health professionals. Rather, health status is more likely to be epitomized by the issues faced every day—the mental disorders, substance abuse, and domestic violence that both reflect the life circumstances of members of various groups and contribution to the community health status.

Increasingly we find that members of groups that are particularly affected by poor health see health problems as symptoms of underlying problems. This is why health status typically does not make the list of the top ten problems they face (even when they are clearly suffering from high morbidity levels). Thus, they tend to assess health status in terms of personal and community safety, adequate housing, access to healthy food, and access to quality schools.

Despite the challenges involved in defining health status, this perspective must be taken into consideration if we are to truly understand the factors that determine the health of a population and allow the implementation of a population health approach.

possible or even appropriate to settle on a single definition of health status. Realizing that no definition will be universally accepted, the following definition is proposed. For our purposes, health status is:

The level of health of a group or population as subjectively assessed by the members of the group and/or objectively assessed through measures that describe the collective health of the group or population.

Health Status Indicators

Having defined health status, analysts must then be able to measure this phenomenon. However, there is no single and straightforward method for quantifying the health status of the population. The challenge becomes one of identifying the indicators that operationalize the definition, calculating the level of health within the population, and establishing a baseline for health status as a basis for assessing its improvement.

Health status can be objectively measured (e.g., through clinical tests) or subjectively measured (e.g., through self-reports by individuals). While the health status of the total population under study is important, it may be necessary to determine the morbidity level for subsets within the population (e.g., subgroups based on geography or demographic attribute) in order to truly understand a population's morbidity patterns.

The degree of granularity with regard to the amount of morbidity is a function of the objectives of the analysis. In some cases an analyst may use a specific clinical reading as the indicator of a disease. A good example of this is the use of the body mass index as a measure of obesity. The BMI has come into use as a meaningful single figure for assessing the health status of an individual and, then, aggregating individuals into an obesity rate for the population under study. The BMI is popular because of the ease with which it can be calculated and the ease of interpretation.

In other cases a category of diseases may be identified as a measure of health status rather than specific diseases. Major groupings of health status indicators are presented below in an effort to reduce confusion. For example, one may determine the overall incidence of acute conditions or the overall prevalence of chronic conditions. This approach might be taken when less specificity is required or when these categories provide a more meaningful view of morbidity levels. Other examples of such categories include: reproductive health problems, childhood diseases and mental health disorders.

Global Measures

In the conceptualization of health status the question arises as to whether health status is an attribute of individuals—who can be subsequently aggregated into a global measure of health—or an attribute of the group that exists independent of the characteristics of the members of that group. Some health status indices are created by collecting data on the health status of individuals, however measured, and aggregating those data to generate a single score or a set of scores that summarize the characteristics of the collective population. For example, a symptom checklist may be administered to individuals and the results combined to generate an "average" that reflects the characteristics of the group. Similarly, a commonly used measure—self-reported health status—applies the same method—that is, eliciting responses on the health status of various individuals and then aggregating the results to determine the proportion of the population that feels that its health is "poor", "fair", "good", "very good", or "excellent". Critiques of this method of measuring health status contend that the collective health status is not being measured, only the sum or average of individual scores.

While self-reported ratings of health status are attractive in their simplicity, some consider them too subjective. Disagreement as to what constitutes health and illness clearly points to the danger of this approach. One respondent's ill-health may be another's normal state, and it is difficult to control for these variations in perception. Recent research has found, in fact, that African-American respondents and white respondents use a different framework for their self-evaluation, thereby limiting the value of comparative data (Brandon & Proctor, 2010).

These concerns have been partially addressed in that a reasonable correlation has been found between self-reports and objective measures of health status. When self-assessments are correlated with responses to a symptom checklist, for example, a relatively strong correlation is evidenced (Wu et al., 2013). That is, respondents with a large number of symptoms (either self-reported or observed) tend to rate their health status lower than those with few identified symptoms. Self-reported health status has even been shown to be a strong predictor of subsequent mortality (Lorem et al., 2020). Box 5.3 presents self-reported ratings of health status for selected demographic groups. Box 5.3 presents an example of data generated through self-reported health assessments.

Other self-reported measures that are sometimes utilized include: poor physical health days and poor mental health days. "Healthy days" are determined by asking people about the number of physically and mentally unhealthy days per month respondents experience. This information is collected through community surveys, most frequently by the National Center for Health Statistics. Two other related indicators for which data are collected in the same manner involve data on frequent physical distress and frequent mental distress.

Outcome Measures: Morbidity

The most direct measure of health status involves the simple counting of cases of recognizable conditions for a specified population or unit of geography. While this approach is straightforward, it raises the question of what to count and where to obtain relevant data. Options with regard to "what" to count include: specific

Box 5.3 Fair or Poor Self-Reported Health Status: By Selected Biosocial Characteristics, United States, 2018

Characteristic	Fair or poor health
Total	9.0%
Age	
Under 18 years	1.7%
18–44 years	6.1%
45–64 years	12.6%
65 and over	22.2%
Sex	
Male	8.8%
Female	9.1%
Race/ethnicity	
White	8.2%
Black	13.5%
Asian	8.2%
American Indian	18.6%
Hispanic	12.3%
Income level	
Below 100% of poverty level	21.0%
100–199% of poverty level	14.6%
200–399% of poverty level	8.5%
400% or more of poverty level	4.1%

Source: National Center for Health Statistics (2020)

indicators for a particular disease, groupings of indicators for a particular disease, narrow categories of diseases, broad categories of diseases or, finally, global indicators that consider *all* available indicators of incidence or prevalence.

In some cases an analyst may use a specific clinical reading as the indicator of a disease. A good example of this is the use of the body mass index (BMI) noted above. The BMI has come into use as a meaningful single figure for assessing the health status of an individual and then aggregating individuals scores to generate an obesity index for the population under study. The BMI is popular because of the ease with which it can be calculated and with which it can be understood.

The level of morbidity is of particular interest to those promoting a population health approach. Morbidity measures are much more salient indicators of health status today than mortality rates. They are more reflective of the social determinants of health and are more directly affected by such factors as poverty, housing instability, food insecurity and other social determinants.

Outcome Measures: Mortality/Life Expectancy

In the past, it has been common to use mortality data as an indicator of health status. The mortality rate was assumed to represent in one figure the general health condition of the population. The widespread availability and quality of mortality data make the death rate a tempting metric. Thus, the trend toward lower mortality rates for the US population in the twentieth century was taken as evidence of improved health status.

Historically, there was a fairly close correlation between common maladies and common causes of death. The immediate cause of death was typically the primary cause of death, with few complicating factors involved. Further, mortality data have long been relatively complete and easily attainable thereby facilitating longitudinal analyses. The connection between mortality and morbidity levels is still recognized today, in that the leading causes of death (e.g., heart disease and cancer) reflect common maladies within the population.

Over time, however, the mortality rate has become a less meaningful proxy for health status. In the United States the mortality rate has dropped to the point that death is a relatively rare event. Further, the correspondence between mortality and morbidity has become diminished. Because of the preponderance of chronic disease, the determination of the cause of death on death certificates is more of a challenge. Chronic diseases typically do not kill people, but some complication (of diabetes, AIDS or cancer for example) is typically the proximate cause of death. This is not to say that mortality analysis cannot provide insights into morbidity patterns, but that the situation is much more complicated than in the past. Contemporary analyses of mortality data require a better understanding of disease processes (and the vagaries of death certificates).

The use of the mortality rate as a proxy for health status is criticized as a convenience for those measuring health status. It is considered a reflection of the medical professional perspective and not necessarily the perspective of the population being assessed. In reality, information on the overall death rate is of limited use (especially in terms of taking ameliorative action); information on the underlying cause of death is required and that raises a number of other issues to be discussed later. In subsequent sections, reference will be made to mortality as a proxy for morbidity with, however, the caveats expressed here.

When examining health status from the perspective of community members, it is doubtful that they will cite causes of death as the key health problems. When health needs assessments are conducted, community respondents are more likely to identify conditions that more directly affect their personal situations than more abstract mortality rates. Thus, respondents are likely to identify obesity, substance abuse and domestic violence, for example, as meaningful metrics for assessing health status.

Another mortality indicator, the infant mortality rate (IMR), is considered by many to be an even better indicator of population health than the overall mortality rate. The premise is that the infant mortality rate is much more than an outcome measure for the healthcare system. Rather, the level of infant mortality is a function of environmental safety, diet, prenatal care, the educational and economic status of the parents, the age of the mother, the occurrence of neglect and abuse, and a number of other factors. Thus, infant mortality is thought to reflect the combined impact of multiple contributors to health and well-being. As with the overall mortality rate, however, infant deaths occur rarely enough that measures of infant mortality have less salience today as indicators of a population's health than they did historically. As with the mortality rate, infant mortality exhibits a high level of disparity when various subpopulations are considered (Matthews & MacDorman, 2013).

The average life expectancy for a population is utilized in the same manner as the mortality rate and is, of course, its inverse. It may even be a preferable indicator to the mortality rate in that it measures life rather than death. It offers the same benefit when it comes to identifying disparities and, in fact, may be more useful in that it reflects historical patterns of health status that have culminated in the current life expectancy profile.

Other Outcome Measures

Some would argue that, in addition to the infant mortality rate noted above, there are a number of outcome measures related to reproductive health that might be considered. Like the infant mortality rate some of measures are thought to be reflective of the social and economic conditions associated with the environments that contribute to unfavorable reproductive health. These include such indicators as: premature births, low-birth-weight births, and miscarriages, along with the level of teen births and births to unmarried women. (Receipt of prenatal care may be considered a utilization measure of some importance under the access/utilization category below.) It is noteworthy that maternal mortality for the US population has experienced an uptick in recent years. As with other mortality indicators, the highest rates are concentrated among certain disadvantaged populations.

There are some categories of outcome measures that are typically neglected but are likely to have considerable importance when health status is being considered from a population health perspective. The level of disability as an indicator of health status typically receives a lot less attention than it should. If anything, the level of disability has become an increasingly important indicator of health status for the US population. According to the Social Security Administration, the proportion of the US population that is classified as disabled has grown substantially over time.

The amount of mental illness is seldom included as a metric for assessing health status. Mental illness is not diagnosed in the same manner as other chronic diseases, and its identification is a much more subjective endeavor. While acquiring accurate data on psychiatric morbidity is more challenging than it is for physical illness, data collected through various sample surveys provide insights into the prevalence of psychiatric disorders in America. Since much of the psychiatric morbidity is undiagnosed, tallies of recorded cases even if available, would not provide the complete picture of what some would consider an epidemic. There is every reason to believe that the level of mental and emotional disorders characterizing the US population is higher than the estimates derived from sample surveys.

Another neglected indicator of health status is the dental health of the population. Part of the reason for this neglect is the lack of understanding of the relationship between dental health and other health problems. A "silent epidemic" of dental and oral diseases is affecting some population groups—a burden of disease that restricts activities in school, work, and home, and often significantly diminishes the quality of life (Bailey et al., 2017). Box 5.4 explores the notion of quality of life as an outcome measure.

Box 5.4: Quality of Life as an Outcome Measure
Quality of life (QOL) is a broad multi-dimensional concept that usually includes subjective evaluations of both positive and negative aspects of life. Although the term "quality of life" has meaning for nearly everyone and every academic discipline, individuals and groups may define it differently. While health is one of the important domains of overall quality of life, other domains to consider include jobs, housing, schools, and neighborhoods. The impact of social determinants on health on one level should be considered along with the impact of life circumstances on another level.

There is growing concern that more people are living longer but with poorer health. A poor quality of life, it is contended, negates the benefits of increased longevity. Health-related quality of life (HRQoL) is a multi-dimensional concept that includes domains related to physical, mental, emotional and social functioning. It goes beyond direct measures of community health such as life expectancy and causes of death and focuses on the impact overall health status has on one's quality of life. The CDC has defined HRQoL as "an individual's or group's perceived physical and mental health over time." Health-related quality of life is viewed as an outcome of the health factors included in the *County Health Rankings*.

Health-related quality of life has traditionally been concerned with those factors that fall within the spheres of influence of healthcare providers and healthcare systems. However, as the population health model has emerged, the quality of life related to other domains has come be seen as important as health-related quality of life. On the community level, HRQOL includes community-level resources, conditions, policies, and practices that influence a population's health perceptions and functional status. As the population health model is refined, greater attention is likely to be paid to not only health-related quality of life but to the quality aspects related to other spheres of existence.

Healthy/Unhealthy Behavior

The fact that lifestyles have become an important contributor to health status has led to a growing emphasis on monitoring health behaviors. "Health behavior" refers to any formal or informal action that is intended consciously or unconsciously to restore, maintain or enhance health. Formal activities include the use of health services for prevention, restoration or enhancement purposes, and these are discussed below in the section on health services utilization. Informal activities include dietary practices and exercise habits, as well as such factors as sleep patterns and the use of auto seatbelts. Tobacco use, alcohol use and substance abuse, along with information on risky sexual behavior, are also relevant metrics.

Environmental Factors

It has become increasingly common to include information on the condition of the environment as health status indicators, especially given the documented relationship between toxic environments and poor health. For example, a clear relationship has been established between proximity to toxic waste concentrations and elevated health risks. Similarly, residents living in proximity to certain industrial operations (e.g., oil refineries) also exhibit higher levels of morbidity. In assessing health status, indicators of air and water quality are considered along with proximity to toxic waste sites. As the health impact assessment movement has gained momentum, the perception of environmental factors has expanded to include housing quality, access to green space, and adequate transportation options.

Social/Economic Factors

Since the first attempts were made to develop a health status index various social and economic attributes have been included. Now that the social determinants of health have been clearly documented there is even more interest in including social and economic variables as proxy measures for health status. To the extent that health problems are increasingly being viewed as *symptoms* of much deeper problems, the social determinants of health are receiving increasing scrutiny.

Prominent among these are socioeconomic measures such as income level and educational attainment. Income may be measured in terms of median household or median family income, and the extent of poverty is increasingly considered a correlate of health status. Marital status and household structure might be considered as well. Single-parent households and households with a large number of children but few resources may serve as proxy indicators. Other factors that might be considered include occupation (or more appropriately occupational level), and employment status (with unemployment obviously being significant).

Cultural/Subcultural Influences

The behaviors (including health behavior), lifestyles and even attitudes of society members are influenced by their cultural milieux. This cultural context influences what people eat, how active they are, what leisure activities they pursue, and the extent to which they participate in healthy or unhealthy behaviors. Few of the decisions individuals make with regard to their lifestyles and health behavior are made as individuals. Decisions are made by members of a group—a group that promotes certain cultural values.

In the extreme it could be argued that there is a subculture of ill-health in which members of certain subgroups have no expectation of good health. Under these circumstances an attitude of accommodation is adopted based on the acceptance of poor health as a fact of life. Rather than attempting to improve health, the goal is to adapt to the situation. A subculture of ill-health would explain why some communities exhibit poor health status generation after generation even in the face of frequent population turnover.

Life Circumstances Indicators

Another perspective involves attention to the life circumstances affecting members of different groups in society. While overlapping somewhat with the categories identified above, life circumstances include factors that have implications for the health and well-being of the members of a population on a daily basis. In addition to household structure and poverty noted above, other factors may include housing instability, food insecurity, unsafe streets and neighborhoods, lack of transportation and lack of social support. These are social determinants of health as they affect individuals and households.

This eclectic grouping of indicators describes the context in which residents spend their lives on the assumption that these factors will contribute to both health status and health behavior. These attributes are linked to such actions as preventive behaviors, accessing health services, complying with medical regimen and other health-related behaviors. Increasingly, it is being found that the life circumstances of groups of patients contribute to some of the undesirable indicators of healthcare utilization (e.g., unnecessary emergency room use, hospital readmission).

Access/Utilization Measures

Access to health services represents an indirect measure of health status and assumes that there is a correlation between the ability to access services and good health. As noted previously, access to care does not necessarily lead to better health but, for purposes of measuring health status, this indicator is commonly used. Access indicators include such measures as the physician-to-population ratio (particularly for primary care physicians), the dental health professional-to-population ratio, the mental health professional-to-population ratio and the hospital bed-to-population ratio. One other important measure of access is the extent to which the population is covered by health insurance, and there is a well-documented relationship between access to insurance and both morbidity and mortality. Utilization measures also include the hospital admission rate, the physician visit/encounter rate, emergency room utilization and similar measures of utilization.

The question that is difficult to answer in this regard is whether utilization of services reflects a higher level of morbidity because there are a lot of sick people needing services (negative indicator) or whether it portends a healthier population because of regular use of health services (positive indicator).

Health Status Rankings

There have been several attempts to create health status rankings that incorporate various indicators and can be universally applied across all geographies and population groups. There are some variations in the approaches taken, but in general they attempt to combine indicators selected from a variety of sources in an understandable format that allows comparisons of the indicators over time and between different communities. Two examples are described below followed by a listing of some other examples.

Perhaps the best known of these rankings is the *County Health Rankings* developed in collaboration between the Robert Wood Johnson Foundation and the University of Wisconsin Population Health Institute. The following goals provide the rationale for the development of the rankings:

- Build awareness of the multiple factors that influence health
- Provide a reliable, sustainable source of local data to communities to help them identify opportunities to improve their health
- Engage and activate local leaders from many sectors in creating sustainable community change, and
- Connect and empower community leaders working to improve health.

As illustrated by the chart in Box 5.5 the data elements comprising the index are grouped into four categories: health behaviors, clinical care, social and economic factors, and physical environment. Each of these are operationalized in the form of two to five indicators. The *Rankings* are compiled using county-level data for most

Box 5.5: County Health Rankings Model

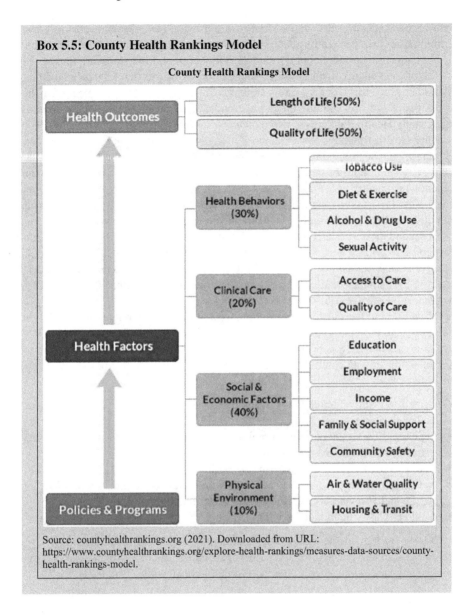

Source: countyhealthrankings.org (2021). Downloaded from URL: https://www.countyhealthrankings.org/explore-health-rankings/measures-data-sources/county-health-rankings-model.

US counties drawn from a variety of national data sources. The annual *County Health Rankings* also asssess "vital health factors", including high school graduation rates, obesity, smoking, unemployment, access to healthy foods, the quality of air and water, income, and teen births.

The annual *Rankings* are intended to provide insights into how health is influenced by where we live, learn, work and play. These rankings show that much of what affects health occurs outside of the doctor's office. From that perspective, many of these indicators appear relevant to a population health approach. These rankings are accompanied by *Roadmaps* that provide guidance and tools to assist communities in understanding data and developing strategies for ameliorative action.

Although the developers of the *Rankings* tout their ability to measure the overall health of each county in all 50 states on the multiple factors that influence health, it should be noted that County Health Rankings do not measure "overall health" in the sense that we understand it in the population health context. The ultimate output of the County Health Rankings is two indicators: length of life and quality of life. The County Health Rankings seek to quantify length of life for county populations by measuring the burden of premature deaths (premature mortality), an important measure of a population's health. Premature deaths are deaths that occur before a person reaches an expected age, for instance, age 75. Measuring premature mortality, rather than overall mortality, highlights the intent of the *County Health Rankings* to focus attention on deaths that could have been prevented and their underlying causes.

A second indicator derived from the County Health Rankings is "years of premature life lost" (YPLL), a concept originally introduced by Hyder et al. (1998). YPLL involves using the number of years of life (life-years) lost due to premature death, defined by a standard cut-off age in a population, to obtain a total sum of the life-years lost before ages 65, 75, or 85 (for example).

In addition to the YPLL measure, the length of life indicator also considers child mortality and infant mortality. Child mortality refers to the number of deaths among children under age 18 per 100,000 population. Infant mortality measures the number of deaths among children less than 1 year of age per 1000 live births.

Other examples of health status ranking include the following:

- United Health Foundation's America's Health Rankings (www.americashealthrankings.org)
- State-level data generated by a major health insurance company based on six indicators and include targeted analyses (e.g., senior report)
- Healthy People 2030 (www.health.gov/healthypeople)
- National-level data on twelve key indicators generated by the Department of Health and Human Services and updated periodically
- Annie E. Casey Foundation's KIDS COUNT (www.datacenter.kidscount.org)

Not-for-profit child advocacy organization provides data at the state, county, city, school district and congressional district for six categories of health indicators (covering 35 separate indicators with a focus on child health).

A New Approach to Health Status

The health status rankings that have been developed by a variety of parties are useful in that they attempt to identify relevant indicators of health status and quantify them. None, however, has been able to generate a single number that represents the health status of a population or geographic area. While these rankings are of some use for tracking changes in a community's health status over time and/or comparing one population to other populations, they fall short of the establishment of a meaningful rating. They generally represent a collection of interrelated, indirectly related and unrelated attributes, making an integrated assessment of health status difficult if not impossible.

Existing health status rankings are criticized on other grounds as well. The question was raised earlier as to whether those attempting to measure health status were truly measuring health status or, to the extent they were, whose vision of health status they were measuring. As noted earlier, many indicators utilized have more salience for the professional's perspective of health status than they do for the healthcare consumer's. The Affordable Care Act, in fact, mandated that health status as considered from the perspective of community members should encourage the consideration of a lay perspective on health and illness and that it reflects their concerns.

Standard metrics used by the healthcare system focus primarily on disease incidence and prevalence, the presence of selected (medical and behavioral) risk factors, reproductive health measures, utilization of health services and measures of mortality. As we argued above, these may not be the metrics that are most important in assessing a population's health status. An emphasis on these factors may translate into unnecessary treatment or the overuse of health services. Additional measures such as the level/type of health insurance, the ability to pay for health-related goods and services, access to transportation, health literacy, and access to prevention resources are also important. These types of metrics are generally beyond the purview of the healthcare system since health professionals have no role (or do not appreciate their role) in addressing them.

A major challenge facing a population health approach involves shifting the dialogue away from the patient to the community as the context for health improvement. While guidance on how to implement a population health approach is being offered by various parties, these "guidelines" seldom get past the first few paragraphs before they start referring to "patients" or individual healthcare consumers. While it's not surprising for health professionals to default to familiar territory, this underscores their lack of understanding of the population health approach. They attempt to force square pegs into round holes by talking about more efficient patient data management, expanded case management activities, personalized patient experiences, wrap around services and a variety of other spinoff activities reflecting a system built on the care of individual patients.

Despite the growing sensitivity to the role of social determinants in health status, some of the most important factors are excluded from commonly used rankings. Housing stability has become an increasingly important consideration with regard to health status and, indeed, some communities have begun addressing the housing problem as a public health issue (Maqbool et al., 2015). Food security is another issue that contributes to poor health, with the existence of "food deserts" in many communities well documented. In many ways, good health starts with adequate nutrition, and many of the ensuing issues stem from a lack of adequate nourishment.

Domestic violence is another contributor to poor health status that is seldom considered when assessing health status.

Some of these issues create a dilemma for those attempting to apply a population health approach. On the one hand, this approach calls for the use of data that reflects the attributes of the population under study. This suggests that aggregate data must be used in order to capture the essence of the total population. However, the use of generally available aggregate data (e.g., mortality rates, certain disease incidence/prevalence rates, reproductive health measures) may not provide the desired insights into the health status of the population. On the other hand, any effort to develop a sense of the level of health from the perspective of the affected parties is likely to involve primary research. While community surveys are likely to generate a different perspective from the top-down view of policy makers, at the end of the day this represents the summed attributes of the sample rather than attributes associated with the group. There is no easy answer to this dilemma and, hopefully, as the population health model is refined, these issues can be resolved.

This situation suggests a need for extensive primary research to elicit data not available elsewhere from populations for which limited data of any type are available. This would involve in-depth research and additional expenditures. However, given what is at stake—and the amount of health resources that are already being wastefully allocated—enhanced data collection efforts cannot be avoided. This topic is discussed in more detailed in the chapter on data needs for population health.

The Importance of Non-Health-Related Data

The population health approach calls for data collection that includes more in-depth analyses, a broader range of data topics, and more frequent data collection. Provisions within the Affordable Care act require that tax-exempt hospitals complete a comprehensive community health needs assessment (CHNA) at least every 3 years. Not only does this provision require that extensive external market data be collected, but it demands that the hospital go beyond the traditional types of data and collect information on the entire community and not just its patient population. The fact that a provider must be accountable not just for the health and well-being of its patients but for the health status of the entire community it serves is a radical idea.

Provisions of the ACA call for not only assessing the health status of the total population but for identifying unmet needs within that population even if those needs are unrelated to services that are typically provided by that hospital. For example, a hospital that does not routinely provide behavioral health services but finds that there are serious unmet needs in that regard within the community must, according to IRS regulations, develop a plan for addressing those unmet needs. Further, at the time of the next CHNA, the hospital, theoretically at least, must document what it has done to address this *community* need.

Clearly, this is a major plank in the population health platform with hospitals now expected to place as much emphasis on consumers in general as they do on their own patients. Further, the hospital will not be allowed to rely exclusively on its own data but must demonstrate that it has accessed resources in the community beyond its own walls. The ACA specifically mandates that the local health department be involved in the CHNA along with other health-related organizations. It further specifies that any organizations inside of and outside of healthcare be consulted to the extent they can provide insights into the needs of the general population.

This leads us to a more radical phenomenon related to data collection: The emphasis on non-health-related data. As will be discussed in more detail in a subsequent chapter, data must be collected on a wide range of topics that historically have not been linked to the health of the population. The recognition of the social determinants of health status has opened the door to the acquisition of data on topics ignored by healthcare organizations in the past. While most analyses include data on the demographic and socioeconomic characteristics of the target population, additional information is now required on the lifestyles of consumers, their social context and cultural milieux, and the life circumstances that have implications for health status and health behavior. In keeping with the population health approach, this information is not collected for individuals per se but for groups within the population.

Even more radical is the notion that data must be collected on topics previously thought to have no implications for health status. Attributes like income, educational level and employment status for the target population would continue to be collected, but now data on the social and physical environment, the availability of affordable and adequate housing, employment options and job training opportunities, access to affordable and healthy food, access to green spaces and recreational activities, access to transportation, and exposure to crime and violence must be considered. The significance of this type of information has been highlighted as it has become increasingly obvious that no level of medical care can overcome poverty, environmental threats, malnutrition and the health implications of a stressful environment.

A population health approach requires a much more extensive understanding not only of existing patients but of the overall community as well as a consideration of data on a wide range of topics that have not historically been considered by healthcare organizations. A subsequent chapter devoted to the social determinants of health will discuss these topics in more detail.

Summary

The ultimate goal of the population health approach is the improvement of the population's health status. However, there is no consensus on how to define "health status", and health professionals regularly use the term without much thought to its meaning. Any health status measure should reflect the attributes of the group independent of the attributes of the individuals that comprise it. To this end, metrics that accurately reflect the collective health of the group must be identified.

The first step toward developing a health status index is establishing a definition of "health." Health may be defined in various ways, and for our purposes "health" is defined as a dynamic process for achieving a state of physical, mental, emotional, intellectual, spiritual and social well-being throughout the lifespan. Like the definition of health itself, health status can be defined in a variety of ways from a variety of perspectives. Realizing that no definition will be universally accepted, health status is defined for our purposes as the level of *health* of a group or population as subjectively assessed by the members of the group and/or objectively assessed through measures of collective health.

Health status can be objectively measured (e.g., through clinical tests) or subjectively measured (e.g., through self-reports by individuals). The most comprehensive approach to measuring the health status of a population is through a "global indicator." Based on survey responses, an assessment of the health status of a targeted population can be made. Other self-reported measures that are sometimes utilized include: poor physical health days and poor mental health days.

The most direct measure of health status involves the simple counting of cases of recognizable conditions for a specified population or unit of geography. The measure may refer to a specific attribute or disease or a category of diseases. Outcome indicators are also utilized with various mortality rates being examples. The infant mortality rate (IMR) is considered by many to be an even better indicator of population health than the overall mortality rate. The average life expectancy for a population is utilized in the same manner and has the advantage of measuring life rather than death while also calling attention to disparities. There is also a number of outcome measures related to reproductive health that might be considered. Other health status measures that are often neglected include the level of disability, the prevalence of mental illness, and the dental health of the population.

Given the importance of lifestyles to health status, health behavior is also considered a useful metric. Health behavior often reflects demographic attributes and may also be influenced by structural factors such as the availability of services and facilities. Access indicators consider the availability of physicians, dental health professionals, and mental health professionals, along with the availability of hospital beds. Access to health insurance is an important component of health status.

Given the importance of socioeconomic factors for health status, measures of income and education are often used as proxy indicators. Other factors that might be considered include occupation (or more appropriately occupational level) and employment status (with unemployment obviously being significant). At the same time, our lifestyles and even our attitudes are influenced by our cultural milieus. Our cultural context influences what we eat, how active we are, what leisure activities we pursue, and the extent of healthy and unhealthy behaviors. A subculture of ill-health leads affected populations to accept poor health as a fact of life and adapt to the situation rather than try to change it. Life circumstances include factors that impinge upon the everyday lives of members of the population and have implications for their health and well-being. Housing insecurity, food insecurity, unsafe streets and neighborhoods, lack of transportation and lack of social support are examples of life circumstances.

There have been several attempts to create health status rankings, and perhaps the best known of the rankings is the *County Health Rankings* in which four categories of factors are considered: health behaviors, clinical care, social and economic factors, and physical environment. The annual *Rankings* are intended to provide insights into how health is influenced by where we live, learn, work and play. While these rankings are useful for tracking changes in a community's health status over time and/or comparing one population to other populations, they fall short of the establishment of a definitive rating that is meaningful. Like most health status indices these two epitomize the challenges involved.

Developments in healthcare call for an innovative approach to community health assessment. The traditional community health needs assessment falls short of what is required for a population health assessment, and a number of changes in assessment methodology are required in order to support multi-sector collaboration for collective impact.

The population health approach goes beyond the scope of most health data initiatives in that extensive non-health-related data are required. Not only does population health require that extensive external market data be collected, but it demands that the assessment go beyond the traditional types of data and collect information on the entire community and not just its patient population. Further, data must be collected on a wide range of topics that historically have not been linked to the health of the population. This includes attributes like income, educational level and employment status for the target population, data on the social and physical environment, the availability of affordable and adequate housing, employment options and job training opportunities, access to affordable and healthy food, access to green spaces and recreational activities, access to transportation, and exposure to crime and violence.

Key Points

- The ultimate goal of any population health initiative is the improvement of the health status of a defined population
- In order to assess the health status of a population, an acceptable definition of health status must be formulated
- In order to formulate a definition of health status there needs to be agreement as to what constitutes health
- Health can be defined in a variety of ways but from a population health perspective it needs to be conceptualized in the broadest terms possible
- While health status can be determined for individuals, the health status of groups is emphasized within the population health context

- Concerns have been raised concerning the appropriateness of the measures of health status traditionally employed, especially since they tend to focus on sickness status rather than health status
- It must be recognized that the perception of health status held by health professionals may differ from that held by the general public
- Health status indicators can take a number of forms from the assessment of a particular disease to aggregate indicators that include a wide range of diseases.
- Traditional metrics used to assess health status such as mortality rates and life expectancy are increasingly less salient
- Where possible "global" measures of health status should be utilized
- Many important indicators are ignored in traditional health status measures (e.g., disability, mental illness, dental health)
- Quality of life is becoming an increasingly important measure of health status
- Despite a long history of the development of health status indices there is no one index that is widely accepted
- Two or more county health ranking systems have been developed for use nationwide but their usefulness is limited for population health purposes
- The data needed for population health analyses is often dated, inaccessible, nonexistent or unavailable below the county level
- Population health analyses require the interface of organizational data and external market data in order to create a complete picture of health status
- Non-health-related data have become increasingly important as the significance of the social determinants of health has been recognized
- Data related to economic conditions, housing, food accessibility, environment, education and other non-health topics must be utilized in population health initiatives

References

Antonovsky, A. (1979). *Health, stress and coping*. Jossey-Bass Publishers.

Aronowitz, R. (2008). Framing disease: An underappreciated mechanism for the social patterning of health. *Social Science and Medicine, 67*(1), 1–9.

Bailey, R. M., Peter, E. L. B. E., Varghese, N. O., et al. (2017). Oral health and quality of life: Current concepts. *Journal of Clinical and Diagnostic Research, 11*(6), ZE21–ZE26.

Brandon, L. J., & Proctor, L. (2010). Comparison of health perceptions and health status in African-Americans and Caucasians. *Journal of the National Medical Association, 102*(7), 590–597.

Conrad, P., & Barker, K. K. (2010). The social construction of illness. *Journal of Health and Social Behavior, 51*(1[supplement]), S67–S79.

countyhealthrankings.org. (2021). Downloaded from URL: https://www.countyhealthrankings.org/explore-health-rankings/measures-data-sources/county-health-rankings-model

Dorian, D., Fiebig, D. G., Johar, M., et al. (2014). Does self-assessed health measure health? *Applied Economics, 47*(2), 180–194.

encyclopedia.com. (2021). *Lay concepts of health and illness*. Downloaded from URL: https://www.encyclopedia.com/education/encyclopedias-almanacs-transcripts-and-maps/lay-concepts-health-and-illness

References

Freund, P. E. S., & McGuire, M. B. (1999). *Health, illness and the social body* (3rd ed.). Prentice Hall.

Gunderson, G., & Pray, L. (2009). *Leading causes of life: Five Fundmentals to change the way you live your life.* Abingdon Press.

Hyder, A. A., Rotilian, G., & Morrow, R. H. (1998). Measuring the burden of disease: Healthy life years. *American Journal of Public Health, 88*(2), 196–202.

Lorem, G., Cook, S., Leon, D.A., et al. (2020). Self-reported health as a predictor of mortality: A cohort study of its relation to other health measurements and observation time. *Scientific Reports* 10(March). Downloaded from URL: https://www.nature.com/articles/s41598-020-61603-0.

Maqbool, N., Viveiros, J., & Ault, M. (2015). *The importance of affordable housing for health.* Center for Housing Policy.

Matthews, T. J., & MacDorman, M. F. (2013). Infant mortality statistics from the 2010 period linked birth/infant death data set. *National Vital Statistics Report, 62*(8), 1–27.

National Center for Health Statistics. (2020). *Health: United States 2019.* National Center for Health Statistics.

O'Reilly, D., & Rosato, M. (2007). *Self-reported health, socio-economic status and area of residence: Understanding the relationships.* Downloaded from URL: http://www.celsius.lshtm.ac.uk/projects/oreillySelfreported.html.

OECD. (2001). *Health at a Glance: 2001.* Downloaded from URL: https://books.google.com/books?id=G6TWAgAAQBAJ&pg=PA20&lpg=PA20&dq=variations+in+self-reported+health+status&source=bl&ots=gpgmFZi8gj&sig=pxbUphzycSKP0v5QrEqLk4QG8Zk&hl=en&sa=X&ved=0ahUKEwiEk_2-_NnOAhWG2SYKHe2tCNwQ6AEIWzAH#v=onepage&q=variations%20in%20self-reported%20health%20status&f=false.

Shelby County (TN) Government. (2015). *Mid-South Regional Greenprint Health Impact Assessment: Preliminary report of baseline conditions.* Downloaded from URL: http://midsouthgreenprint.org/wp-content/uploads/2015/02/Greenprint-HIA-Preliminary-Report-Final-10-3-13.pdf

Snead, C. M. (2007). Self-rated health. In G. Ritzer (Ed.), *Blackwell encyclopedia of sociology.* Blackwell Publishing.

Wu, S., Wang, R., Zhao, Y., et al. (2013). The relationship between self-rated health and objective health status: A population-based study. *BMC Public Health, 13*, 320.

Additional Resources

America's Health Rankings (annual) at www.americashealthrankings.org/learn/reports/2020-annual-report.

Annie E. Casey Foundation, Kids Count at www.datacenter.kidscount.org

Antonovsky, A. (1987). *Unraveling the mystery of health: How people manage stress and stay well.* Jossey-Bass Publishers.

Behavioral Risk Factor Surveillance System (BRFSS) at www.cdc.gov/brfss.

Centers for Disease Control and Prevention (Weekly). *Morbidity and Mortality Weekly Report (MMWR)* at www.cdc.gov/mmwr/.

Healthy People 2030 at www.health.gov/healthypeople.

National Center for Health Statistics at www.cdc.gov/nchs.

Peters, C. M. (2021). *Checklist: Review of symptoms.* Downloaded from URL: https://www.charlespetersmd.com/Review%20of%20Systems%202.pdf

Robert Wood Johnson Foundation at www.rwjf.org.

Thomas, R. K. (2020). *Health services planning* (3rd ed.). Springer.

Tomenson, B., Essau, C., Jacobi, F., et al. (2013). Total somatic symptom score as a predictor of health outcome in somatic symptom disorders. *British Journal of Psychiatry, 203*, 373–380.

Chapter 6
The Social Determinants of Health and Illness

Health professionals now realize that contemporary health problems have their roots in social conditions rather than being a function of biological pathology or genetics. This shift in disease etiology has greatly reduced the importance of the historical causes of disease onset and brought sources of sickness such as lifestyles, demographic attributes, and life circumstances to the fore. These factors are affected in turn by such social determinants as poverty, housing instability, food insecurity, and unhealthy environments. This chapter examines the underlying causes of ill-health and the contribution of these factors to the health disparities exhibited by the US population.

In this chapter, the reader will:

- Learn about changes in the cause of most common diseases with an emphasis on the shift away from a biological etiology to a social one.
- Explore the issue of life circumstances and how they are the manifestation of social determinants at the individual and household level.
- Review the manner in which lifestyle has contributed to America's changing health status.
- Discover the nature of the social determinants of health and how they affect health status at the group level.
- Be exposed to the various categories of social determinants and trace the role each contributes to community health status.

Introduction

There is growing recognition of the contribution of social factors to the level of ill-health within a population and to the health disparities that exist between various groups within society. This realization has been a major factor in the emergence of the population health movement. As biological pathogens and genetics have waned as etiological factors, social factors have come to the fore. While we could claim to be "victims" of pathogens or genetics, we are not blameless when it comes to contemporary causes of ill health.

As individuals and as a society we are, in fact, responsible for most of the health problems that currently affect us. As individuals we affect our own health through the lifestyles we pursue. These lifestyles are "social" to the extent that they are mediated through the groups of which we are members. We all face pressure to conform to the lifestyles characteristics of these groups often without being aware of their influence.

As a society we have encouraged unhealthy lifestyles through the promotion (and even the subsidization) of unhealthy—but profitable—food choices. We have also allowed an unacceptable level of environmental degradation. Environmental pollutants contribute to the high rate of cancer and air pollution to the rise in chronic obstructive pulmonary disease. We have contaminated our soil and water with lead and other chemicals, with the recent lead poisoning tragedy in Flint, Michigan, representing the tip of the iceberg. We have tolerated an unacceptable level of housing deterioration, with a large segment of the population forced to live in unsafe and unhealthy housing.

At a deeper level we have allowed—if not outright fostered—the emergence of a level of socioeconomic inequality perhaps never experienced by the US population. As more and more financial resources are concentrated among the wealthiest in society, lower- and working-class populations have access to fewer resources. This translates into unhealthy lifestyles and a lack of access to health services thereby creating a perpetual cycle of financial distress and ill-health for these segments of society.

As the impact of social factors on health status has become documented, the argument is increasingly being made that the health conditions exhibited by a population are not the *problems* per se but are *symptoms* of underlying problems. Thus, the morbidity levels exhibited by various populations are a reflection of the social determinants of health and illness that are, in effect, the true problems. The presence of disease can thus be seen as the manifestation of these underlying conditions. This perspective is supported by research that suggests that disadvantaged populations are likely to identify as "health problems" such factors as lack of food, inadequate housing, and unsafe streets.

Critics of the US healthcare system point out that we have historically treated these symptoms while not addressing the true cause of the problems. Putting a band-aid on the wound is of limited usefulness if the underlying infection is not addressed. An approach that addresses symptoms without affecting a true cure is clearly ineffective when it comes to improving population health. This explains the fact that there is no correlation between health resources expended and health status. Thus, we now acknowledge that better access to health insurance does not guarantee access to care. Access to care does not assure utilization of services. Utilization of services does not necessarily foster better patient outcomes and by itself clearly does not contribute to improved population health.

Our system has labored under the delusion that more care means better health and that the health status of the population will be improved by providing greater access to health services. It is hard to ignore the fallacy of this perspective. Providers are well aware of the high rate of recidivism despite the best efforts of the medical community. Patients return for care repeatedly because their symptoms were treated but not the underlying disease. Research on hospital readmissions has found, for example, that readmission has little to do with the care that was received but almost everything to do with the conditions associated with the patient prior to admission and after discharge from medical care (Hui et al., 2014).

Improvement in population health will require attention to the root causes of ill-health within the population. Over 20 years ago healthcare analysts initially noted the impact of social determinants on health and illness (Evans et al., 1994). This emergent viewpoint was described as a "common focus on trying to understand the determinants of health of populations." Foreseeing the breadth of the population health approach, this work brought together research findings from epidemiology, biomedical science, psychology, sociology, economics, political science and history. While, as seen below, our understanding of the social determinants of health and illness has been significantly advanced since then, we still have a lot to learn about the connection between social conditions and health status.

Intermediate Causes

While there are deep-rooted social conditions that influence a population's health status, there are some intermediate or proximate influences that might be considered first. Factors like poverty, limited education, lack of job opportunities and similar factors may ultimately be blamed for variations in health status, but these factors are typically not routine daily considerations. There are other more mundane circumstances that reflect these underlying determinants that have a more immediate impact at the individual and household levels.

These conditions might be described as "life circumstances" to distinguish them from more deep-rooted social determinants. Life circumstances include the conditions of everyday living that constrain people's activities and influence their behavior. These might include household structure (e.g., living alone or in overcrowded conditions), housing adequacy, neighborhood safety, and access to resources and other factors that provide a context for understanding both health status and health behavior. These are the factors that do not necessarily represent traumatic forms of stress but the everyday stresses that accumulate over time. Box 6.1 provides further detail on life circumstances and their implications.

> **Box 6.1: Life Circumstances and Health**
> There is growing concern among healthcare providers, third-party payers and policy makers over the poor outcomes that are being generated by our healthcare system. Even with access to the world's most advanced technology and best-trained specialists, disappointing outcomes are often recorded. Further, there are significant disparities in the outcomes for different groups with similar conditions. Members of different racial groups, for example, with similar health conditions, the same level of acuity, and the same treatment in the same health facilities, may record different outcomes (Hopper, 2011). Findings of this type suggest that there are factors other than the quality of medical treatment that contribute to differential outcomes.
>
> Increasingly, characteristics attributable to patients before and after medical treatment are being analyzed for their effect on clinical outcomes. The "life circumstances" of patients and consumers are increasingly being seen as important drivers of health status, health behavior and healthcare outcomes. While there is no consensus with regard to what should be considered as life circumstances at this time, it is clear that certain attributes and conditions affect individual patients and consumers as well as families and social groups.
>
> Conditions identified by Peek (2014) include: unemployment, lack of job opportunities, substandard housing, the absence of health insurance, and low educational attainment. In addition, ethnic group membership, language proficiency and even religious affiliation can represent aspects of life circumstances. These attributes are frequently incorporated into assessments of health disparities within communities and can become deep-rooted attributes that provide an on-going negative backdrop for the lives of affected individuals and households (Ellaway, 2014).
>
> Additional life circumstances attributes likely to affect households include family stability, housing security (as opposed to housing quality), the safety of the living environment and surrounding community, the quality of the physical environment, and access to affordable healthy food (Pace, 2014). Other factors include access to transportation, personal assistance and support resources, and information that informs individual health and well-being.
>
> Collectively, life circumstances factors can offer insights into the variations in observed health status and health outcomes. A recent study noting the effect of life circumstances on the risk of death was completed by Puterman et al. (2020). In actuality, life circumstances may represent more important targets for remedial actions than the delivery of additional health services (Pederson et al., 2011). Clearly, the impact of the delivery of clinical services is limited by the circumstances that affected the patient prior to and after the receipt of clinical services. Given the impact that life circumstances appear to have, it could be argued that putting a clinic on every corner would not improve health status if important life circumstance issues are not addressed.

(continued)

> **Box 6.1** (continued)
> Increasingly, an understanding of the social and environmental factors affecting individuals and groups of patients, employees and consumers is required in order to: (1) identify the context in which the patient or consumer functions; and (2) anticipate the impact of the context on the therapeutic process. While the healthcare system can do little by itself to change the contextual life circumstances of patients and consumers within its service area, early and accurate intelligence on these risk factors can contribute to more effective operation of the healthcare system.

One aspect of life conditions that has received increasing attention is adverse childhood experiences (ACES). These include the trauma to which young children are exposed to in their homes or communities that have implications for their mental and emotional development. Children that are exposed to domestic violence, physical, emotional or sexual abuse, or even the routine negative effects of poverty, unstable housing, food insecurity and other adverse conditions are likely to suffer long-term and even life-long consequences (Cronholm et al. (2015).

Some of these intermediate factors could be encapsulated under the heading of "lifestyle" since this term covers a range of attitudes, preferences and behaviors that may be thought to contribute to one's health status and, ultimately, to the health status of groups within the population. Some aspects of lifestyle have been heavily scrutinized and clearly linked to health status. Factors such as dietary habits, participation in exercise, sleep adequacy and the avoidance of harmful substances are clearly linked to variations in health status. While these might be considered aspects of personal lifestyles they are still very much influenced by the groups in which individuals participate. It could be argued that some participate in these behaviors out of necessity (e.g., food deserts, lack of green space) and that issue is discussed below. At the same time members of certain subpopulations are likely to exhibit these characteristics even if they did have access to healthy foods and exercise facilities.

The use and abuse of tobacco, alcohol and drugs (legal and illegal) are clearly aspects of the lifestyles of certain subpopulations. Even to the extent that members of these groups are aware of the dangers of substance abuse, they may be encouraged by their peers to participate in these unhealthy activities. The same may be said for risk-taking behaviors and risky sexual activities. Even wearing automobile seatbelts may be discouraged as "not cool" by members of some subpopulations. More recently, the reluctance to wear facemasks in the midst of a pandemic often reflects group influences. Box 6.2 discusses the use of lifestyle segmentation to study the impact of lifestyles on health status and health behavior.

While the examples above refer to activities reflecting the volition of the actors, many aspects of lifestyle are imposed upon society members who have no ability to resist. While poverty may be viewed from a broad perspective to the extent that it affects a wide spectrum of life conditions, as an intermediate contributor it takes the

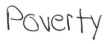

Box 6.2: Lifestyle Segmentation and Health
In an attempt to quantify lifestyle differences a variety of psychographic classification systems have been developed. The intent is to describe a population in terms of its lifestyle attributes, develop a profile of the population as a basis for segmenting it into meaningful subgroups, segment the population based on the clustering of attributes, and assign an appropriate label to the psychographic cluster associated with that segment. Lifestyle clusters are generated based on the analysis of hundreds of different variables.

Once a psychographic cluster is established it becomes possible to (1) assign clusters to any group or even any household and (2) associate a wide range of characteristics with each cluster. Thus, if a household or group is assigned to the "Pools and Patios" cluster it is possible to determine its characteristics in terms of age, race/ethnicity, income and educational level, and community type among others. More important, however, is the ability to profile the target group in terms of various lifestyle attributes—consumer behaviors, exercise patterns, recreational activities, dietary preferences and so forth—that might contribute to health status.

Although health professionals have been slow to associate health-related variables with psychographic clusters, an increasing amount of information has become available in this regard. More obvious applications are the association of alcohol and drug abuse and various mental disorders with certain lifestyle groups. Even more common conditions, however, can often be associated with specific lifestyle clusters. Patterns of distribution for diabetes, asthma, and heart disease, along with various disabilities, for example, correlate with psychographic patterns. An example where psychographics trump demographics might be in the case of heart disease—where two populations may display similar age and sex distributions but vary significantly in terms of heart disease morbidity and mortality. While lifestyles might not account for all of the difference, evidence suggests that life-long patterns of diet, exercise and tobacco and alcohol abuse—i.e., lifestyle attributes—are more significant than advanced age in shaping morbidity patterns with regard to heart disease.

Lifestyles have also been found to influence health behavior independent of other characteristics. Members of certain lifestyle clusters may be thought of as "traditionalists" when it comes to healthcare, emphasizing the use of conventional services. Others might be considered "early adopters" and be willing to try new and different therapies. Healthcare consumers likely to use alternative therapies can often be distinguished from those preferring more conventional services by their psychographic cluster. Those pursuing healthy lifestyles typically fall into different psychographic clusters than those who exhibit unhealthy behaviors. All of these considerations suggest a role for psychographic analysis when developing a population health model.

form of the inability to afford food (or at least healthy food), to afford adequate housing, or to pay the utility bill—much less the ability to afford a fitness center membership fee.

At a secondary level the lack of financial resources creates a multiplier effect in that the dearth of resources means that there is no money for the childcare necessary to allow the individual to go to work or to school or for the transportation necessary to travel to work or school or to a job training program. The lack of money for food noted above also carries over to the work or school setting where it has been demonstrated that hungry or malnourished children and adults cannot perform schoolwork or job activities effectively (Hickson et al., n.d.; Brown et al., 2007).

The lack of financial resources has implications for health behavior as well as health status. Aside from its impact on access to healthy foods and exercise options, there is no money for basic prevention items such as soap and toothpaste. Importantly, there is no money available to purchase health insurance or to pay for health services when the need arises. As a result, members of certain populations are unable to participate in preventive activities or to access necessary health services. Even if basic care could be obtained from a free clinic or hospital emergency room, the ability to purchase necessary drugs may be limited. Thus, a financial exigency becomes transformed into an aspect of lifestyle.

Lifestyles also affect health behavior in several direct and indirect ways. A clear example relates to food preferences. Youth and many adults adopt a "fast-food lifestyle" and seldom eat any other type of food. To do so would risk ridicule from their peers. Healthy foods once promoted by certain subcultures (e.g., the greens and vegetables associated with African- American culture) are eschewed in favor of inexpensive but unhealthy processed foods. The churches patronized by members of certain subcultures are notorious for their unhealthy church supper fare. Mexican immigrants may give up corn-based food products for more "American" wheat-based products with negative consequences for their health (Giuntella, 2012).

One implication for people living under these circumstances is the low priority placed on personal health. In actuality, most of the US population displays a cavalier attitude toward their health despite the much ballyhooed fitness movement. These problems are particularly acute among specific subpopulations. While we are frequently exposed to health promotional materials, the mere distribution of information on healthy lifestyles appears to have little impact. In fact, research (Beck, 2016) has found that less than 3% of Americans exhibit what would be considered a healthy lifestyle (i.e., appropriate diet and exercise, avoidance of unhealthy activities).

Large segments of the population, in fact, have little interest in health and wellness. A study (Thomas, 2009) of an established African-American community in a southern city found that the residents were divided into three groups in terms of their interest in health and wellness (as determined through a consumer database): (1) little interest; (2) almost no interest; and (3) no interest whatsoever. It is absurd, of course, to suppose that the residents would not like to be healthy but, as a practical matter, they had other issues that they considered much more pressing.

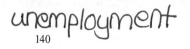

One factor affecting certain subpopulations is a lack of employment. Unemployment is another proximate contributor to poor health status and, aside from the obvious financial exigencies caused by unemployment, the impact of this on health status has been well documented. Research has shown that unemployed people are more likely to have poor health habits, characterized by excess drinking, smoking, lack of exercise, and a sedentary lifestyle. The fear of unemployment has been linked to increased cholesterol levels. Studies from around the world have found people who had been unemployed in prior years had higher mortality rates than people never unemployed, with men much more likely to be affected. Further, unemployment increased long-term mortality when other risk factors were controlled for (Halliday, 2014).

Unemployment is associated with a range of increased health problems (Strully, 2009). For individuals with no prior health problems, being fired or laid off increased the risk of fair or poor health by 83% in one study. Previous unemployment was linked to a significant increase in acute myocardial infarction. The longer and more frequently people are unemployed, the greater the cumulative risk. Research in Sweden (Voss et al., 2004) indicated that the higher death rates of previously unemployed individuals (followed over a 24-year period) were related to higher rates of suicide, accidents, cancer and cardiovascular disease. The fact that these health risks continue for 24 years suggests that unemployment is a potentially dangerous life event. Indeed, the risks associated with unemployment may be of the same magnitude—or greater—as smoking, diabetes and hypertension. Unemployment serves as an additional source of stress for subpopulations that are already living under stressful conditions.

The Influence of Stress on Health Status

When an individual experiences stress, certain hormones are released, such as catecholamines and cortisol. Cortisol, the primary stress hormone, increases sugars (glucose) in the bloodstream, enhances the brain's use of glucose, and increases the availability of substances that repair tissues. Cortisol also curbs functions that would be nonessential or detrimental in a fight-or-flight situation. It alters immune system responses and suppresses the digestive system, the reproductive system and growth processes. Cortisol levels are increasingly used to measure stress, and research has tied elevated cortisol levels to a number of health conditions.

Given that everyone is exposed to stress the question is raised with regard to its idiosyncratic effects. The fact that some people get sick and others do not reflects the existence of factors that "trigger" various diseases. This is significant for the health status of the population since most "diseases of civilization" are stress induced. One explanation of observed differences in the distribution of disease has been offered by Antonovsky (1979) who argued that certain people (or, in our case, certain groups of people) benefit from a sense of coherence—the conviction that no matter how bad the situation that it will eventually have a positive outcome. Not surprisingly, such an attitude is not likely to be exhibited by disadvantaged populations facing inordinate stress.

Box 6.3: Health Conditions Influenced by Stress
The following health conditions (among others) are thought to be triggered or exacerbated by stress:

- Obesity
- Heart disease
- High blood pressure
- Diabetes
- Asthma
- Menstrual problems
- Acne and other skin problems
- Digestive problems
- Various mental disorders
- Rheumatoid arthritis
- Sleep disorders

While there is a tendency to consider stress as an individual condition, in reality stressful conditions affect groups of people in a "wholesale" manner. Members of minority populations or poverty-stricken communities all face stress of various types. For example, research on differences in clinical outcomes for whites and blacks when acuity levels and treatment modality are controlled suggests that the observed differences reflect a lifetime of unremitting stress on the part of the latter (Abdullah et al., 2014).

The negative life circumstances described above all have the potential to contribute to the stress experienced by members of disadvantaged groups. Indeed, there is growing evidence that the everyday stressors faced by members of certain groups are more significant than major traumatic but infrequent stressful events. Box 6.3 lists important conditions that are often attributed to high rates of stress.

Root Causes

Social determinants of health are factors that reflect conditions in society and can affect the health and well-being of individuals and populations. They include the attributes of society and culture that directly or indirectly impact health status and health behavior. The intermediate causes discussed above are thought to be more directly impactful on individuals while the social determinants discussed in this section have a more indirect impact on population health.

Social determinants of health are "the structural determinants and conditions in which people are born, grow, live, work and age" (Heiman & Artiga, 2015). A growing body of research has found that these social determinants affect the likelihood of being exposed to health risks, of contracting a health condition, of receiving adequate medical care, and of having a favorable clinical outcome. The health status and life chances of various groups in society are reflections of social determinants

Box 6.4: Social Determinants of Health

Economic Stability	Neighborhood and Physical Environment	Education	Food	Community and Social Context	Health Care System
Employment	Housing	Literacy	Hunger	Social integration	Health coverage
Income	Transportation	Language	Access to healthy options	Support systems	Provider availability
Expenses	Safety	Early childhood education		Community engagement	Provider linguistic and cultural competency
Debt	Parks	Vocational training		Discrimination	
Medical bills	Playgrounds				
Support	Walkability	Higher education			Quality of care

Health Outcomes
Mortality, Morbidity, Life Expectancy, Health Care Expenditures, Health Status, Functional Limitations

Source: Kaiser Family Foundation.

that account for a significant proportion of deaths every year (Galea et al., 2011). While there are various conceptualizations of categories of social determinants, the approach developed by the Kaiser Family Foundation (Box 6.4) is used for illustration purposes. The discussion below roughly follows this format.

Economic Instability   SES

Economic success is a primary value in American society, and financial status has an inordinate impact on the health status and health behavior of members of various groups. Income is the indicator that most directly measures material resources, although wealth is sometimes employed in a similar fashion. Income can influence health by its direct effect on living standards, and while we typically think of income as an individual or family attribute, it is the economic status of various population subgroups that has relevance for population health.

On virtually every indicator of health status we find a disadvantage for the less affluent. As income decreases, the prevalence of both acute and chronic conditions increases. Interestingly, in a society that has become characterized by chronic health conditions, acute disorders remain surprisingly common among lower income groups. In fact, the disease profile of many low-income communities more closely resembles that of a less developed nation than it does the United States. Not only are there more episodes of certain types of both acute and chronic conditions recorded as income decreases, but the severity of the conditions is likely to be greater when income is lower. Not surprisingly, members of lower-income groups assess themselves as being in poorer health than do the more affluent (National Center for Health Statistics, 2020).

While the levels of both acute and chronic conditions increase as income decreases, morbidity differences based on income are particularly distinct for chronic conditions. For the lowest income group (those with household incomes less than $35,000) prevalence rates are higher for heart disease, diabetes, emphysema, kidney disease, and arthritis than for those with incomes greater than $35,000 (National Center for Health Statistics, 2012). Higher rates are also recorded among the lowest income groups for most chronic respiratory conditions. Note that, if the lowest income group is broken down further (e.g., Into <$15,000, $15,000–$24,999, etc.), the disparities exhibited would be greater at the lowest income levels.

The long-term impact of poverty on a population is as significant as its immediate effects. It has been found that living in poverty in childhood can have detrimental health effects later in life (Evans & Kim, 2007). Interestingly, the relationship between income and health status remains even in the face of improved health behaviors on the part of the lower income groups suggesting a permanence to the adverse effects of poverty.

While absolute poverty creates a health burden for individuals, relative poverty has a more perverse effect on groups within society. Wide income gaps between social groups in developed societies have consequences for health, not so much because of material deprivation but because of its psychosocial effects. The psychosocial processes associated with this lack of social cohesion ultimately affect the health of all regardless of their economic status. The poor can become socially marginalized and therefore less likely to adhere to the norms of that society, resulting in greater levels of crime and personal violence (Marmot, 2015). Living under poverty conditions adds a qualitative dimension that exacerbates its impact on other social determinants of health status. This helps to explain the fact that the use of health services does not translate into better health for members of disadvantaged groups.

Analysis of economic and health data for the last 50 years reveals that the narrowing of the black-white gap in economic status was associated with a parallel narrowing of the black-white gap in health status; similarly, a widening of the racial gap in SES is now associated with a widening gap in health. From the late 1960s to the mid-1970s, as a result of the gains of the civil rights movement, there was some narrowing of the black-white gap in income. There was a corresponding narrowing of the racial gap in health status. During the early 1980s, the health status of economically vulnerable populations worsened in several states in the wake of substantial changes in social and economic policies at the national level.

Neighborhood and Physical Environment

A growing body of research suggests that the best predictor of health and well-being is a person's ZIP Code of residence (Heiman, 2014). The impact on health status of the conditions characterizing the community in which one lives, works and plays cannot be overstated. Not only does the environment have an immediate effect on the health status of residents but an impact that can last for years to come and even have multi-generational effects has been observed (Chetty et al., 2014).

Most experts on the health effects of social factors agree that where you live can shape your health in many important ways. The physical features, social relationships, services and opportunities available in neighborhoods can either enhance or constrain an individual's choices. The overwhelming weight of evidence indicates that both features of neighborhoods and the characteristics of individual residents influence health. One study that compared heart disease among people living in different neighborhoods found that individuals who lived in the most socioeconomically disadvantaged neighborhoods were more likely to develop heart disease than socioeconomically similar individuals who lived in the most advantaged neighborhoods (Robert Wood Johnson Foundation, 2015).

Neighborhoods can influence health in many ways (Cubbin et al., 2008). First—and perhaps most obvious—is through the physical characteristics of neighborhoods. The "built environment" influences the healthiness of the circumstances in which individuals find themselves and creates constraints related to health-producing resources. For example, proximity to supermarkets (which typically sell fresh produce) has been linked to less obesity, while proximity to small convenience stores (which generally do not sell fresh produce) has been linked to a higher rate of obesity (Pereira et al., 2005).

The built environment has a major influence on physical activity. Current urban design and transport systems favor automobile use over walking and limit opportunities for physical activity (Dannenberg et al., 2003). Street patterns that present pedestrian obstacles constrain activities that may lead to better health. Walkability is determined by the physical and built environment (e.g., sidewalks and greenery) as well as the social environment (e.g., crime rates, norms regarding control of dogs and their waste), with the physical environment interacting with the social environment to affect health status. A growing body of public health research, for example, suggests that even perceptions of neighborhood safety are linked to health outcomes (Ziersch et al., 2005).

The physical environment can represent a direct threat to the health of residents. Aspects of the physical environment that can adversely affect health include: poor air and water quality and/or proximity to concentrations of toxic and/or hazardous substances; substandard housing conditions exposing residents to lead paint, mold, dust or pest infestation; lack of access to nutritious foods and safe places to exercise combined with ready access to fast food outlets and liquor stores (Cubbin et al., 2008).

Many studies have found a relationship between disadvantaged neighborhoods and health status even after controlling for individual characteristics, reinforcing the contention that these are not attributes of individuals themselves but reflect community characteristics. Children may be particularly vulnerable to unhealthy conditions in neighborhoods, with consequences for health in childhood and extending later in life. Individuals in minority racial or ethnic groups also are more likely to live in poor neighborhoods; nearly half of all blacks live in poor neighborhoods, compared with only one in ten whites. Among families with similar incomes, blacks and Hispanics live in neighborhoods with higher concentrations of poverty than whites. There are a number of aspects of the neighborhood environment that affect the health and well-being of residents and several of these are discussed below. Box 6.5 discusses factors that may contribute to hospital readmissions.

Box 6.5: Social Factors and Hospital Readmission
The Medicare program finances most of the health services consumed by the nation's senior citizens. The Centers for Medicare and Medicaid (CMS) is the agency with responsibility for management of the Medicare program. In the process of seeking ways in which to contain costs, CMS officials identified hospital readmissions as a potential problem area. It was felt that a hospital readmission for the same condition within 28 days after discharge was an indicator of less than ideal care and a target for cost reduction.

On the assumption that hospital readmissions represented a deficiency in the system, the CMS readmission reduction program was implemented in October 2012 as part of the Patient Protection and Affordable Care Act. Under this initiative CMS calculates each hospital's readmission performance over a 3-year period, targeting conditions such as acute myocardial infarction, heart failure and pneumonia. If a hospital had a readmission ratio that was worse than the national average, its Medicare reimbursement is docked up to 2%. The maximum penalty rose to 3% in fiscal 2015. The methodology took into account certain individual factors, such as the presence of co-morbidities that disproportionately affect certain patient groups but ignored any social determinants.

A number of studies have suggested that the premise driving the CMS readmission reduction program is faulty—that readmissions reflect factors other than the quality of care provided by the facility. A recent study by Truven Health Analytics (2014) found that race and unemployment were particularly strong predictors of higher readmission rates. Unemployment was found to contribute to about 18% of a community's readmissions, with about 6% related to poverty among the elderly. The chances of a black patient being readmitted were almost 15% higher than they were for a white patient.

Another study (Hui et al., 2014) looked specifically at the effect of community socioeconomic status on readmission rates. This study used inpatient data from an urban teaching hospital to examine how individual characteristics and neighborhood socioeconomic status influenced the likelihood of readmission. Patients living in high-poverty neighborhoods were 24% more likely than others to be readmitted, after adjusting for demographic characteristics and clinical conditions. Married patients were at significantly reduced risk of readmission, which suggests that they had more social support than unmarried patients.

It appears that attributes and experiences exhibited by patients prior to their admission to care and after discharge may play an inordinate role in hospital readmission. Socioeconomic conditions—such as poverty, low levels of literacy, limited English proficiency, minimal social support, poor living conditions and limited community resources—appear to have direct and significant impacts on avoidable hospital readmissions. These and previous findings that document socioeconomic disparities in readmission raise the question of whether CMS's readmission measures and associated financial

(continued)

> **Box 6.5** (continued)
>
> penalties should be adjusted for the effects of factors beyond hospital influence such as neighborhood poverty and lack of social support. .
>
> In response to these findings, legislation has been proposed that would encourage CMS to take these non-clinical factors into consideration. The Hospital Readmissions Program Accuracy and Accountability Act would require that CMS account for patient socioeconomic status when calculating risk-adjusted readmissions penalties. CMS officials, however, have raised some concerns about a practice that treats some categories of patients differently from others and argues that there are steps that hospitals can take to address these non-clinical factors. No doubt this issue will continue to be debated among health professionals and policy makers in the future.
>
> Sources: Hui et al. (2014), Rice (2016), and Truven Health Analytics (2014)

Housing Access and Quality — Housing

Housing is an important determinant of health, and access to adequate, affordable housing can affect how healthy a person is (Egerter et al., 2008). People spend most of their time indoors, at home, especially young children, who are particularly vulnerable to threats in the home environment (Braveman et al., 2011). As a result, housing adequacy has long been recognized as a public health issue.

Substandard housing affects multiple dimensions of health. Poor housing conditions contribute to increased exposure to biological (e.g., allergens), chemical (e.g., lead) and physical (e.g., thermal stress) hazards, which directly affect physiological and biochemical processes. Stress induced by substandard housing may also play a role in undermining health by increasing the allostatic load on the body. For example, excessive noise (common in poorly insulated housing units) has been associated with sleep deprivation that leads to psychological stress.

Although lead levels in the blood of young children have been declining, recent incidents suggest that there may be a resurgence in lead poisoning and that the metrics used may understate the extent of the problem. An estimated half million young children in the United States have blood lead levels high enough to adversely affect their intelligence, behavior, and development (Centers for Disease Control and Prevention, 2016). Most lead exposure occurs in the home, particularly in homes built before 1978 that often contain lead-based paint and lead in the plumbing systems. Deteriorating paint in older homes is the primary source of lead exposure for children, who ingest paint chips and inhale lead-contaminated dust. A quarter of the nation's housing—24 million homes—is estimated to have significant lead-based paint hazards.

Substandard housing conditions such as water leaks, poor ventilation, dirty carpets and pest infestation can lead to an increase in mold, mites and other allergens associated with poor health. Indoor allergens and damp housing conditions play an important role in the development and exacerbation of respiratory conditions including asthma, which currently affects over 20 million Americans and is the most common chronic disease among children (Platts-Mills et al., 1997). Approximately 40% of diagnosed asthma among children is believed to be attributable to residential exposures.

Exposure to very high or very low indoor temperatures can be detrimental to health. Cold indoor conditions have been associated with poorer health, and extreme low and high temperatures have been associated with increased mortality, especially among vulnerable populations such as the elderly. Housing can be a source of exposure to various carcinogenic air pollutants. Radon, a natural radioactive gas released from the ground, has been associated with lung cancer; an estimated one in 15 homes has elevated radon levels. Residential exposure to environmental tobacco smoke, pollutants from heating and cooking with gas, volatile organic compounds and asbestos have been linked with respiratory illness and some types of cancer.

Concerns over the impact of housing on health have increased as the quality of and access to affordable housing has become more of a challenge. An increasing body of evidence has associated housing quality with morbidity from infectious diseases, chronic illnesses, injuries, poor nutrition, and mental disorders. Features of substandard housing, including lack of safe drinking water, absence of hot water for washing, ineffective waste disposal, intrusion by disease vectors (e.g., insects and rats) and inadequate food storage, features identified as contributing to the spread of infectious diseases. Damp, cold, and moldy housing is associated with asthma and other chronic respiratory symptoms, even after potentially confounding factors such as income, social class, smoking, crowding, and unemployment are controlled for.

Pest infestations, through their association with asthma, provide another linkage between substandard housing and chronic illness. Cockroaches can cause allergic sensitization and have emerged as an important asthma trigger in inner-city neighborhoods. Children with asthma who are sensitized and exposed to cockroaches are at elevated risk for hospitalization. Mouse allergen also acts as a clinically important cause of allergy and asthma morbidity. Inadequate food storage and disposal facilities provide cockroaches and rodents with opportunities to obtain food. Dead spaces in walls harbor pests and permit circulation among apartments in multiunit dwellings.

Exposure to toxic substances found in homes can result in chronic health problems. The association between indoor tobacco smoke and respiratory disease is well documented (American Cancer Society, 2016). Poor ventilation may increase exposure to smoke, and poorly functioning appliances have been associated with asthma symptoms. Exposure to volatile organic compounds (emitted by particle board and floor coverings) may be associated with asthma and "sick building syndrome".

Poorly functioning heating systems can cause headache due to carbon monoxide, whereas higher levels result in acute intoxication. Asbestos exposure (from deteriorating insulation) can cause mesothelioma and lung cancer. Polyvinyl chloride flooring and textile wall materials have been associated with bronchial obstruction during the first two years of life.

A lack of affordable housing has been linked to inadequate nutrition, especially among children. Relatively expensive housing may force low-income tenants to use more of their resources to obtain shelter, leaving less for other necessities such as food. Renters (which include most low-income citizens) are now paying well over 30% of their income for housing and related expenses (governing.com, 2016), thereby increasing the likelihood of food insecurity. Low-income children whose families were on a waiting list to obtain housing subsidies exhibited more undernutrition and decreased growth than children whose families had obtained a housing subsidy (Meyers et al., 1995).

Not surprisingly, substandard housing may also adversely affect mental health, although the evidence is more tentative. Excessive indoor temperature has been linked with irritability and social intolerance. Damp, moldy, and cold indoor conditions may be associated with anxiety and depression. Homelessness and living in substandard, temporary housing have been related to behavioral problems among children. Substandard housing conditions may lead to social isolation because occupants are reluctant to invite guests into their homes. High-rise buildings may inhibit social interaction because they lack common spaces.

Exposure to substandard housing is not evenly distributed across the US populations. Members of minority groups and disadvantaged populations are disproportionately affected. People with low income are more likely to live in overcrowded homes and be disproportionately exposed to a wide range of associated health risks. Injuries occur more commonly in low-income households because of substandard conditions and a lack of resources to repair them. Clutter stemming from lack of storage space and hazardous cooking facilities also contribute to increased risk of injury from fire. Homes of people with low income are more likely to be too warm or too cool because they are less well insulated.

Transportation

Transportation may not often be associated with health conditions but it affects community health along a number of dimensions. There is growing consensus that the US transportation system can be harmful to our health and well-being (Robert Wood Johnson Foundation, 2012). Motorized transportation modes dominate in our society, leading to increased air pollution, traffic crashes, and decreased physical activity. Major highways often run through or adjacent to low-income neighborhoods, neighborhoods that are more likely to have minority residents and be disproportionately affected by poor air quality and noise pollution. Young children are particularly affected.

More than 45 million people in the United States live, work, or attend school within 300 feet of a major road, airport or railroad making the health impacts of roadway traffic a growing concern (Environmental Protection Agency, 2014). Proximity to a major roadway places residents at higher risk for asthma and other respiratory illnesses, cardiovascular disease, pre-term births, and premature death. A recent survey of the studies on the effect of traffic emissions on pregnancy outcomes has linked exposure to emissions to adverse effects on gestational duration and possibly intrauterine growth (Pereira et al., 2010).

It is well documented that patterns of physical activity are influenced by the physical and built environments, with features of the built environment such as mixed land use, well-connected street networks and high residential density positively associated with higher levels of physical activity. Our current transportation system contributes to physical inactivity—each additional hour spent in a car per day is associated with an increase in the likelihood of obesity. On the other hand, use of public transportation is associated with greater physical activity based on a review of of recent research (Rissel et al., 2012). Walking or bicycling as a form of transportation or walking to public transportation stations, such as bus stops, also count toward meeting the daily physical activity recommendations. Analysis by federal agencies found that there is a significant reduction in mortality associated with active transportation.

Transportation barriers are often cited as barriers to healthcare access. Transportation barriers lead to rescheduled or missed appointments, delayed care, and missed or delayed medication use. These consequences may lead to poorer management of chronic illness and thus poorer health outcomes. A synthesis of the literature on the prevalence of transportation barriers to healthcare access (Syed et al., 2013) found that access to transportation is an important barrier, particularly for those with lower incomes or the under/uninsured.

A review of previous research by Syed et al. (2013) found lack of access to a vehicle to be a barrier that could result in missing a cancer treatment. Further, patients who lived in neighborhoods where households were less likely to have access to a vehicle were significantly less likely to receive first line chemotherapy. Lack of private transportation to medical care was found to increase the likelihood of not having a regular source of care. Patients who did not use private transportation were also more likely to delay care. This was a more significant barrier than excessive distance, expense, or the inconvenience of public transportation.

Access to transportation is particularly important for those with chronic diseases (Syed et al., 2013). Chronic disease care requires regular clinician visits, medication access, and changes to treatment plans. However, without transportation, delays in clinical interventions can lead to a lack of appropriate medical treatment, chronic disease exacerbation or unmet healthcare needs. Box 6.6 provides an overview of the relationship between access to transportation and health.

Patients with transportation barriers carry a greater burden of disease which may, in part, reflect the relationship between poverty and transportation availability. This situation has become more obvious with the movement of disadvantaged populations into America's suburbs (Kneebone & Garr, 2010). While there are some advantages to suburban living over inner-city living, access to transportation is not

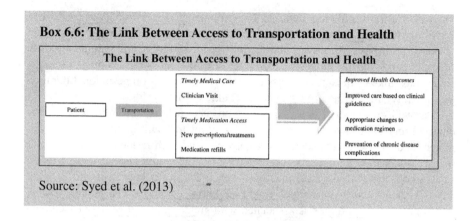

Box 6.6: The Link Between Access to Transportation and Health

Source: Syed et al. (2013)

one of them. The "suburbanization of poverty" has had the effect of decreasing access to health facilities and services.

Health impact assessments are useful in helping policy makers understand the health effects of proposed laws and programs yet to date they have little influence on transportation policy and planning. Health costs typically are not included in transportation decision-making. Currently 80% of federal transportation funding goes to building highways and improving road infrastructures, creating a situation that works against a healthy lifestyle (American Public Health Association, 2010).

Education

The relationship between educational attainment and health status has been well documented. Those at higher educational levels are likely to rate themselves as being in better health than those with less education (National Center for Health Statistics, 2020). The better educated report fewer episodes of acute conditions and fewer chronic conditions than the poorly educated (National Center for Health Statistics, 2012). The prevalence of heart disease (e.g., coronary heart disease, hypertension) increases as educational level decreases. The same pattern—higher rates with declining education—holds for chronic respiratory conditions, arthritis and diabetes.

The relationship between educational level and mental illness, like that for physical illness, appears to be fairly clear cut. Adults with less than a high school education report the highest rates of sadness, hopelessness and worthlessness while those with at least a bachelor's degree report the lowest rates. Further, the poorly educated are more likely to report feelings of nervousness and restlessness. As the level of education increases, there appears to be an increase in the prevalence but a decrease in the severity of disorders. The better educated appear to be more characterized by neurotic conditions, while the less educated appear to be more frequently psychotic. The presence of psychiatric symptoms can exacerbate stress which in turn can induce physical symptoms.

The level of disability exhibits a clear pattern with regard to educational attainment (National Center for Health Statistics, 2020). An analysis of data from the National Health Interview Survey found an inverse relationship between educational levels and chronic conditions, limitation of activities, and number of bed days for disability.

The pattern with regard to mortality also resembles that exhibited for income. The death rate for the poorly educated is much higher than that for those with higher educational achievement. According to NCHS data, the risk of mortality for those with a high school education is 60% higher than that for those with a graduate degree (University of Pennsylvania, 2020). Indeed, recent research indicates an increase in mortality among poorly educated US citizens (Olshanky, 2012). The poorly educated are likely to be characterized by lifestyle-related deaths such as homicides and accidents. Education, in fact, has been shown to demonstrate a stronger association with mortality than does income (Rogers et al., 2000).

Infant mortality, once a leading cause of death, has been virtually eliminated from the groups with the highest educational levels, with the poorly educated accounting for the bulk of infant deaths. The correlation between educational level and infant mortality rates is reflected in differences in low birth-weight babies and premature births for those at different educational levels. Babies born to women who did not complete high school are almost twice as likely to die in their first year than babies born to women who did.

As with income, the relationship does not necessarily reflect the level of education per se but the differential consequences of varying educational levels. Those with less education are likely to be more affected by financial insecurity, poor housing conditions, and unsafe environments, all contributing to an increase in morbidity levels. Box 6.7 illustrates the relationship between educational level and perceived health status.

Additional years of education are not only associated with better health status, but they contribute to healthier behaviors. An additional 4 years of education has been found to cut the likelihood of smoking in half and reduce the likelihood of alcohol abuse by more than 60%. The risk of obesity is reduced by more than 20% with the additional years of education.

Food Insecurity

Food insecurity refers to the inability to afford nutritionally adequate and safe foods. Most adults living in food-insecure households report being unable to afford balanced meals, concern about the adequacy of their food supply, running out of food, and cutting the size of meals or skipping meals. At the most severe levels of food

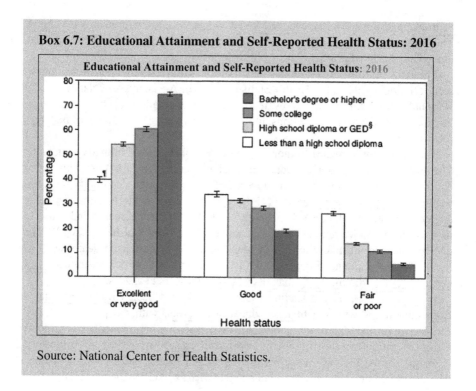

Box 6.7: Educational Attainment and Self-Reported Health Status: 2016

Source: National Center for Health Statistics.

insecurity, many adults report not eating for an entire day. While some episodes of food insecurity may be short in duration, the dietary changes associated with food insecurity may persist over extended periods due to repeated food shortages (Seligman et al., 2010). During the past two decades policy makers and those responsible for conducting research have come to appreciate the connection between food insecurity and the conditions, manifestations, and ramifications of ill health. Among other things, the implication is that hunger, in addition to being a symptom of food insecurity, is also a part of the panoply of conditions that signal compromised health status (Schroeder, 2016).

Undernourishment and malnutrition are two conditions widely agreed to be the results of hunger and food insecurity. Among children, conditions that coincide with the latter include weight loss, fatigue, stunting of growth, and frequent colds. Studies have shown that undernourished pregnant women are more likely to bear babies with low birth weight, and these babies are subsequently more likely to experience developmental delays that can lead to learning problems (Groce et al., 2014). Moreover, hunger and food insecurity worsen the effects of all diseases and can accelerate degenerative conditions, especially among the elderly. Hunger and food insecurity create psychological responses such as anxiety, hostility, and negative perceptions of self-worth. In an energy- and resource-constrained world, infectious conditions can be expected to become more prevalent.

Where people live has a dramatic effect on their health and access to affordable and healthy food. Residents who live far away from grocery stores and cannot access healthy foods are considered to live in "food deserts." The availability of supermarkets is associated with socioeconomic status (Cummins & Macintyre, 2005). Low-income and minority neighborhoods have fewer chain supermarkets and produce stores (Powell, 2007). Many residents only have access to convenience stores that offer no healthy foods. The result is less variety and poorer quality of foods in low-income neighborhoods (Sloane et al., 2003). The only available restaurants may be "fast food" establishments. Higher consumption of fast foods is associated with a decrease in nutrient intake and diet quality and an increase in energy intake, weight gain, and insulin resistance (Pereira et al., 2005). Box 6.8 illustrates the extent of food deserts across the nation.

A lack of access to affordable healthy foods has laid the groundwork for the current epidemic of obesity. Obesity underlies the growing diabetes epidemic, with all the co-morbid disorders that entails: heart disease, kidney failure, leg amputations, and blindness. Healthcare for obese individuals costs more than for normal-weight individuals, and the costs rise with increasing levels of obesity. The annual healthcare costs for people who are extremely obese are almost twice those of normal-weight people.

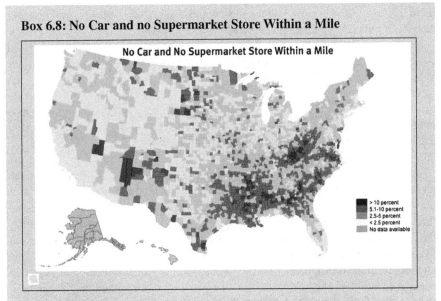

Box 6.8: No Car and no Supermarket Store Within a Mile

Source: U.S. Department of Agriculture; Center for Disease Control and Prevention (2010)

The population health model looks at environmental conditions that contribute to the obesity epidemic through their effects on food consumption. The supersizing of cheap sources of energy-dense food and the proliferation of fast-food outlets pit healthy food choices against convenience and getting "the most bang for your buck." The food industry's marketing of foods that exploit evolutionarily programmed human preferences for sugar and fat affects food preferences and their associated caloric intake. There is particular concern about the marketing of food like sweetened cereals, beverages, and snack foods to children (Kumanyika & Grier, 2006).

Community and Social Context

Health status is influenced by the social environments of neighborhoods—that is, by characteristics of the social relationships among their residents, including the degree of mutual trust and feelings of connectedness among neighbors (Cubbin et al., 2008). A supportive community has been found to contribute to good health while communities that foster isolation, disassociation, and lack of social support are detrimental to health. Residents of "close-knit" neighborhoods may be more likely to work together to achieve common goals, to exchange information, and to maintain informal social controls, all of which can directly or indirectly influence health. Neighborhoods in which residents lack mutual trust have been linked with higher homicide rates. Less closely-knit neighborhoods and higher levels of social disorder have been linked to anxiety and depression.

A society with wide gaps between rich and poor produces low levels of social cohesion which is important for coping with stress. The psychosocial processes associated with this lack of social cohesion ultimately affect the health of *all*, rich and poor alike. The poor become socially marginalized and are therefore less likely to adhere to the norms of society, resulting in greater levels of crime and violence. In societies with extreme income inequality high proportions of the population are excluded from full social participation (Marmot, 2015) leading them to develop alternative (and often unhealthy) lifestyles.

It can be argued that persistent on-going discrimination is a factor in the health problems associated with members of various subgroups within the population. A growing body of evidence suggests that persistent discrimination leads to higher levels of stress which in turn can lead to physical health problems (American Psychological Association, 2016). The aforementioned lack of social cohesion limits the ability to cope with higher stress. The fact that health disparities remain even after controlling for socioeconomic status suggests that discrimination represents a residual factor affecting health status. Parents who report that their neighborhood is unsafe may limit their children's time in outdoor independent play, which can decrease the child's opportunities for physical activity. Children of parents who believe their neighborhood is unsafe are also more likely to be overweight.

Furthermore, evidence suggests that individuals' sense of neighborhood safety is associated with the extent to which they participate in and interact with their community (de Jesus et al., 2010). Studies examining the role of neighborhood factors on health demonstrate that higher levels of safety are associated with higher respondent perceptions of social cohesion and better health outcomes. This research demonstrates that "the degree to which an individual is interconnected and embedded in a community—is vital to an individual's health and well-being…"

Social network structure tends to vary by socioeconomic status (SES), and the social networks of those with lower incomes tend to be more place-based, be homogeneously low income, contain more close relationships, and involve more overlapping relations. Conventional wisdom suggests that lower-income populations are more relation-oriented since this is about the only resource available to them. For example, Child (2016) examined the social networks in a low-income neighborhood and found that those who lived in these neighborhoods, rather than being involved in more intense and strong relationships, tended to have weaker relationships than those in middle-income areas. Thus, even existing relationships may be too weak to offer beneficial social support, and these relationships are made even more tenuous due to frequent changes of residence. Box 6.9 presents data on the relationship between race and ethnicity and neighborhood perception.

Children living in single-mother households are nearly twice as likely to live in a neighborhood that is described as unsafe as are children living with two biological or adoptive parents. Children living at or below the poverty line are more than three times as likely as children living above 200% of the poverty level to live in a neighborhood described as never or only sometimes safe.

Residential Segregation

Perhaps the most significant aspect of the community context is the persistent (and in some cases increasing) residential segregation exhibited by many communities. Although this phenomenon was not cited specifically in the Kaiser framework, it has come to be seen as a major consideration with regard to health status. In fact, the 2016 *County Health Rankings* report added a new measure on residential segregation to illustrate the extent to which populations are isolated from the larger society (Shwarz, 2016).

Segregation is a fundamental cause of differences in health status between African Americans and whites because it shapes socioeconomic conditions for blacks not only at the individual and household levels but also at the neighborhood and community levels (Williams & Collins, 2001). The evidence suggests that segregation is a key determinant of racial differences in socioeconomic mobility and, additionally, can foster social and physical risks in residential environments that adversely affect health. Indeed, residential segregation based on race is a fundamental cause of racial disparities in health.

Box 6.9: Percentage of Parents Who Report Children are Living in Unsafe Neighborhoods,* by Race and Hispanic Origin, 2003, 2007 and 2011/12

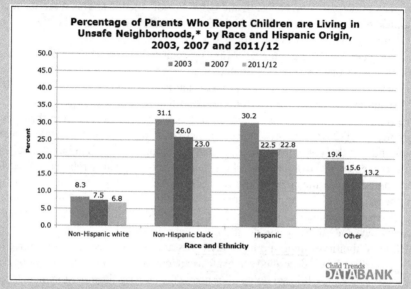

Source: Child Trends' original analyses of data from the National Survey of Children's Health
*Children in unsafe neighborhoods referes to children whose parents responded "never" or "sometimes safe"
when asked "How often do you feel the child is safe in your community or neighborhood?"

The degree of residential segregation remains extremely high for most African Americans and their situation is unique. Although numerically there are more poor whites than poor African Americans in the US, most poor white people are residentially located next to non-poor people, while most poor African Americans are concentrated in high poverty neighborhoods.

Although most immigrant groups have experienced some residential segregation in the United States, no immigrant group has ever lived under the high levels of segregation that currently exist for the African American population. In most immigrant ghettos, the ethnic immigrant group did not constitute a majority of the population of that area, and most members of European ethnic groups did not live in immigrant enclaves. Extreme and persistent residential segregation has truncated the socioeconomic mobility of African Americans and remains a central mechanism through which racial inequality is created and reinforced.

Residential segregation, especially the separation of whites and blacks or Hispanics in the same community, continues to have lasting implications for the well-being of people of color and the health of a community. In many US counties and cities, neighborhoods with little diversity are commonplace. When neighborhoods are segregated, so too are schools, public services, jobs and other kinds of opportunities that affect health. Segregation can also adversely affect health by creating a broad range of pathogenic residential conditions that can induce adverse effects on health status (Williams & Collins, 2001). Measures of segregation appear to capture some of the effects of racism at the area level, and these community-level effects are one reason for the persistence of racial differences in health status even after controls are introduced for individual variations in socioeconomic status.

A growing number of studies using multilevel analyses indicate that social and economic characteristics of residential areas are associated with a broad range of health outcomes independent of individual indicators of socioeconomic status. Numerous studies have found that people residing in disadvantaged neighborhoods have a higher incidence of heart disease than people who live in more advantaged neighborhoods. Several studies have specifically operationalized residential segregation and related the level of segregation to rates of morbidity and mortality. This body of research has found that residential segregation is related to elevated risks of cause-specific and overall adult mortality, infant mortality, and tuberculosis. (Arcaya & Schnake-Mahl, 2017).

An investigation of segregation also sheds light on the racial differences in some health outcomes that have strong environmental components. African Americans are much more likely than whites to be victims of all types of crime, including homicide, and several studies have found that segregation is positively associated with the risk of being a victim of homicide for blacks. Irrespective of racial status, the homicide rate is strongly influenced by socioeconomic status. These dramatic racial differences may reflect an important area effect, and research on the causes of urban violence clearly suggests that the elevated homicide rate for African-Americans is a consequence of residential segregation (Peterson & Krivo, 1993). The elevated rates of violent crime and homicide for African-Americans are determined by the structural conditions of their residential contexts.

Residential segregation by race also leads to unequal access for most blacks to a broad range of services provided by municipal authorities. Political leaders have been more likely to cut spending and services in poor neighborhoods, in general, and African American neighborhoods, in particular, than in more affluent areas. Poor people and members of minority groups are less active politically than their more economically and socially advantaged peers, and elected officials are less likely to encounter vigorous opposition when services are reduced in the areas in which large numbers of poor people and people of color live.

Criminal Justice

The criminal justice system is another contributor to health status that was not included within the Kaiser framework. As a nation, we have tried to lock our problems away and are now seeing the harmful impact of mass incarceration on our society at-large (Benjamin, 2015). The United States has the largest prison population in the world by a large margin. More than 60% of the nation's 2.3 million prisoners are people of color. Nearly one-third of federal prisoners are Hispanic, and the number of women in prison is rising. Sixteen states put more people behind bars than in college housing.

Mass incarceration of people of color further exemplifies how structural factors perpetuate racialized health disparities. Current estimates are that one in three black men will be behind bars at some point in their lifetime (Alexander, 2010). The mass incarceration of blacks is largely the result of institutional policies in our police and judicial systems, which includes aggressive enforcement of low-level drug crimes and mandatory harsh sentencing laws that disproportionately affect Blacks. The consequences of mass incarceration extend beyond a prison sentence. Once released, individuals with a criminal record lose eligibility for social programs (Roberts, 2004), experience voter disenfranchisement, and face discrimination when seeking housing and employment, all of which are deleterious for the health and well-being of individuals, families, and communities.

Epidemiologic studies have confirmed that jail and prison inmates have a higher burden of chronic diseases such as hypertension, asthma, and cervical cancer than the general population (Binswanger et al., 2009). Furthermore, inmates are particularly at risk for substance use disorders, psychiatric disorders, victimization, and infectious diseases, including hepatitis C, HIV, and tuberculosis (American Association of Family Practitioners, 2017). Despite the prevalence of poor health status among both minorities and inmates, the effect of criminal justice involvement on population health disparities has been largely overlooked in research on population health disparities.

Criminal justice involvement may be associated with health outcomes through direct or indirect effects (Binswanger et al., 2012). Because individuals engaged with the criminal justice system are already at risk for poor health outcomes, the health screening and care provided by jails and prisons could have an important impact on racial/ethnic healthcare disparities. While jails and prisons may provide access to care due to constitutional mandates, the quality of care in correctional facilities is variable and has been poorly measured. Further, a large proportion of those released from prison are characterized by significant health problems. Probationers and parolees, who represent the largest proportion of criminal justice involved populations, suffer from inadequate access to care and risk deterioration in health status and death (Binswanger et al., 2012).

Prisons are overcrowded with people who have mental illness, drug addictions and little education, and prisoners generally receive inadequate therapy for their conditions. Half of all people in prison are parents, with their families suffering the consequences. The average prison sentence is nearly 10 years, and prisoners are often inappropriately cared for while there. After release, few options exist within their communities, further reducing the likelihood of successful rehabilitation.

In addition to health effects on criminal justice-involved individuals, the system is likely to impact the health of families and communities, predominantly in urban areas (Binswanger et al., 2012). The adverse effects of criminalization of drug users on health involve decreased access to health benefits, housing, and employment, as well as subsequent impacts on families and communities. Rates of sexually transmitted diseases and teenage pregnancy have been shown to be associated with community incarceration rates. Urban neighborhoods whose inhabitants have high rates of incarceration, and many returning inmates experience a phenomenon similar to "forced migration" which disrupts social, family, and sexual networks and has secondary effects on the health of the community.

Summary

Social determinants of health are factors that reflect conditions in society that directly or indirectly affect the health and well-being of individuals and populations. They include factors like socioeconomic status, education, the physical environment, employment, and social support networks, as well as access to healthcare. The health status and life chances of various groups in society are reflections of social determinants that account for a significant proportion of deaths every year.

The main categories of social determinants identified by the Kaiser Family Foundation include: economic stability, neighborhood and physical environment, education, food, and community and social context. Other social determinants to be considered include residential segregation and the criminal justice system.

Health professionals now realize that contemporary health problems have their roots in social conditions rather than being a function of biological pathology or genetics. This shift in disease etiology has greatly reduced the importance of the historical causes of disease onset and brought sources of sickness such as lifestyles, demographic attributes, and life circumstances to the fore. While we could claim to be "victims" of pathogens or genetics, we are not blameless when it comes to contemporary causes of ill health.

As individuals and as a society we are, in fact, responsible for most of the health problems that currently affect us. As a society we have encouraged unhealthy lifestyles through the promotion of unhealthy food choices. We have allowed an unacceptable level of environmental degradation. We have tolerated an unacceptable level of housing deterioration, with a large segment of the population forced to live in unsafe and unhealthy housing. We have also allowed the emergence of a level of socioeconomic inequality perhaps never experienced by the US population. As more and more financial resources are concentrated among the wealthiest in society, lower- and working-class populations have access to fewer resources. This translates into unhealthy lifestyles and a lack of access to health services thereby creating a perpetual cycle of financial distress and ill-health.

As the impact of social factors on health status has become documented, the argument is increasingly being made that the health conditions exhibited by a population are not the *problems* per se but are *symptoms* of underlying problems. Critics of the US healthcare system point out that we have been treating these symptoms while not addressing the underlying problems.

Improvement in population health will require attention to the root causes of ill-health. The first step in this process is to identify the factors that immediately influence the health status of the population in question and, beyond that, to identify the underlying social determinants that have a significant if less direct impact on health status. Life circumstances include the conditions of everyday living that constrain people's activities and influence their behavior. Some of these factors could be encapsulated under the heading of "lifestyle" since this term covers a range of attitudes, preferences and behaviors that may be thought to contribute to one's health status and, ultimately, to the health status of groups within the population.

Studies are emerging that suggest that many of the differences in the observed onset of physical and mental disorders and variations in the progression of disease, clinical outcomes and even mortality rates are a function of differences in the level of chronic stress, all other factors being equal. This is significant for the health status of the population since most "diseases of civilization" are stress induced. While there is a tendency to consider stress as an individual condition, in reality stressful conditions affect groups of people in a "wholesale" manner. Members of minority populations or poverty-stricken communities, for example, all face stress of various types.

Key Points

- Historical contributors to ill-health like genetics and biological pathogens have become less important as the nature of disease has changed.
- Rather than being "victims" of nature, society members are responsible for most of the ill-health that affects society.
- Existing health conditions should be thought of as "symptoms" rather than problems, with social determinants ultimately being the source of most health problems.
- Life circumstances reflect the conditions under which members of society live and contribute to differences in health status and health behavior.
- Stress contributes to the onset of ill-health, and many of the "diseases of civilization" are triggered or exacerbated by stress.
- Several categories of social determinants have been identified, each making its own contribution to ill-health.
- Economic instability is a major contribution with poverty being a primary driver of ill-health and unemployment directly impacting health status.

- The neighborhood and social context affect the health status of those living in unsafe or unhealthy communities.
- Housing insecurity is an important contributor to ill-health, and inadequate housing directly affects the health of residents.
- Limited educational attainment and poor job skills are associated with poor health status.
- Food insecurity is a major contributor to poor health and has a spillover effect on one's ability to hold a job or obtain an education.
- Communities that lack social cohesion also exhibit poor health status, with residents of disadvantaged communities often lacking social support.
- Residential segregation is a major contributor to health disparities, and the discrimination implicit in segregated housing contributes to poor health.
- Mass incarceration is another factor contributing to health disparities, with minorities disproportionately affected by incarceration and related threats to health.

References

Alexander, M. (2010). *The new Jim crow: Mass incarceration in the age of colorblindness*. The New Press.

Abdullah, S. A., Dekker, R., Tovar, E., et al. (2014). Examination of the potential association of stress with morbidity and mortality outcomes in patient with heart failure. *GE Open Med*. Downloaded from URL: https://www.ncbi.nlm.nih.gov/pmc/articles/PMC4523379/#:~:text=Stress%2C%20variably%20defined%20as%20psychological,in%20patients%20with%20cardiovascular%20diseases.&text=Others%2C%20with%20large%20sample%20sizes,rates%20related%20to%20cardiovascular%20disease

American Association of Family Practitioners. (2017). *Incarceration and health: A family medicine perspective*. Downloaded from URL: https://www.aafp.org/about/policies/all/incarceration.html#during

American Cancer Society. (2016). *Health risks of second-hand smoke*. Downloaded from URL: http://www.cancer.org/cancer/cancercauses/tobaccocancer/secondhand-smoke

American Public Health Association. (2010). *The hidden health costs of transportation*. Downloaded from URL: https://www.apha.org/~/media/files/pdf/factsheets/hidden_health_costs_transportation.ashx

American Psychological Association. (2016). *Stress in America: The impact of discrimination*. Downloaded from URL: http://www.apa.org/news/press/releases/stress/2015/impact-of-discrimination.pdf

Antonovsky, A. (1979). *Health, stress and coping*. Jossey-Bass Publishers.

Arcaya, M. C., & Schnake-Mahl, A. (2017). *Health in the Segregated City*. Downloaded from URL: https://furmancenter.org/research/iri/essay/health-in-the-segregated-city#:~:text=We%20highlight%20three%20salient%20facets,system%2C%20which%20is%20associated%20with

Beck, J. (2016). Less than 3% of Americans live a healthy lifestyle. *The Atlantic*. Downloaded from URL: http://www.theatlantic.com/health/archive/2016/03/less-than-3-percent-of-americans-live-a-healthy-lifestyle/475065/

Benjamin, G. (2015). *Why our Justice System is a hazard to our health*. Downloaded from URL: http://www.centerforhealthjournalism.org/2015/09/14/why-our-justice-system-hazard-our-health

Binswanger, I. A., Krueger, P. M., & Steiner, J. F. (2009). Prevalence of chronic medical conditions among jail and prison inmates in the USA compared with the general population. *Journal of Epidemiology and Community Health, 63*(11), 912–919.

Binswanger, I. A., Redmond, N., Steiner, J. F., et al. (2012). Health disparities and the criminal justice system: An agenda for further research and action. *Journal of Urban Health, 89*(1), 98–107.

Braveman, P., Dekker, M., Egerter, S., et al. (2011). *Housing and health.* Donlodaed from URL: http://www.rwjf.org/en/library/research/2011/05/housing-and-health.html

Brown, J., Shepard, D., Martin, T, et al. (2007). *The economic cost of domestic hunger: Estimated annual burden to the United States.* Downloaded from URL: http://www.sodexofoundation.org/hunger_us/newsroom/studies/hungerstudies/costofhunger.asp

Centers for Disease Control and Prevention. (2016). *Lead.* Downloaded from URL: http://www.cdc.gov/nceh/lead/

Chetty, R., et al. (2014). Where is the land of opportunity? The geography of intergenerational mobility in the United States. *The Quarterly Journal of Economics, 129*(4), 1553–1623.

Child, S. (2016). *Social capital and social networks: The importance of social ties for health among residents of disadvantaged communities.* Unpublished dissertation. https://scholarcommons.se.edu/etd/3848

Cronholm, P. F., Forke, C. M., Wade, R., et al. (2015). Adverse childhood experiences: Expanding the concept of adversity. *American Journal of Prevention Medicine, 49*, 354–361.

Cubbin, C., Pedregon, V., Egerter, S., et al (2008). *Where we live matters for our health: Neighborhoods and health.* Downloaded from URL: http://www.commissiononhealth.org/PDF/888f4a18-eb90-45be-a2f8-159e84a55a4c/Issue%20Brief%203%20Sept%2008%20-%20Neighborhoods%20and%20Health.pdf

Cummins, S., & Macintyre, S. (2005). Food environments and obesity—Neighbourhood or nation. *International Journal of Epidemiology, 35*(1), 100–104.

Dannenberg, A. L., Jackson, R. J., Frumkin, H., et al. (2003). The impact of community design and land-use choices on public health: A scientific research agenda. *American Journal of Public Health, 93*(9), 1500–1508.

De Jesus, M., Puleo, E., Shelton, R. C., et al. (2010). Associations between perceived social environment and neighborhood safety: Health implications. *Health & Place, 16*(5), 1007–1013.

Egerter, S., Sadegh-Nobari, T., Dekker, M., et al. (2008). *Where we live matters for our health: The links between housing and health.* Downloaded from URL: http://www.commissiononhealth.org/PDF/e6244e9e-f630-4285-9ad7-16016dd7e493/Issue%20Brief%202%20Sept%2008%20-%20Housing%20and%20Health.pdf

Ellaway, A. (2014). The impact of the local social and physical environment on wellbeing. In E. Burton & R. Cooper (Eds.), *Wellbeing and the environment Vol. 2.* Wiley-Blackwell.

Evans, R. G., Barer, M. L., & Marmor, T. R. (Eds.). (1994). *Why are some people healthy and others not? The determinants of health of populations.* Aldine de Gruyter.

Evans, G. W., & Kim, P. (2007). Childhood poverty and health: Cumulative risk exposure and stress dysregulation. *Psychological Science, 18*(11), 953–957.

Environmental Protection Agency. (2014). *Near roadway air pollution and health: Frequently asked questions.* Downloaded from URL: https://nepis.epa.gov/Exe/ZyPDF.cgi/P100NFFD.PDF?Dockey=P100NFFD.PDF

Galea, S., et al. (2011). Estimated deaths attributable to social factors in the United States. *American Journal of Public Health, 101*(8), 1456–1465.

Giuntella, O. (2012). *Why does the health of immigrants deteriorate?* Downloaded from URL: https://www.dartmouth.edu/~neudc2012/docs/paper_232.pdf

governing.com. (2016). *Housing affordability burden For U.S. cities.* Downloaded from URL: http://www.governing.com/gov-data/economy-finance/housing-affordability-by-city-income-rental-costs.html

Groce, N., Challenger, E., Berman-Bieler, R., et al. (2014). Malnutrition and disability: Unexplored opportunities for collaboration. *Paediatrics and International Child Health, 34*(4), 308–314.

References

Halliday, T. (2014). Unemployment and mortality: Evidence from the PSID. *Social Science & Medicine, 113*, 15–22.

Heiman, H. J. (2014). *Why ZIP codes matter: Advancing health equity in all policies.* Downloaded from URL: http://www.rwjf.org/en/culture-of-health/2014/12/why_zip_codes_matter.html

Heiman, H. J., & Artiga, S. (2015). *Beyond health care: The role of social determinants in promoting health and health equity.* Downloaded from URL: http://kff.org/disparities-policy/issue-brief/beyond-health-care-the-role-of-social-determinants-in-promoting-health-and-health-equity/

Hickson, M., Ettinger de Cuba, S., Weiss, I., et al. (n.d.). *Too hungry to learn: Food insecurity and school readiness.* Downloaded from URL: http://www.childrenshealthwatch.org/wp-content/uploads/toohungrytolearn_report.pdf

Hopper, K. (2011). *Disparities in Cardiac Rehab.* Unpublished presentation. Downloaded from URL: http://www.aacvpr.org/Portals/0/events_edu/annualmeeting11/2011%20Online%20Syllabus%20PPT/BO31Hopper.pdf

Hui, J., Gonsahn, M. D., & Nerenz, D. R. (2014). Socioeconomic status and readmissions: Evidence from an urban teaching hospital. *Health Affairs, 33*(5), 778–785.

Kneebone, E., & Garr, E. (2010). *The Suburbanization of Poverty: Trends in Metropolitan America, 2000 to 2008.* Downloaded from URL: https://www.brookings.edu/wp-content/uploads/2016/06/0120_poverty_paper.pdf

Kumanyika, S. K., & Grier, S. (2006). Targeting interventions for ethnic minority and low-income populations. *The Future of Children, 16*(1), 187–207.

Marmot, M. (2015). *The health gap.* Bloomsbury.

Meyers, A., Frank, D. A., Roos, N., et al. (1995). Housing subsidies and pediatric undernutrition. *Archives of Pediatric and Adolescent Medicine, 149*, 1079–1084.

National Center for Health Statistics. (2020). *Health: United States 2019.* National Center for Health Statistics.

Olshansky, S. J., Antonucci, T., Berkman, L., et al. (2012). Differences in life expectancy due to race and educational differences are widening, and many may not catch up. *Health Affairs, 31*(8). Downloaded from URL: https://www.healthaffairs.org/doi/abs/10.1377/hlthaff.2011.0746

Pace, K. (2014). *Get to root causes: Address poor health outcomes through a health equity lens".* Michigan University Extension webpage (Jan. 24). Downloaded from URL: http://msue.anr.msu.edu/news/get_to_root_causes_address_poor_health_outcomes_through_a_health_equity_lens

Pedersen, P. V., Gronbaek, M., & Curtis, T. (2011). Associations between deprived life circumstances, wellbeing and self-rated health in a socially marginalized population. *The European Journal of Public Health, 22*(5), 647–652.

Peek, M. (2014). Poverty's association with poor health outcomes and health disparities. *Health Affairs.* Downloaded from URL: http://healthaffairs.org/blog/2014/10/30/povertys-association-with-poor-health-outcomes-and-health-disparities/

Pereira, M. A., Kartashov, A. I., Ebbeling, C. B., et al. (2005). Fast-food habits, weight gain, and insulin resistance (the CARDIA study): 15-year prospective analysis. *Lancet, 365*, 36–42.

Pereira, G. et al. (2010). *Residential exposure to traffic emissions and adverse pregnancy outcomes.* Downloaded from URL: http://sapiens.revues.org/966?gathStatIcon=true

Peterson, R. D., & Krivo, L. J. (1993). Racial segregation and black urban homicide. *Social Forces, 71*(4), 1001–1026.

Platts-Mills, T. A. E., Vervloet, D., Thomas, W. R., et al. (1997). Indoor allergens and asthma: Report of the third international workshop. *Journal of Allergy and Clinical Immunology, 100*, S1–S24.

Powell, L. M. (2007). Food store availability and neighborhood characteristics in the United States. *Preventive Medicine, 44*, 189–195.

Puterman, E., Weiss, J., Hives, B. A., et al. (2020). Predicting mortality from 57 economic, behavioral, social, and psychological factors. *Proceedings of the National Academy of Sciences, 117*(28), 16273–16282.

Rice, S. (2016). Bill would adjust readmissions for socio-economic factors. *Modern Healthcare.* Downloaded from URL: http://www.modernhealthcare.com/article/20140620/NEWS/306209964

Rissel, C., Curac, N., Greenaway, M., et al. (2012). Physical activity associated with public transport use—A review and modelling of potential benefits. *International Journal of Environmental Research and Public Health, 9*(7), 2454–2478.

Robert Wood Johnson Foundation. (2015). *How do neighborhood conditions shape health?* Robert Wood Johnson Foundation.

Roberts, D. E. (2004). The social and moral cost of mass incarceration in African American communities. *Stanford Law Review, 56*(5), 1271–1305.

Rogers, R. G., Hummer, R. A., & Nam, C. B. (2000). *Living and dying in the USA: Behavioral, health and social differentials of adult mortality.* Academic.

Robert Wood Johnson Foundation. (2012). *Health policy snapshot public health and prevention: How does transportation impact health?* Downloaded from URL: http://www.rwjf.org/content/dam/farm/reports/issue_briefs/2012/rwjf402311

Schroeder, B. (2016). *Health and Food Security.* Downloaded from URL: http://www.resilience.org/stories/2011-02-01/health-and-food-security

Seligman, H. K., Laraia, B. A., & Kushel, M. B. (2010). Food insecurity is associated with chronic disease among low-income NHANES participants. *Journal of Nutrition, 140*(2), 304–310.

Shwarz, D. F. (2016). *What's the connection between residential segregation and health?* Downloaded from URL: http://www.rwjf.org/en/culture-of-health/2016/03/what_s_the_connectio.html

Sloane, D. C., Diamant, A. L., Lewis, L. B., et al. (2003). REACH Coalition of the African American Building a legacy of health project improving the nutritional resource environment for healthy living through community-based participatory research. *Journal of General Internal Medicine, 18*, 568–575.

Strully, K. W. (2009). Job loss and health in the U.S. labor market. *Demography, 46*(2), 221–246.

Syed, S. T., Gerber, B. S., & Sharp, L. K. (2013). Traveling towards disease: Transportation barriers to health care access. *Journal of Community Health, 38*(5), 976–993.

Thomas, R. K. (2009). *Orange mound community assessment.* Health and Performances Resources.

Truven Health Analytics. (2014). *Truven Health Analytics study finds as many as 12 percent of excess hospital readmissions are attributable to race, employment, education.* Downloaded from URL: https://truvenhealth.com/news-and-events/press-releases/detail/prid/9/as-many-as-12-percent-of-excess-hospital-readmissions-are-attributable-to-race-employment

University of Pennsylvania. (2020). *The increasing mortality gap by education.* Downloaded from URL: https://budgetmodel.wharton.upenn.edu/issues/2020/7/6/mortality-gap-by-education#:~:text=Summary%3A%20Over%20the%20last%20two,18%20percent%20lower%20mortality%20rate

Voss, M., Nylen, L., Floderus, B., et al. (2004). Unemployment and early cause-specific mortality: A study based on the Swedish twin registry. *American Journal of Public Health, 94*(12), 2155–2161.

Williams, D. R., & Collins, C. (2001). Racial residential segregation: A fundamental cause of racial disparities in health. *Public Health Reports, 116*, 404–416.

Ziersch, A. M., Baum, F. E., MacDougall, C., et al. (2005). Neighborhood life and social capital: The implications for health. *Social Science & Medicine, 60*(1), 71–86.

Additional Resources

American SPCC. (2018). *Adverse childhood experiences (ACES) are a significant risk factor for substance use disorders and can impact prevention efforts.* Downloaded from URL: https://americanspcc.org/adverse-childhood-experiences-aces-are-a-significant-risk-factor-for-substance-use-disorders-and-can-impact-prevention-efforts/

Centers for Medicare and Medicaid Services. (2020). *Hospital Readmissions Reduction Program (HRRP).* Downloaded from URL: https://www.cms.gov/Medicare/Medicare-Fee-for-Service-Payment/AcuteInpatientPPS/Readmissions-Reduction-Program

Clarke, P., Morenoff, J., Debbink, M., et al. (2013) Cumulative exposure to neighborhood context: Consequences for health transitions over the adult life course. *Research on Aging.* Published on-line January 2, 2013.

Corporation for Supportive Housing. (2014). *Housing is the Best Medicine: Supportive Housing and the Social Determinants of Health.* Downloaded from URL: http://www.csh.org/wp-content/uploads/2014/07/SocialDeterminantsofHealth_2014.pdf

National Association of Community Health Centers. PRAPARE application for assessing the social determinants of health at https://www.nachc.org/research-and-data/prapare/.

Robert Wood Johnson Foundation (2015). Making the case for linking community development and health. : Robert Wood Johnson Foundation.

Taylor, L. (2018). Housing and health: An overview of the literature. *Health Affairs Health Policy Brief.* Downloaded from URL: https://www.healthaffairs.org/do/10.1377/hpb20180313.396577/full/

U.S. Department of Agriculture. (2020). *Food access research Atlas* at https://www.ers.usda.gov/data-products/food-access-research-atlas/

Chapter 7
Paying the Piper: Health Disparities

The developments that have been discussed in previous chapters have had a wide range of consequences for American society and for various subgroups within it. Perhaps the most significant consequence has been the emergence, persistence and even augmentation of dramatic health disparities among various segments of the population. Changing patterns of morbidity have clearly had the effect of putting members of certain subgroups at a health disadvantage. This chapter describes the nature of health disparities, who is affected by them, and why the existence of disparities calls for a population health approach.

In this chapter the reader will:

- Be exposed to the definition and characteristics of health disparities
- Learn about the factors that have contributed to the emergence of health disparities
- Examine the variety of ways in which health disparities manifest themselves
- Gain knowledge of the populations that are most affected by health disparities
- Receive information on the health conditions most associated with health disparities
- Be exposed to the impact of health disparities on the lives of those affected

© The Author(s), under exclusive license to Springer Nature Switzerland AG 2021
R. K. Thomas, *Population Health and the Future of Healthcare*,
https://doi.org/10.1007/978-3-030-83887-4_7

Introduction

Previous chapters have chronicled the trends related to population change and the developments within healthcare that have dramatically impacted the nation's health. These trends have contributed to a situation in which social factors have become the primary determinants of health status. As social factors have supplanted biological and genetic determinants of health and illness, the patterns of morbidity for the US population have been significantly affected. These "modern" causes of health problems have not only shifted the nature of the health conditions faced by the population but have contributed to the emergence of distinctive patterns of morbidity. While biologically generated illnesses were no respecter of age, sex, race or any other demographic attribute, "diseases of civilization" are relatively selective in their choice of "victim." Thus, contemporary patterns of morbidity are associated with variations in the demographic attributes of various subpopulations.

Health disparities are, according to the National Institutes of Health, differences in the incidence, prevalence, mortality and burden of disease and other adverse conditions that exist among specific populations in the US (National Institutes of Health, 2011). Differences become "disparities" when they reflect disadvantages inherent in the status of affected parties and/or are the consequences of an inequitable and/or discriminatory system.

Disparities in health status are certainly nothing new for our population, and as long as statistics have been generated variations in mortality rates and life expectancy have been observed. Throughout our history the poor, members of minority groups, immigrants, and other marginal populations in US society have experienced higher death rates and shorter life expectancy.

Despite these historical differences in mortality rates, members of disadvantaged groups suffered from essentially the same conditions and causes of death as those in more advantaged groups. Biologically generated illnesses were not discriminatory, and everyone in society was at essentially the same risk of infection from communicable diseases—particularly those taking epidemic form. As the standard of living improved and public health measures were implemented, Americans enjoyed better health overall.

While there was general overall improvement in the health status of the US population during the twentieth century, not all subpopulations benefited equally from these positive developments. Emerging patterns of disease distribution created an unprecedented situation with regard to epidemiological differences between subgroups in society. As acute conditions gave way to chronic conditions, clear-cut patterns of morbidity distribution began to emerge. Unlike communicable diseases the ascendant chronic conditions were selective in their victims, with some populations and/or geographic areas affected more than others. While the mortality gap became less of an issue, the morbidity gap grew at a dramatic rate. These new patterns of disease distribution were not related to differential exposure to biological pathogens but were a function of the social conditions that selectively affected various population groups.

The Stratification of Health Conditions

The emergence, persistence and even augmentation of dramatic disparities in the health status of various segments of the US population has become a growing concern for health professionals. The changes observed in morbidity patterns during the last half of the twentieth century included the redistribution of disease within the population along demographic lines. Clear patterns of distribution emerged that involved the concentration of various health problems among certain demographic subgroups.

The selectivity exhibited by diseases of civilization resulted in patterns of disease distribution along racial and ethnic dimensions, income and educational lines, and even in terms of sociocultural factors such as marital status, occupation and religion. As a result, a distinctive disease configuration could be identified for most demographic subgroups. The morbidity profile for low-income African Americans, for example, came to look a lot different from that of affluent white Americans, the health conditions of poor, white rural residents came to look a lot different from those of upwardly mobile urban residents, and the health status of second- and third-generation immigrants came to look a lot different from that of newly arrived immigrants.

At the same time, the US population has experienced the stratification of health conditions along demographic dimensions. While most chronic conditions in contemporary societies are widespread throughout the population, they are likely to be concentrated more among certain groups than others, creating a unique disease-specific pattern. While diabetes, for example, affects all demographic groups to a certain extent, some groups exhibit higher rates of prevalence and mortality than others. Similarly, heart disease as the leading cause of death is widespread throughout the population but has a greater impact on certain subpopulations.

The patterns of morbidity distribution that have emerged are of such a significance that they are not just viewed as "differences" but as "disparities". The latter more negative term reflects the fact that members of some groups are increasingly affected by the emerging diseases. The social determinants of health have a disproportionate impact on certain subpopulations—the poor, minorities, immigrants, the poorly educated and other "vulnerable" populations.

This development has contributed to the bifurcation of the population in terms of health status, into a portion of the population that, while not totally free of chronic conditions, maintains relatively high health status and another portion of the population that faces an inordinate share of chronic problems and adverse health conditions. The sections that follow describe the causes and the nature of health disparities, identify the groups that are most affected, and discuss the role of health disparities in the emergence of the population health approach.

While these patterns of disease distribution by themselves are not inherently discriminatory, the fact that certain disadvantaged groups are characterized by higher rates for most contemporary conditions than other groups is noteworthy. The factor driving the discussion in this chapter is the fact that, as these differences have become disparities, they take on certain connotations that are transferred to the populations that are adversely affected. Because of persistent health disparities, it is not unreasonable to now *expect* certain subgroups to suffer from differential morbidity and mortality rates. Once these disparities are established, they tend to be self-perpetuating and passed from generation to generation.

Health Metrics Associated with Disparities

The existence of health disparities within the US population was identified by epidemiologist based on observed differences in health status for different populations as measured by a variety of metrics. If a subpopulation was identified as characterized by an unusually poor score on a measure of health status, this could be written off as an aberration or attributed to some unusual attribute of that population. However, when poor scores are recorded for a number of different metrics, it could be argued that poor health status is an inherent trait of that population. When that population is considered to be disadvantaged, that difference then becomes a disparity. The following factors are considered metrics that could be used to establish differences with provide the basis for a determination of disparity.

To the extent that self-reported health status reflects underlying morbidity within the population, there are clear disparities that exist between various groups on this measure. This discrepancy exists along a number of dimensions (Centers for Disease Control and Prevention, 2000). The racial and ethnic disparity is substantial, with African Americans reporting much less favorable health status than whites. African Americans are nearly twice as likely as whites to report only poor or fair health status; American Indians are more than twice likely. (Differences in self-assessed health status should be interpreted with caution, it should be recalled, since there are indications that members of different racial groups may use different criteria for assessing their own health status [Brandon & Proctor, 2010]). Disparities in perceived health status are also noteworthy with regard to income and education, with the poorest and least educated subgroups exhibiting the lowest health status.

When the reported number of unhealthy days is considered, significant disparities are found. American Indians report the most unhealthy days followed by Hispanics and African Americans (Centers for Disease Control and Prevention, 2000). Lower income residents report more average unhealthy days, with the reported number for the poorest twice that for the most affluent. Residents of states with larger inequalities in reported number of healthy days also report fewer healthy days on average. The least educated also exhibit disparities for this measure, reporting many more unhealthy days on the average than the college educated. The unemployed report twice the number of unhealthy days as the employed, and those without health insurance exhibit a slightly higher level of unhealthy days than those with insurance.

With regard to poor mental health days, American Indians reported the highest level, followed by African Americans and, at a distance, Hispanics. Those in the lowest income category reported twice the number of poor mental health days as the affluent, while the least educated reported one and one-half times the number days as the best educated. The unemployed had a high average of poor mental health days, twice that of the employed. People without health coverage were considerably more likely to suffer poor mental health days a month than people with health coverage (Centers for Disease Control and Prevention, 2000).

Although the importance of mortality as a measure of health status has less relevance today, it is still commonly used as an indicator of health status. When it comes to examining disparities it does have some usefulness. At one time in the recent past, every racial and ethnic minority reported higher death rates than whites. We find now that for all-cause mortality only African Americans report a higher mortality rate than whites. The African-American mortality rate (particularly for males) has remained consistently higher than the white rate even though the spread is less today than in the past. When mortality rates are examined for specific causes, we find that African Americans record higher mortality rates for virtually every cause of death.

When it comes to infant mortality—which some consider to be a better measure of health status than overall mortality—African Americans stand out for their high rates. In 2011, the highest infant mortality rate was recorded for African Americans, followed by American Indians and Hispanics (Matthews & MacDorman, 2013). Similarly, when it comes to maternal mortality, much of the maternal mortality (and particularly the recent uptick) can be attributed primarily to the black population.

When aggregate measures of chronic conditions are considered significant disparities are found based on race. Numerous studies have found that African Americans and Hispanics, and people in lower socioeconomic groups are much more likely to suffer from these diseases and have worse outcomes (Crook & Peters, 2008). While a significant proportion of the total population is characterized by chronic disease, the disparities are more obvious when the presence of multiple chronic conditions is noted. African Americans and American Indians are more likely to report multiple chronic conditions than other racial and ethnic groups (Ward et al., 2014).

Differences in disease-specific morbidity exist between various racial and ethnic groups, with the epidemiology of cancer reflecting this phenomenon. Different groups suffer from different types of cancer. Colon/rectal cancer, breast cancer, and bladder cancer, for example, affect certain groups disproportionately. On the other hand, lung, prostate, stomach, and esophageal cancer are more prevalent among other groups (National Center for Health Statistics, 2012). Some conditions (e.g., HIV/AIDS and sexually transmitted infections) may be more common among certain groups by a factor of ten or more (Mead et al., 2008). Respiratory diseases unequally affect the socioeconomically disadvantaged and some ethnic minorities.

Obesity might be considered a "sentinel" condition due to its implications for other health problems. While the entire US population exhibits increasing levels of obesity, the impact is greater for some groups than for others (National Center for Health Statistics, 2016). Among adults (20+ years) the obesity rate for African

Americans is 50% higher than for whites and the rate for Hispanics is one-third higher. The rate of obesity for the lowest income group is considerably higher than that for the highest income group. Obesity rates for children follow a similar pattern, with the rates for 2–5-year-old African Americans twice that for whites while the rate for Hispanics is three times higher. For children 6–12 years the rate for African Americans is 65% higher and for Hispanics nearly twice as high. For children 12–19 years, the rates of obesity for both African Americans and Hispanics is 25% higher than for whites. Rates based on income for children follow the same patterns observed for adults: obesity increases with poverty despite the age of the child.

When reproductive health issues (other than infant mortality) are considered, it is found that certain racial and ethnic groups exhibit disparities in various measures. When low birth weight is considered, all monitored racial and ethnic groups exhibit higher rates than whites (Child Health USA, 2013). The highest rates for low birth-weight babies are found for African Americans, followed at a distance by American Indians, Hispanics and Asian Americans. Similarly, when rates for premature births are examined, a similar pattern is found.

When the prevalence of disabilities is examined, there are disparities along a number of dimensions regardless of what measure is used (Centers for Disease Control and Prevention, 2000). In terms of racial and ethnic disparities, American Indians reported the most disability, followed by African Americans and Hispanics. Those in the lowest income category report a disability level three times that of the most affluent, while the least educated exhibit three times the disability as the most educated. The unemployed report disability levels 3 to 4 times those for the employed, and disability rates for those without health insurance are 50% higher than those who are insured.

The contribution of lifestyles to health disparities cannot be overstated, with tobacco use in particular associated with differentials in morbidity and mortality (Centers for Disease Control and Prevention, 2006). Despite overall declines in cigarette smoking, disparities in smoking rates persist among certain racial/ethnic minority groups, particularly among American Indians/Alaska Natives. Smoking rates decline significantly with increasing income and educational attainment, leaving the poorest and least educated to carry the burden of lifestyle-related morbidity. Smokers are nearly twice as likely as non-smokers to suffer from activity limitations, report poor mental health days, and report nearly one and a half times the number of unhealthy days overall. Heavy drinkers are slightly more likely to suffer limited activity than light drinkers or teetotalers and report poor mental health days at a rate one-third higher. While lack of exercise is less of a predictor of morbidity than smoking and drinking, it is found that smokers, heavy drinkers and those who do not get exercise have more unhealthy days, poor mental health days, and more limited activity days.

The Causes of Health Disparities

The reasons for the existence of disparities in their various forms within the US population are numerous and complex. The very diversity of the population almost guarantees that different subgroups will exhibit different characteristics. Differences in lifestyles further result in differential exposure to health risks. The lifestyles associated with different groups contribute to the process whereby differences become disparities. Health disparities are also affected by economic status, lack of healthcare access, health literacy, cultural beliefs, social and family situations, governmental policies and inordinate risk exposure for vulnerable populations.

The influence of social factors can be clearly observed, and there are some factors that especially stand out for their contribution to health disparities. Galea and colleagues recently estimated that of the 2.5 million deaths in the United States, more than 145,000 were attributable to low education in 2010 (Krueger et al., 2015), 176,000 to racial segregation (Pardo & Prakash, 2011), 162,000 to weak social support, 133,000 to individual-level poverty, and 119,000 to income inequality (Galea et al., 2011).

Without completely reiterating the various social determinants of health described in the previous chapter, the Kaiser framework is generally followed below in outlining the contributors to observed disparities. Poverty, with both direct and indirect implications for health status, has been associated with every measure of health status and, in fact, overrides the impact of other important determinants such as race and ethnicity. The link between poverty and mortality has been previously noted, with infant mortality and maternal mortality essentially monopolized by the poor.

Poverty and Health Disparities

Poverty does not arise *sui generis*, of course, but is the end-result of a combination of contributing factors. The level of poverty characterizing the US population cannot easily be attributed to a few specific factors. It reflects the long-term impact of individual and institutional racism. The immediate cause may be a lack of job skills (or even work ethic) or the unavailability of accessible and suitable jobs. However, the roots of poverty can be traced back generations to a time when certain groups were denied access to the educational opportunities requisite for job acquisition.

The ultimate factor in the existence of poverty is more deeply rooted and reflects the discriminatory aspects imbedded in each US institution. As well described by Wilkerson in *Caste* (2020), at the end of the day, race (or "caste" from her perspective) trumps other attributes, thereby assuring disparities in all societal realms.

Poverty rates reflect a lack of education and job skills as well as the dearth of available jobs—all, of course, contributors to health disparities in their own right. As noted earlier, poverty triggers more immediate contributors to ill-health—from poor diets to inadequate housing to simply an unsafe, unhealthy daily existence. These factors contribute to the establishment of a negative feedback loop. For example, poverty results in poor nutrition and exposure to harmful aspects of the environment. These exposures lead to poor health status on the part of the affected groups. Poor health status in turn limits one's ability to attend school or keep a job. These factors then reinforce the conditions of poverty which then lead to poor health and so forth.

Poverty, of course, is not limited to any one group but is more concentrated in some rather than others. Thus, African Americans, Hispanics and some other ethnic groups tend to exhibit an inordinate level of poverty (and, hence, health disparities). Yet, recent research has uncovered disparities affecting even some segments of presumably "advantaged" populations. A review of mortality data over the past 20 years has found increasing mortality and declining life expectancy among some segments of the non-Hispanic white population (Olshansky et al., 2012). Those affected by this phenomenon are primarily poorly educated, low-income whites, thereby supporting the notion that poverty trumps most other attributes.

One of the implications of a poverty-level existence that contributes to disparities is its impact on one's personal priorities. Poverty-level populations seldom have the luxury of placing a high priority on their health, and, when questioned concerning their priorities, their health is likely to be far down the list. There are too many other pressing needs to be addressed. Members of such groups are often quoted as saying: "I can't afford to be sick." All other factors aside, the low priority placed on health by members of disadvantaged populations virtually assures poor health status.

The inevitability of disparities reflects the fact that poor health is accepted as the normal state of affairs for poverty-level populations. There appears to be a "subculture of ill-health" that emerges in certain communities that reinforces the normalcy of ill-health and has the effect of perpetuating disparities. Once established these subcultures appear to persist decade after decade and generation after generation regardless of who moves in or out of the community. Even if other factors contribute to the onset of illness, the subculture of ill-health serves to perpetuate health problems and "institutionalize" ill-health as a normal state. Box 7.1 describes the subculture of ill-health and its implications for health status.

Environmental Conditions and Health Disparities

The nature of the physical and social environments is a major consideration when examining health disparities. Disadvantaged populations are more likely to reside in areas characterized by polluted air, soil and water. Proximity to toxic waste

> **Box 7.1: The Subculture of Ill-Health**
> It has been observed that communities that exhibit poor health status often tend to perpetually maintain this status over a long period of time. There appears to be a "subculture of ill-health" that emerges in certain communities

(continued)

Box 7.1 (continued)

that reinforces the normalcy of ill-health and has the effect of perpetuating disparities. The inevitability of disparities reflects the fact that poor health is accepted as the normal state of affairs for poverty-level populations and poor health status becomes a self-fulling prophecy. Once established these subcultures appear to persist decade after decade and generation after generation regardless of who moves in or out of the community. The subculture of ill-health serves to perpetuate health problems and "institutionalize" ill-health as a normal state. This involves the development of values and norms that allow the population to accommodate perpetual ill-health. Not only do these conditions appear impervious to change, but now appear to have expanded their impact to increasingly younger cohorts within the African-American population over time. There is no illusion that one can have good health, and ill-health is accepted as inevitable. Rather than seeking ways to be healthier—a pipe dream—actions focus on making the best of an inevitably bad system. Ill-health is normalized as a survival mechanism.

This subculture of ill-health involves a cultural framework that emphasizes adapting to illness and disability, utilizing the healthcare system to support this adaptive mechanism, and developing a value system, supported by normative behaviors, that emphasizes accommodation, adaptation, and compensation. This system is abetted by social support systems that do not encourage health improvement much less cure or rehabilitation.

The table below compares the attributes of a subculture of ill-health to the manner in which mainstream America responds to the onset of health problems.

Culture of Ill-Health	Mainstream Society
Survival	Maintenance/enhancement
Accommodation/adaptation	Management
Passivity	Activism
Nurturance	Instrumentalism
Maintenance/deterioration reduction	Restoration
Pessimism	Optimism
Hopelessness	Hopefulness
Uselessness	Sense of purpose
Self-demeanment	Self-actualization
Denial/avoidance	Prevention
Present orientation	Future orientation

Once a subculture of ill-health has become established, it becomes self-perpetuating. Values and norms evolve to support it, and peer pressure materializes to encourage adherence to the cultural artifices that shore up the subculture.

concentrations and other sources of pollutants is a common condition of life for poverty populations, and they have the cancer rates to prove it (Kay & Katz, 2012). Disadvantaged populations are likely to live in areas of crumbling infrastructure and deteriorating housing. Vacant lots with their concomitant negative aspects contribute to an unhealthy environment. A lack of green space and the presence of unsafe streets prevent physical activity, carry the threat of danger, and contribute to higher levels of stress. Substandard housing constitutes a health risk in its own right, with dilapidated structures contributing to an unhealthy environment. Health disparities found to be associated with environmental stress include childhood asthma, hypertension, substance abuse, diabetes, obesity and depressive symptoms (Quinn et al., 2010; Lee et al., 2009; Braveman, 2009).

Housing conditions represent a major factor with regard to the environment, and housing insecurity has been identified as a major social determinant of health. Lack of access to permanent affordable housing is a major concern for millions of Americans and contributes to poor health in a number of ways. Members of disadvantaged populations live under the constant threat of loss of housing and must devote an inordinate amount of their income to housing expenses, thereby limiting their ability to pay for necessities (e.g., food, healthcare). Housing insecurity often means frequent moves with accompanying health implications. Homelessness contributes to poor health with chronic disease and mental disorders a common feature of the homeless. Children are particularly susceptible to the impact of homelessness.

High levels of housing deterioration and abandonment create a negative environment, while the constant turnover characterizing many such neighborhoods is not conducive to social cohesion. Excessive residential turnover can diminish neighborhood social ties and weaken neighborhood institutions by disrupting neighbors' participation in social life. High residential instability, combined with concentrated disadvantage, limits the ability of residents to prevent threats to their health and safety.

Education and Health Disparities

As noted previously, a lack of education is a major contributor to poverty and, hence, to poor health. There are also some direct implications for health from a lack of education. For one thing, members of affected populations are thought to be characterized by low "health literacy". They often lack a basic understanding of health risks, appropriate health practices, and/or available health resources. Members of certain racial and ethnic minorities and the poor often lack an awareness of common chronic diseases and their risk factors. This often results in a delay in diagnosis and, hence, more advanced disease states to contend with (Crook & Peters, 2008). It is not only a lack of formal education that fosters low health literacy, but the isolation and lack of interface with the larger society characteristic of disadvantaged populations. It is not surprising that there is limited knowledge of such topics since there is no obvious source from which this information can be obtained for these populations. It is not likely that members of disadvantaged groups will make "good choices" if they do not know that choices exist.

Food Insecurity and Health Disparities

Food insecurity was noted as a common condition for certain subsets of the population, and on a day-to-day basis this is perhaps one of the most direct contributors to poor health. Poverty-level populations often do not have access to healthy food even if they can afford it. Living in a food desert means that access is limited to cheap, unhealthy food and fast-food restaurants. Lack of adequate nutrition has a multiplier effect, limiting the ability of affected populations to attend school or work or to perform adequately when they do attend.

Residential Segregation and Health Disparities

The persistent residential segregation noted in previous chapters is also a factor in the introduction of disparities. Segregation invariably involves low health literacy and limited exposure to the information and resources required to maintain good health. High levels of morbidity and disability within most segregated communities establish the foundation for a culture of ill-health that emphasizes accommodation of an irresolvable situation rather than a proactive search for health. Segregation, thus, not only provides a fertile ground for the emergence of health disparities but serves to exacerbate the conditions that do emerge. And, as noted by Galea et al. above, an estimated 176,000 deaths can be attributed to segregation (and that was over 15 years ago).

Community and Social Context and Health Disparities

While the neighborhood environment was noted above there is another aspect of "community" that needs to be considered. Beyond the physical and social environments there is the issue of the social "atmosphere" of the community. This includes the "sense of community" that exists, the presence of social networks, and the level of social cohesion. While many disadvantaged neighborhoods are noteworthy for their level of social integration and sources of social support, these are more the exception than the rule. Disadvantaged neighborhoods are more often than not characterized by a high level of social disorganization—often driven by housing insecurity. Increasingly, members of such communities do not know their neighbors, do not or cannot participate in community organizations, and are reluctant to move about in their own neighborhoods.

Lifestyles, although not specifically called out in the Kaiser framework, also contribute to disparities in morbidity, with subgroups within society pursuing varying lifestyles that have consequences for their health status—either positive or negative. Noteworthy are those subgroups whose members are involved in unhealthy, risky, or otherwise health-negative behaviors. As previously noted, unhealthy lifestyles may not be a matter of choice; they may simply reflect the life circumstances in which members of certain populations find themselves. To the extent that unhealthy or risky behavior is a matter of choice, these actions may take the form of coping behavior in the face of overwhelming stress. In other cases, lifestyles may reflect cultural preferences that, in contemporary society, become health liabilities.

Many neighborhoods suffering from a lack of social integration may be peopled by recent immigrants. Acculturative stress involves feelings of tension and anxiety arising from efforts to adapt to the orientation and values of the dominant culture (American Psychological Association, 2017). It can have an influence on physical and mental health disparities such as hypertension and depression. Acculturation stress has been found to be significantly associated with substance dependence and anxiety disorders. Empirical studies on immigrant adolescents and the children of immigrants have found that acculturative stress increased depressive symptoms. Regardless of age at immigration, foreign-born women experience more depressive symptoms than native-born women during early adulthood (Potochnick & Perreiara, 2011).

Crime and Criminal Justice and Health Disparities

US incarceration policies and programs have a disproportionate impact on urban communities, especially black and Latino ones. Health conditions that are overrepresented within incarcerated populations include substance abuse, human immunodeficiency virus (HIV) and other infectious diseases, mental illness, chronic disease, and reproductive health problems upon release (Freudenberg, 2001). Nascent patterns of morbidity are solidified as members of already disadvantaged groups are exposed to the illness-promoting effects of incarceration. These individuals typically return to communities that are not only characterized by ill-health but lack the resources to address the former prisoners often advanced disease states.

Ultimately, the role of discrimination in health disparities cannot be overlooked. Although scholars have been slow to link discrimination to poor health status there is a growing body of information to document this relationship. A review of research by Williams and Mohammed (2009) revealed a relationship between a lifetime of discrimination and poorer health status. While much of the black/white disparity is attributed to socioeconomic status differences, Sims et al. (2012) found that, after adjustment for age, gender, and socioeconomic status, a lifetime of stress and the burden of discrimination were associated with greater hypertension prevalence. Research has also found that discrimination can have an impact on pregnancy outcomes for minority women (Canady et al., 2010).

Groups that Exhibit Disparities

When the various racial and ethnic groups in the United States are examined in terms of health status, significant differences are found. The major distinction is between whites and blacks, with Hispanics, Asian-Americans and American Indians manifesting less distinct health status characteristics (National Center for Health Statistics, 2016). Other groups that suffer from significant disparities are described along with certain population segments defined in terms of demographics such as the impoverished and poorly educated. Box 7.2 describes some vulnerable populations that are particularly prone to health disparities.

Box 7.2: Vulnerable Populations

Vulnerable populations (from a healthcare perspective) are those segments of the population that are at inordinate health risk due to their particular attributes. They are relatively more susceptible to various health conditions than the less vulnerable. Vulnerable populations include the economically disadvantaged, racial and ethnic minorities, the uninsured, low-income children, the elderly, the homeless, and those with other chronic health conditions. The vulnerable may also include rural residents, who often encounter barriers to accessing healthcare services. The vulnerability of people in these categories may be exacerbated by race, ethnicity, age, sex, and factors such as income, insurance coverage (or lack thereof), and absence of a usual source of care. Their health and healthcare problems intersect with social factors, including housing quality, poverty, and educational attainment.

Although each vulnerable sub-population can be small in size, as a group these subpopulations represent a substantial number of persons at inordinate risk. Certain settings have high concentrations of at-risk populations, including nursing homes, correctional facilities, and homeless shelters. Infectious diseases that emerge from such settings or within these populations can eventually spread to the general population.

The health domains of vulnerable populations can be divided into three categories: physical, psychological, and social. Those with physical needs include high-risk mothers and infants, the chronically ill and disabled, and persons living with HIV/AIDS. In the psychological domain, vulnerable populations include those with chronic mental conditions, such as schizophrenia, bipolar disorder, major depression, and attention-deficit/hyperactivity disorder, as well as those with a history of alcohol and/or substance abuse. In the social realm, vulnerable populations include those living in abusive families, the homeless, immigrants, and refugees. The most vulnerable may be affected by more than one domain and have multiple problems, facing more significant comorbidities and cumulative risks.

(continued)

> **Box 7.2** (continued)
>
> The numbers of these vulnerable populations are increasing, not only as the ranks of the uninsured have grown, but as the population ages. For instance, the number of individuals with chronic medical conditions has risen from 125 million in 2000 to 141 million in 2012, with an overall increase to 171 million people expected by 2030.
>
> Shi and Stevens (2010) evaluated data on 32,374 adults from the 2000 National Health Interview Survey and identified three risk factors for poor access to healthcare: low income, lack of health insurance, and lack of regular care. They found that those without insurance were seven times less likely to get the healthcare they need and 4.5 times more likely to not fill a prescription. Meanwhile, adults with low incomes were more likely to delay or not receive necessary medical, dental, and mental healthcare and to not fill prescriptions. Overall, researchers found that about 1 of 5 US adults has multiple risk factors for unmet health needs, creating up to a fivefold difference in the rates of these unmet needs, such as delayed medical care between those with the greatest number of risk factors and those with the least.
>
> Sources: American Journal of Managed Care (2006), Shi and Stevens (2010)

On virtually every indicator African Americans exhibit poorer health status than whites. While less than 9% of whites assessed their health as fair or poor in 2014, the figure for blacks was nearly 14%. Compared to whites African Americans have higher rates of many types of acute and chronic conditions, with the differences more profound for chronic problems. The number of symptoms, the number of illness episodes, and the severity of the conditions all place African Americans at a health status disadvantage. Although relatively more prone to acute health conditions, African Americans actually suffer higher rates of both acute and conditions than whites. African Americans represent 12% of the population, for example, but account for 28% of the diagnosed hypertension (Lloyd-Jones et al., 2010).

Overall, African Americans exhibit higher incidence and prevalence rates for a wide variety of health conditions (Thomas, 2015). They have a 70% higher rate for skin conditions, 44% higher for acute urinary conditions, 36% higher for digestive tract conditions, 53% higher for diabetes, and 20% higher for hypertension. African Americans represent 12% of the population but account for 28% of the diagnosed hypertension (Lloyd-Jones et al., 2010). The morbidity disadvantage for African Americans is reflected in the proportion overweight or obese, with a rate of 69% recorded for this group compared to 54% for whites (Mead et al., 2008). Even at higher income levels, African Americans still report higher levels of chronic disease than comparable whites. African-American children have 81% more childhood diseases than white children, and black children are more likely to be hospitalized and die from asthma.

In terms of all-cause mortality, only African Americans stand out. The age-adjusted mortality rate for the white population was 7.3 deaths per 1000 population in 2014, compared to a rate of 8.6 for blacks (National Center for Health Statistics, 2016). Age-adjusted mortality rates for other groups in 2014 were 5.2 for Hispanics, 5.9 for American Indians and 4.1 for Asian-Americans. African Americans are characterized by higher mortality risks at nearly all ages and for nearly all causes (Rogers et al., 2000).

All things being equal, African Americans who contracted life-threatening diseases are more at risk of death than are whites with the same conditions. (See, for example, American Lung Association, 2011). Black men and women are much more likely to die of heart disease and stroke than their white counterparts. Coronary heart disease and stroke are not only leading causes of death in the United States, but also account for the largest proportion of inequality in life expectancy between whites and blacks, despite the existence of low-cost, highly effective preventive treatment. There are also large racial/ethnic disparities in preventable hospitalizations, with blacks experiencing a rate more than double that of whites.

What is of more significance, however, are persistent disparities in infant mortality and, now, in maternal mortality. While the infant mortality rate is unacceptably high for the entire population (relative to other similar countries), infant mortality is concentrated within the African-American population. Maternal mortality—a cause of death long thought essentially banished from modern societies—has experienced an uptick in the United States. Again, this phenomenon is not randomly distributed but is exhibited by the African-American population at a rate three times the average. Infants born to black women are 1.5 to 3 times more likely to die than infants born to women of other races/ethnicities.

Common conditions that may be easily resolved for whites and/or the more affluent, for example, often result in complications for African Americans. In the case of endometrial cancer, for example, blacks are at greater risk of mortality than women in any other racial or ethnic group, regardless of the stage of the cancer (Cote et al., 2015). Hypertension is by far most prevalent among blacks (42% vs 29% among whites), while Mexican-Americans are least likely to have their hypertension under control. Mortality disparities for some health conditions actually exceed the morbidity disparity. For example, African-American men report a 50% higher prevalence rate for prostate cancer but a 100% higher mortality rate from this condition than do white males (Harvard Health Publications, 2016).

The distribution of mental illness with regard to race and ethnicity has been of great interest to researchers and health professionals. Historically, it was believed that blacks and certain other racial and ethnic groups in US society were characterized by worse mental health status than whites. Even after the scientific study of mental illness became established, evidence was developed that suggested higher rates of mental disorder among these non-white groups. African Americans were most often singled out and depicted as a group as being disproportionately characterized by psychotic disorders.

Although historically African Americans have been thought to suffer from an inordinate amount of mental illness, researchers now believe that the impression of higher rates of mental disorder among blacks and certain other racial and ethnic groups is a function of at least three factors: (a) collection of data historically from public mental institutions; (b) a middle-class bias in the diagnosis of mental disorders; and (c) a failure to consider important intervening variables such as social class (Murali & Oyebode, 2004). Another study argues that differences in types of mental pathology make comparisons based on race problematic (Riolo et al., 2005).

The major national study on psychiatric morbidity (Kessler et al., 2003) found that African Americans were 30% *less* likely to experience *any* mental disorder over their lifetimes compared to whites. To the extent that differences do exist, the disparity appears to be not in prevalence but in types of disorders. Blacks seem to be characterized by more severe forms of disorders (e.g., psychoses), and whites by milder forms (e.g., neuroses), although this same study indicated that blacks were 40% less likely to experience a major depression disorder over their lifetimes.

Indicators of disability also are found to be higher among African Americans. Data from the 2010 National Health Interview Survey indicated that 12.2% of the white population had some limitation due to disability, compared to 16.5% of the African-American population (National Center for Health Statistics, 2011). African Americans are characterized by higher levels of disability than whites, whether measured by the actual presence of handicaps or by such proxy measures as work-loss days and bed-restricted days.

Of the major racial and ethnic groups, Hispanics exhibit the greatest disparities after African Americans (Centers for Disease Control and Prevention, 2004). Hispanics bear a disproportionate burden of disease, injury, death, and disability when compared with non-Hispanic whites. When affected by disease, Hispanics are more likely to get sicker, have serious complications and even die from them (Families USA, 2014). Hispanics are 50% more likely than whites to assess their health status as poor or fair.

In 2012, Hispanic adults in the United States were twice as likely as non-Hispanic whites to be obese, leading to a 65% higher rate of diabetes. They were also twice as likely to have asthma, six times as likely to have tuberculosis, 15% more likely to have liver disease, and 55% more likely to suffer from end-stage renal disease. Hispanics (mostly males) exhibited an HIV infection rate two-and-a-half times that of non-Hispanic whites, while Hispanic females reported a 45% higher rate for cervical cancer. When Hispanics contracted certain conditions they are more likely to die from them than their non-Hispanic white counterparts (Families USA, 2014). For HIV the death rate is 250% higher, for diabetes 45% higher and for cervical cancer 40% higher.

Hispanic children in 2012 also recorded a high level of disparities, including a 30% higher infant mortality rate, 35% more obesity, and 60% more depression. During 1999–2000, Mexican Americans aged 20–74 years reported higher rates of overweight and obesity (7% higher for males and 32% higher for females) than non-Hispanic whites; Mexican-American youths aged 12–19 years also reported higher rates of overweight (112% higher for males and 59% higher for females). These disparities are exacerbated by the fact that twice the proportion of Hispanics lack health insurance compared to non-Hispanic whites.

In 2001, Hispanics experienced more age-adjusted years of potential life lost before age 75 years per 100,000 population than non-Hispanic whites for stroke (18% more), chronic liver disease and cirrhosis (62% more), diabetes (41% more), human immunodeficiency virus (HIV) disease (168% more), and homicide (128% more); in 2000, Hispanics had higher age-adjusted incidence for cancers of the cervix (152% higher) and stomach (63% higher for males and 150% higher for females). These figures reflect the fact that the leading causes of death among Hispanics vary from those for non-Hispanic whites, with Hispanics more likely to die from lifestyle-related conditions (e.g., diabetes, HIV).

Overall, the health status of Hispanics appears to be improving relative to non-Hispanic whites while increasing the gap between African Americans and Hispanics. Hispanics already exhibit a low mortality rate (and greater life expectancy) than native-born whites despite poor health status on some indicators.

In many ways, American Indians/Alaskan Natives exhibit worse health status than other racial and ethnic groups. They are given less attention, however, because their numbers are smaller, and they tend to be more isolated from mainstream US society. The American Indian and Alaska Native people have long experienced lower health status when compared with other Americans (Office of Minority Health, 2016). Lower life expectancy and the disproportionate disease burden exist are attributed to inadequate education, disproportionate poverty, discrimination in the delivery of health services, and cultural differences.

The proportion of American Indians/Alaskan Natives suffering from 2–3 chronic conditions is 25% higher than that for whites, and the HIV prevalence is 50% higher and increasing. For children, the asthma rate is one-third higher. The rate of psychological distress is 65% higher than for whites. Lifestyle plays a role and the use of illicit drugs is one-and-a-half times that of whites with the combined effect of these factors resulting in the highest disability rate of any racial or ethnic group.

American Indians and Alaska Natives experience a high rate of reproductive health problems. The infant mortality rate is one-and-a-half times that of whites. This high rate is partly explained by the facts that pre-term births occur 30% more often among this group, low birth weight deliveries are slightly higher, the teen birth rate is twice as high, and the proportion of births to unmarried women is nearly twice as high.

While the overall mortality rate for American Indians/Alaskan Natives has dropped below that for whites, there are still conditions for which this group exhibits higher rates. These include accidents, chronic liver disease, septicemia and diabetes, as well as suicide and homicide (Office of Minority Health, 2016). American Indians have a particularly high rate of suicide during adolescence and early adulthood, making it comparable to whites but significantly higher than other racial and ethnic groups. Interestingly, Native Americans have made the greatest gains of any group in reducing mortality in recent years. Native Americans record the lowest mortality for cancer of any group but by far the highest mortality rates for diabetes, suicide, and accidents. American Indians and Alaska Natives born today have a life expectancy that is 4.4 years less than the US averages.

Given the higher health status enjoyed by most Americans, the lingering health disparities of American Indians and Alaska Natives are troubling. One contributor to persistent disparities might be an uninsurance rate twice that of whites and a larger proportion of people with no regular source of care (National Center for Health Statistics, 2016).

Certain immigrant groups appear to be especially vulnerable to health disparities. This fact is somewhat ironic in that recently arrived immigrants are typically in better health than native-born Americans. The disparities arise after a period of residence in the U.S., perhaps eventually being mediated over a period of time. The factors that affect immigrants' vulnerability include socioeconomic background, immigration status, limited English proficiency, governmental policies related to access to publicly funded healthcare, residential segregation, and the stigma and marginalization associated with immigrant status (Derose et al., 2007). Research suggests that it is not baseline differences in health status that explain observed disparities but access to health insurance, access to health services and the manner in which the healthcare system treats immigrants. Variations in immigration and acculturation experiences also play a role.

Much of the mortality advantage characterizing Asian-Americans and Hispanics has been attributed to the foreign born among these populations. Subsequent generations of Asian-Americans and Hispanics, it seems, do not fare as well in comparative mortality analyses.

Migrant farm workers tend to be particularly vulnerable to health disparities due to a number of factors. Migrant and seasonal agricultural workers (MSAWs) perform work that is often dangerous or at the very least unhealthy, they live in inadequate housing that is health threatening, and they have no health insurance and essentially no means of obtaining care. These populations experience serious health problems including diabetes, malnutrition, infectious diseases, pesticide poisoning, and injuries from work-related machinery. These critical health issues are exacerbated by the migratory culture of this population, which makes it difficult to develop a relationship with a healthcare provider, observe treatment regimens, and maintain their health records. The very fact of constant migration itself contributes to poor health status.

The MSAW population presents a unique challenge when it comes to addressing health disparities in that it is essentially invisible. There are no data collection efforts focused on determining the size, distribution or characteristics of this population. According to the National Center for Farmworker Health (2015), approximately 42% of farmworkers are migrant workers and 58% are seasonal farmworkers. Both of these population groups are predominantly Hispanic/Latino, and a large majority of Hispanic/Latino farmworkers were born in Mexico. MSAW populations also include whites, African Americans, Haitians, and Asians. More than half (52%) of all farmworkers in the United States are unauthorized residents.

Prisoners represent another vulnerable population, and this is a significant concern given the size of the incarcerated population. Health conditions that are overrepresented in incarcerated populations include substance abuse, human immunodeficiency virus (HIV) and other infectious diseases, perpetration and victimization by violence, mental illness, chronic disease, and reproductive health problems (Freudenberg, 2001).

Disparities in health status are as striking based on income as they are for race and ethnicity. Poverty is the social determinant most commonly linked to health disparities, even overriding the influence of race and ethnicity (Thomas, 2015). Those in the lowest identified income group (<$35,000) are more than four times as likely to report only poor or fair health that those in the highest income group ($100,000+). If the lowest income category were to be further broken down, the differences would be even more glaring. Those in the lowest income category (at or below poverty level) exhibit an age-adjusted rate of chronic disease more than twice that of the most affluent. The physician diagnosed prevalence of diabetes is twice as high for the poorest cohort, as is the amount of chronic pain. The rates for depression and serious psychological distress among poverty-level adults is four times that of the most affluent (yet treatment rates for mental disorders among the poor are much lower).

The levels of both acute and chronic conditions increase as income decreases. Morbidity differences based on income are particularly distinct for chronic conditions. For the lowest income group (those with household incomes less than $35,000) the prevalence rate is higher for heart disease than for those in the highest income group (those with household incomes of $100,000 or more). Similar disparities are noted for diabetes, emphysema, kidney disease, and arthritis (National Center for Health Statistics, 2012). Higher rates are also recorded among the lowest income groups for most chronic respiratory conditions.

It is hard to overstate the contribution of income to health disparities. Some 14% of premature deaths among whites and 30% of premature deaths among blacks between 1960 and 2002 would not have occurred if everyone had experienced the mortality rates of whites in the highest income quintile (Centers for Disease Control and Prevention, 2006). Other research has found that 25% of all deaths in Virginia between 1996 and 2002 would have been averted if the mortality rates of the five most affluent counties and cities had applied statewide. Further, those living on incomes of less than 200% of the federal poverty level lost more than 400 million quality-adjusted life-years between 1997 and 2002, meaning that poverty had a larger effect than tobacco use and obesity. (Woolf & Braveman, 2012). Children of low economic status (as determined by Medicaid use) with cystic fibrosis have lower forced vital capacity, height, and weight, and a greater chance of exacerbations. They have nearly four times the adjusted risk of death compared with children not on Medicaid. The obesity rate for children in poverty is 40% higher than that for more affluent children. There is evidence now that this "white advantage" is disappearing, and Box 7.3 discusse this topic.

Not only are there more episodes of certain types of both acute and chronic conditions recorded as income decreases, but the severity of the conditions is likely to be greater when income is lower. In fact, the rate of preventable hospitalizations increases as income decreases. When afflicted by acute conditions, the poor tend to have more prolonged episodes characterized by greater severity. Interestingly, in a society that has become characterized by chronic health conditions, acute disorders

Box 7.3: The Diminishing White Health Advantage

Virtually every discussion of health disparities begins with the premise that the white population in the United States has higher health status than other racial and ethnic groups. Whites have historically been noteworthy for their low level of morbidity and mortality and have been able to avoid the worst aspects of ill-health as long as records have been kept. Not only have whites been less exposed to many of the factors associated with ill health, but they have had the advantage of relatively better access to services. Further, they have been able to take advantage of available health services due to their ability to pay. Indeed, assessments of health status generally use the white rate as the standard against which other racial and ethnic groups are measured.

While there is ample evidence of poorer health status relative to the white population on the part of certain racial and ethnic minorities, there is growing evidence that the white health advantage is disappearing (even though whites report higher self-assessed health status than all groups but Asian-Americans). Given the increased age of the non-Hispanic white population some decline in health status relative to other younger groups should be expected. However, when age-adjusted rates are examined the evidence for declining white health status remains and is especially noteworthy for non-Hispanic whites.

The primary source of data on comparative health status is *Health, United States 2016*, a compendium that incorporates a wide range of statistics generated or compiled by the National Center for Health Statistics and other organizations. Statistics presented on morbidity and mortality are particularly suited for this analysis. The groups considered for this review are whites, non-Hispanic whites, blacks or African Americans, Asian-Americans, American Indians/Alaskan Natives, and Hispanics. Data are not available for all groups for all indicators, and, in many cases, non-Hispanic whites are not broken out from the white umbrella category.

When the incidence and prevalence of various conditions are considered, it appears that the white population is losing ground relative to other groups. A higher proportion of whites report one or more chronic conditions than any other racial or ethnic group, with whites more likely to suffer from a chronic disease and/or a disability than any group except African Americans. When rates for specific diseases are considered, it is found that whites exhibit the highest rate of all groups for heart disease, certain cancers and high cholesterol. While whites are second to African Americans in overall cancer rates, they rank highest on the prevalence of urinary/bladder cancer, non-Hodgkin lymphoma, and leukemia. Among children representing the various racial and ethnic groups, white children exhibit the highest rates for ADHD, serious emotional or behavioral disorders, respiratory allergies and food allergies. To the extent that consumption of prescription drugs indicates higher morbidity, a higher proportion of whites report use of one or more prescription drugs than members of other groups.

(continued)

Box 7.3 (continued)

Some observers have suggested that fragmented evidence of a declining health advantage for whites does not carry as much weight as the continued mortality advantage held by whites. However, that mortality advantage appears to be evaporating with each successive mortality report. For the 2012–14 period, it is found that, except for African Americans, whites exhibit higher mortality rates for heart disease, stroke, and cancer; non-Hispanic whites exhibit higher rates than all groups for chronic lower respiratory disease, influenza/pneumonia and Alzheimer's disease. Newly released data on deaths from opioid overdose/poisoning finds higher rates for whites than for other racial and ethnic groups. Only American Indian males report higher suicide rates than white males, and white males are second to African Americans in firearms-related mortality. While whites have long been considered sheltered from the tragedy of infant mortality, it is now found that both Asian-Americans and Hispanics report lower infant death rates.

When age-adjusted all-cause mortality is considered for 2016, the white population is characterized by a rate of 729/100,000 (749 for non-Hispanic whites) compared to 526 for Hispanics, and 394 for Asian-Americans. Only African Americans (883) and American Indians (800) exhibit a higher death rate than whites. Indeed a review of mortality data over the past 30 years has found increasing mortality and declining life expectancy among some segments of the non-Hispanic white population (Olshansky et al., 2012). Those affected by this phenomenon are primarily poorly educated, low-income whites, thereby supporting the notion that poverty trumps most other attributes. Rates of drug-induced deaths increased between 2003 and 2007 among men and women of all race/ethnicities, with the exception of Hispanics, and rates are highest among non-Hispanic whites. Prescription drug abuse now kills more persons than illicit drugs, a reversal of the situation 15–20 years ago. It appears now that adverse trends in mortality for the white population may extend well beyond these disadvantaged white groups.

remain surprisingly common among the lower income groups. In fact, the disease profile of many low-income communities more closely resembles that of a less developed nation than it does the United States. Interestingly, the relationship between income and health status remains even in the face of improved health behaviors on the part of the lower income groups (Lantz et al., 1998). The most disadvantaged group overall is poverty-level African-American males.

More striking yet, is the difference in self-reported health status between the best and worst educated within the population—with those with high school educations or less five times as likely as those with a bachelor's degree to report only poor or fair health status. The least educated reported much lower health status than the best educated. The former report 20% more chronic pain than the latter, and the obesity level for those with only a high school degree is 40% higher than those with a college degree. The least educated also reported a higher level of depression than the better educated.

Rates of preventable hospitalizations increase as incomes decrease, reflecting the inability of members of certain groups to obtain timely healthcare. Obviously, the poorly educated are not as clearly defined a subpopulation as the poor or African Americans and American Indians. However, many subpopulations are characterized by all three of the characteristics—minority group status, poverty and low education—creating a "perfect storm" when it comes to low health status.

Those lacking health insurance are also considered at risk for health disparities. Although persons throughout society may experience a lack of insurance, this disadvantage is concentrated among certain groups. While access to insurance does not guarantee access to care (and at the end of the day may not even contribute to better health), available statistics indicate that the uninsured face higher rates of morbidity and mortality. The list of conditions and procedures for which being uninsured is associated with poorer outcomes and higher mortality includes: cardiac valve surgery, surgery for colorectal cancer, breast cancer treatment, and abdominal aortic aneurysms (Gorski, 2012). Uninsured persons are only about half as likely to have hypertension under control as those with insurance, regardless of type. It is further found that the uninsured exhibit a much higher level of depression than the insured. Indeed, it is argued that the US records 45,000 deaths a year that can be attributed to a lack of insurance although this figure is hard to verify (Factcheck.org, 2016). It is clear from mortality data, however, that the risk of death is 35% higher for the uninsured (Rogers et al., 2000).

One other contributing factor that would encompass many of the vulnerabilities already described is residential segregation. To the extent that one's ZIP Code is the best predictor of one's health status, it could be argued that community of residence represents an interface of minority concentration, economic hardship, low health literacy, and lack of insurance that contributes to health disparities. While residential segregation may not be the immediate cause of health disparities it perhaps provides the setting where all of these factors can converge.

It might be argued that any one attribute is not sufficient to create health disparities. Being African-American by itself does not guarantee poor health status. Similarly, there are people living in some rural areas with poverty-level incomes who do not suffer from disparities. Education and income are elements of a web of social and economic conditions that affect health (and influence each other) in complex ways over a lifetime. These conditions include employment, wealth, neighborhood characteristics, and social policies as well as culture and beliefs about health.

It may be that it is a combination of attributes that come together to trigger health disparities. This suggests that the relationship between disparities in morbidity and various demographic attributes is complicated, and observed relationships often require considerable parsing to derive the true association. Sociologist David Williams (2005) reviewed several years' worth of health experiences for whites and African Americans and examined a wide range of factors to determine their correlation with morbidity. He found, like most everyone else, a clear disparity in health status between whites and African Americans. However, when he held income constant, *most* of the disparity between whites and African Americans disappeared. However, there was still some residual disparity that could not be explained by socioeconomic differences.

That raises the question: How do we account for the fact that being African-American carries an increased health risk. Is it racism? A lifetime of being a second-class citizen? The persistent stress of day-to-day survival? This dimension of disparity-causing factors is only now being explored in depth, and a recent review of research by Williams and Mohammed (2009) has revealed a relationship between a lifetime of discrimination and its associated stress and poorer health status.

Trends in Health Disparities

The existence of health disparties has long been recognized as an issue, going back to the War on Poverty in the 1960s. Since then, considerable effort—money, facilities, services—has been directed toward reducing identified disparities and particularly those associated with poverty. In retrospect it could be argued that much of the effort was misplaced, and certainly a population health perspective would have augured a different approach for previous initiatives—one that would have addressed the causes rather than the symptoms.

As a result of (or in spite of) these efforts, some progress has been made in reducing identified disparities at least based on some indicators during the latter part of the twentieth century. Even so, disparities in the health of minority and disadvantaged populations have persisted. Since the 1960s, the mortality rate for blacks has been 50% higher than that for whites, and the infant mortality rate for blacks has been twice as high as that for whites. Health disparities exist even in healthcare systems that offer patients similar access to care, such as the Department of Veterans Affairs (Woolf & Bravemen, 2012). A comparative study at a large hospital system found that blacks and whites with similar health conditions and identitical treatment exhibited quite different outcomes that could not be attributed to differences in the care received (Hopper, 2011). Recently studies on hospital readmission rates have been found to be primarily a function of non-clinical factors—particularly the life circumstances of the patients independent of their clinical experience (Hui et al., 2014). These studies suggest that disparities exist independent of the formal healthcare setting.

An examination of trends in selected measures of disability (i.e., severe headache, low back pain, neck pain) between 1997 and 2014, found the disparity between blacks and whites remained the same or increased for two of the three measures, the disparity between the lowest income group and highest increased or remained the same for all three conditions and the disparity between the least educated and best increased or remained the same for two of the three measures (National Center for Health Statistics, 2016).The disability rate for the poorest is nearly twice as high as that for the most affluent. The prevalence of asthma is 11.2% for children in families living below the poverty level compared with 8.7% for children in families earning 200% above the poverty level.

The interaction of various social determinants has been noted above, and alarming disparities persist among racial groups and between the well-educated and those with less education. Olshansky et al., 2012) found that in 2008 US adult men and women with fewer than 12 years of education had life expectancies not much better than those of all adults in the 1950s and 1960s. When race and education are combined, the disparity is even more striking. In 2008 white US men and women with 16 years or more of schooling had life expectancies far greater than black Americans with fewer than 12 years of education—14.2 years more for white men than black men, and 10.3 years more for white women than black women. These gaps have widened over time and reinforce the notion of "two Americas" with very different life chances based on race and education.

Another relatively important cause of death for blacks is infant mortality. Although infant mortality has been dramatically reduced as a cause of death in the United States in this century, it continues to be a serious health threat for many groups of nonwhites. The infant mortality rate for African Americans in 2007 was two and a half times that for whites, 13.2 per 1000 live births versus 5.6 (Matthews & MacDorman, 2011). The rates for both groups have declined since the late 1980s, with the gap between the two actually narrowing in recent years. Exhibit 7.4 presents trends in infant mortality by race and ethnicity. As can be seen, little decrease in the gap between African Americans and other racial and ethnic groups with regard to infant mortality has been observed through 2013.

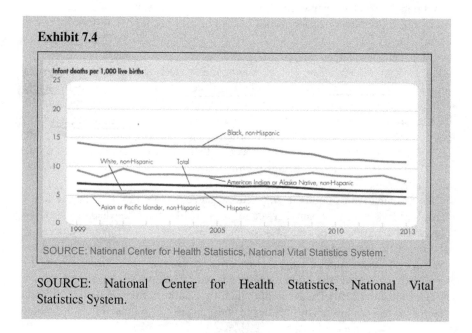

Exhibit 7.4

SOURCE: National Center for Health Statistics, National Vital Statistics System.

Although the gap in infant mortality has narrowed between whites and other racial and ethnic groups over time, this raises the question of the meaning of observed differences. For example, is an African-American infant mortality rate that is two times the rate for whites in 2013 a meaningful improvement over a rate two-and-one-half times as high in 1999? Can this be considered enough improvement over a 15-year period to consider the gap narrowed? It could be argued that this falls short of any reasonable expectations and is not such a meaningful improvement.

Other racial and ethnic groups display quite disparate trends in regard to infant death. Certain Asian American groups, for example, report much lower than average infant mortality, while Hispanics as a group record infant mortality rates between those of whites and blacks. Native Americans and native Alaskans historically have recorded very high infant mortality rates; however, since the 1950s, their rates have come to resemble the US average. Infant mortality rates for selected groups are 5.5/1000 live births for Hispanics, 9.2 for American Indians and 4.8 for Asian-Americans (Matthews & MacDorman, 2011). The Hispanic infant mortality rate is something of an anomaly, given the relatively poor health status of this population and this group's lower level of access to health services. The low Hispanic infant mortality rate is generally attributed to the emphasis on family in this culture. Indeed, it could be argued that factors outside of healthcare are responsible for the confluence of infant mortality rates. Questions remain as to the relative impact of individual choices and social determinants, and Box 7.4 addresses this issue.

Box 7.4: Who's Responsible: The Individual or Society?
An important consideration, and one that is germane to the very concept of population health, is the extent to which health disparities are attributes of individuals or to groups (or at least individuals as members of groups). The American ethos places inordinate onus on personal responsibility, and our society is quick to blame individuals when they do not live up to societal standards. "Society made me do it" is the derisive put-down that is sarcastically voiced by critics of those who fall short of societal expectations.

For a quarter of a century the US population has been led to believe that if we eat properly, exercise, avoid smoking and otherwise lead a healthy lifestyle most health problems can be avoided. The emphasis of health education has been on influencing behavior by educating the population with regard to healthy living. This approach has placed the onus on the individual without regard to other considerations or even the ability of individuals to pursue desirable goals. Countless millions of Americans have been shamed for their inability to pursue healthy lifestyles and obtain optimal health despite being given the information they need to improve their health.

An alternative approach has been to penalize individuals for their unhealthy behavior. This has included everything from raising taxes on tobacco products to charging higher insurance premiums for those who smoke or otherwise do

(continued)

> **Box 7.4** (continued)
>
> not pursue healthy lifestyles. While there have been some positive results from some of these efforts (e.g., smoking cessation), most of them have had little impact on individual behavior. At the end of the day, people's behavior is more driven by the expectations of their social group than by an increase in "sin taxes".
>
> Our attempts to improve health status heretofore have proceeded as if poor health status was an individual attribute that could be addressed by getting John Doe to eat less, exercise more and stop smoking. We now realize that there are serious barriers to health improvement at the individual level and that individual attributes today have little impact on one's risk of experiencing health disparities. The victim continues to be blamed even as we realize that, as long as we eat the processed products that the food industry foists on us, there is little hope of improving the health status of individuals or the overall health status of the population. Indeed, an estimated 100,000 lives are lost in the United States every year due to excess salt consumption (even though individuals have cut back on its use); the fact of the matter is that nearly 80% of our salt intake comes from processed foods and restaurants (He et al., 2013).
>
> When the causes of ill-health are a polluted environment, exclusion from jobs and educational opportunities, residential segregation, and unhealthy food options it is hard to single out any individual for blame. The *raison d'etre* for the population health movement is the fact that health disparities affect groups of people within the population, and neither the actions of the individual nor the efforts of clinical medicine can positively impact population health. If the problem is at the group level then the solution must be at the group level. As discussed in later chapters, efforts must be undertaken to influence the conditions affecting populations and not conditions affecting individuals. This means directing efforts to the causes of ill-health and not the effects.

Summary

Developments over the past several years in healthcare and society have resulted in a reconfiguration of morbidity patterns. The major consequence has been the developments of patterns of disease distribution that reflect demographic and geographic attributes. While acute conditions were more or less randomly distributed within the population, chronic conditions tend to sort themselves out in terms of population attributes. On the one hand we find that certain conditions are more prevalent among certain groups within the population than other groups. While much of the population is affected by chronic disease, the concentration is greater among the least advantaged and most vulnerable populations. Thus, both morbidity and mortality are unequally distributed within the population, with the poor, minority group members and those otherwise disadvantaged the most affected. On the other hand, we find that certain groups within the population are characterized by high levels of morbidity no matter what indicator is examined. At the same time, we see that health conditions tend to cluster in terms of geography as well as in terms of demographic attributes. Thus, the ZIP Code of residence becomes the best indicator of health status.

One of the consequences of the resorting of health conditions among population groups is a pattern of health disparity. Differences in morbidity and mortality are nothing new but the patterns that are exhibited today that reflect demographic and geographic concentrations have converted these differences into "disparities." Differences become "disparities" when they reflect disadvantages inherent in the status of affected parties and/or are the consequences of an inequitable and/or discriminatory system. Disparities can exist with regard to health status, with regard to access to healthcare resources, and in terms of differential treatments. The latter two factors contribute directly and indirectly to the disparities observed in health status. While the existence of disparities is not new, their scope as a major feature of the healthcare landscape has more recently been recognized. The fact that disparities persist among population subgroups serves as an indictment of our healthcare system and offers additional support for a population health approach.

Disparities can be measured using the various metrics and indicators discussed earlier in this book. These would include global measures of health status, morbidity in terms of the incidence and prevalence of acute and chronic conditions, the prevalence of mental illness and the level of disability found for various subgroups. Less commonly used but nevertheless important indicators that reflect disparities are measures of reproductive health, oral health and substance abuse. Although less significant for our discussion here, the healthcare system itself contributes to health disparities through unequal access to health insurance, healthcare resources and effective treatment. Disparities are perpetuated through missed and inappropriate diagnoses and less than optimal therapies.

African Americans tend to exhibit the highest level of disparities and exhibit the lowest level of health status on virtually every indicator. Despite some improvement with regard to certain metrics, this population has continued to exhibit disparities at a time when improvement is being noted for virtually every other racial and ethnic group. Hispanics tend to suffer from health disparities more than any other racial and ethnic group, although nowhere near the level of African Americans. American Indians/Alaska Natives also suffer disproportionately from disparities but receive less attention because of their small numbers and relative isolation. Disparities are also observed for low-income populations and for the poorly educated. In fact, it has been asserted that income and education may, in fact, trump race and ethnic as predictors of disparity. The combination of race and poverty creates a perfect storm of health disparities with low-income African-American males representing the height of disparity. Although *some* improvement on the part of *some* subgroups has been observed, part of this can be attributed ironically to a decline in the health status of non-Hispanic whites. Perhaps more than any other factor, health disparities remain a serious issue and underscore the importance of a population health approach.

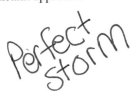

Key Points

- Beginning during the last years of the twentieth century a number of developments occurred to change the healthcare environment
- The population was experiencing a rapid process of aging with an accompanying shift from a predominance of acute conditions to a predominance of chronic conditions
- The emergence of chronic conditions resulted in a reconfiguration of morbidity patterns within the population
- Diseases were increasingly sorted out in terms of demographic attributes and geographic location
- As a result, various chronic conditions came to affect some populations more than others and be more concentrated in some geographic locations more than others
- Some of the variations simply reflected differences in distribution patterns, but those that reflected the impact of social factors came to be seen as "disparities"
- Disparities have been identified in terms of morbidity and mortality, with the metrics used including global measures, disease incidence and prevalence, and disability rates
- Although there is reason to downplay the usefulness of mortality measures, clear disparities in death rates remain among various groups especially as related to infant and maternal mortality
- Some less frequently utilized measures such as reproductive health and oral health also reflect disparities
- Beyond health status, disparities have been observed in terms of access to health resources (including health insurance), the manner in which different groups of patients are perceived, and the manner in which they are treated.
- Specific chronic diseases tend to cluster within certain groups creating a clear-cut pattern of morbidity distribution
- African Americans exhibit the highest level of disparity with this group reporting unfavorable rates for virtually every measure of disparity
- Hispanics as a group exhibit the most disparities after African Americans, although nothing like those exhibited by African Americans
- American Indians/Alaska Natives also exhibit disparities for a number of metrics but this group is often overlooked
- Significant disparities also exist with regard to income and education, with the poorest and least educated reporting disparities as significant as those for race
- Some reduction in disparities has been noted for various racial and ethnic minorities (except for African Americans), although some of this improvement reflects a decline in the health status of non-Hispanic whites
- Limited improvement can be observed in the gap between the poor and affluent and between the least and best educated

References

American Journal of Managed Care. (2006). *Vulnerable populations: Who are they?* Downloaded from URL: http://www.ajmc.com/publications/supplement/2006/2006-11-vol12-n13suppl/nov06-2390ps348-s352/

American Lung Association. (2011). *Trends in asthma morbidity and mortality*. American Lung Association.

American Psychological Association. (2017). *Stress and health disparities*. Downloaded from URL: https://www.apa.org/pi/health-disparities/resources/stress-report.pdf

Brandon, L. J., & Proctor, L. (2010). Comparison of health perceptions and health status in African Americans and Caucasians. *Journal of the National Medical Association, 102*(7), 590–597.

Braveman, P. (2009). A health disparities perspective on obesity research. *Preventing Chronic Disease: Public Health Research, Practice, & Policy, 6*(3), A91–A97.

Canady, R., Bullen, B., Holzman, C., Broman, C., & Tian, Y. (2010). Discrimination and symptoms of depression in pregnancy among African American and white women. *Women's Health Issues, 18*(4), 292–300.

Centers for Disease Control and Prevention. (2000). *Measuring healthy days*. Centers for Disease Control and Prevention.

Centers for Disease Control and Prevention. (2004). Health disparities experienced by Hispanics—United States. *Mortality and Morbidity Weekly Report, 53*(40), 935–937.

Centers for Disease Control and Prevention. (2006). *The power of prevention*. Downloaded from URL: https://www.cdc.gov/chronicdisease/pdf/2009-power-of-prevention.pdf

Child Health USA. (2013). *Low Birth Weight*. Downloaded from URL: https://mchb.hrsa.gov/chusa13/perinatal-health-status-indicators/p/low-birth-weight.html

Cote, M. L., Ruterbursch, J. J., Olsen, S. H., et al. (2015). The growing burden of endometrial cancer: A major racial disparity affecting Black Women. *Cancer Epidemiology, Biomarkers and Prevention*. Downloaded from URL: http://cebp.aacrjournals.org/content/early/2015/08/10/1055-9965.EPI-15-0316.abstract?fdn

Crook, E. R., & Peters, M. (2008). Health disparities in chronic diseases: Where the money is. *American Journal of Medical Science, 335*(4), 266–270.

Derose, K. P., Escarce, J. J., & Lurie, N. (2007). Immigrants and health care: Sources of vulnerability. *Health Affairs, 26*(5), 1258–1268.

Factcheck.org. (2016). *Dying from lack of insurance*. Downloaded from URL: http://www.factcheck.org/2009/09/dying-from-lack-of-insurance/

Families USA. (2014). *Latino health disparities compared to Non-hispanic Whites*. Downloaded from URL: familiesusa.org/product/latino-health-disparities-compared-non-hispanic whites

Freudenberg, N. (2001). Jails, prisons, and the health of urban populations: A review of the impact of the correctional system on community health. *Journal of Urban Health, 78*(2), 214–235.

Galea, S., Tracy, M., Hoggatt, K. J., et al. (2011). Estimated deaths attributable to social factors in the United States. *American Journal of Public Health, 101*(8), 1456–1465.

Gorski, D. (2012). Mortality and lack of health insurance. *Science Based Medicine*. Downloaded from URL: https://www.sciencebasedmedicine.org/health-insurance-and-mortality/

Harvard Health Publications. (2016). *Prostate cancer risks in African Americans*. Downloaded from URL: http://www.harvardprostateknowledge.org/prostate-cancer-risk-in-African Americans.

He, F. G., Li, J., & MacGregor, G. A. (2013). Effect of longer term modest salt reduction on blood pressure: Cochrane systematic review and meta-analysis of randomised trials. *British Medical Journal, 346*, f1325.

Hopper, K. (2011). *Disparities in Cardiac Rehab*. Unpublished presentation. Downloaded from URL: http://www.aacvpr.org/Portals/0/events_edu/annualmeeting11/2011%20Online%20Syllabus%20PPT/BO31Hopper.pdf

Hui, J., Gonsahn, M. D., & Nerenz, D. R. (2014). Socioeconomic status and readmissions: Evidence from an urban teaching hospital. *Health Affairs, 33*, 5778–5785.

Jackson, J. S., Knight, K. M., & Rafferty, J. A. (2010). Race and unhealthy behaviors: Chronic stress, the HPA Axis, and physical and mental health disparities over the life course. *American Journal of Public Health, 100*(5), 933–939.

Kay, J., & Katz, C. (2012). Pollution, poverty, people of color: The Factory on the hill. *Environmental Health News.* Downloaded from URL: http://www.environmentalhealthnews.org/ehs/news/2012/pollution-poverty-and-people-of-color-richmond-day-1

Kessler, R. C., Berglund, P., Demler, O., et al. (2003). The epidemiology of major depressive disorder: Results from the National Comorbidity Survey Replication (NCS-R). *Journal of the American Medical Association, 289*(23), 3095–3105.

Kruger, P. M., Tran, M. K., Hummer, R. A., et al. (2015). Mortality attributable to low levels of education in the United States. *Plus One, 10*(7).

Lantz, P. M., House, J. S., Lepkowski, J. M., et al. (1998). Socioeconomic factors, health behaviors, and mortality results from a nationally representative prospective study of US adults. *Journal of the American Medical Association, 279*(21), 1703–1708.

Lee, H., Harris, K., Gordon-Larsen, P., & P. (2009). Life course perspectives on the links between poverty and obesity during the transition to young adulthood. *Population Research and Policy Review, 28*(4), 505–532.

Lloyd-Jones, D., Adams, R. J., Brown, T. M., et al. (2010). Heart disease and stroke statistics—2010 update: A report from the American Heart Association. *Circulation, 121*, e46–e15.

Matthews, T. J., & MacDorman, M. F. (2011). Infant mortality statistics from the 2007 period linked birth/infant death data set. *National Vital Statistics Report, 59*(6), 1–30.

Matthews, T. J., & MacDorman, M. F. (2013). Infant mortality statistics from the 2010 period linked birth/infant death data set. *National Vital Statistics Report, 62*(8), 1–26.

Mead, H., Cartright-Smith, L., Jones, K., et al. (2008). *Racial and Ethnic Disparities in U.S. Health Care: A Chartbook.* Downloaded from URL: http://www.commonwealthfund.org/Publications/Chartbooks/2008/Mar/Racial-and-Ethnic-Disparities-in-U-S%2D%2DHealth-Care%2D%2DA-Chartbook.aspx

Murali, V., & Oyebode, F. (2004). Poverty, social inequality and mental health. *Advances in Psychiatric Treatment, 10*, 216–224.

National Center for Farmworker Health. (2015). *Farmworkers' Health Work Sheet.* Downloaded from URL: https://www.farmworkerjustice.org/sites/default/files/NawsHealthFactSheet_FINAL.pdf

National Center for Health Statistics (2011). Summary health statistics for the U.S. population: National Health Interview Survey, 2010. : National Center for Health Statistics.

National Center for Health Statistics. (2012). *Health United States, 2011.* National Center for Health Statistics.

National Center for Health Statistics. (2016). *Health United States, 2015.* National Center for Health Statistics.

National Institutes of Health. (2011). *NIH announces Institute on Minority Health and Health Disparities.* Downloaded from URL: https://www.nih.gov/news-events/news-releases/nih-announces-institute-minority-health-health-disparities

Office of Minority Health. (2016). *Profile: American Indian and Alaska Native.* Downloaded from URL: https://minorityhealth.hhs.gov/omh/browse.aspx?lvl=3&lvlid=62

Olshansky, S. J., Antonucci, T., Berkman, L., et al. (2012). Differences in life expectancy due to race and educational differences are widening, and many may not catch up. *Health Affairs, 31*(8), 1803–1813.

Pardo, F., & Prakash, S. (2011). Racial Segregation Kills More Than Lung Cancer. *American Civil Liberties Union blog.* Downloaded from URL: https://www.aclu.org/blog/smart-justice/mass-incarceration/racial-segregation-kills-more-lung-cancer

Potochnick, S. R., & Perreira, K. M. (2011). Depression and anxiety among first-generation immigrant Latino youth: Key correlates and implications for future research. *Journal of Nervous and Mental Disease, 198*(7), 470–477.

References

Riolo, S. A., Nguyen, T. A., Greden, J. F., et al. (2005). Prevalence of depression by race/ethnicity: Findings from the National Health and nutrition examination survey III. *American Journal of Public Health, 95*(6), 998–1000.

Quinn, K., Kaufman, J., Siddiqi, A., & Yeatts, K. (2010). Stress and the City: Housing stressors are associated with respiratory health among low socioeconomic status Chicago children. *Journal of Urban Health, 87*(4), 688–702.

Rogers, R. G., Hummer, R. A., & Nam, C. B. (2000). *Living and dying in the USA*. Academic.

Shi, L., & Stevens, G. D. (2010). *Vulnerable populations in the United States* (2nd ed.). Jossey-Bass.

Sims, M., Diez-Roux, A. V., Dudley, A., et al. (2012). Perceived discrimination and hypertension among African Americans in the Jackson heart study. *American Journal of Public Health, 102*(Suppl 2), S258–S265.

Thomas, R. K. (2015). *In sickness and in health: Disease and disability in contemporary America*. Springer.

Ward, B. W., Schiller, J. S., & Goodman, R. A. (2014). Multiple chronic conditions among US adults: A 2012 update. *Preview of Chronic Disease*. Downloaded from URL: https://www.cdc.gov/pcd/issues/2014/13_0389.htm

Wilkerson, I. (2020). *Caste*. Penguin Random House.

Williams, D. R. (2005). The health of U.S. racial and ethnic populations. *Journal of Gerontology: Series B, 60B*(Special Issue II), 53–62.

Williams, D. R., & Mohammed, S. A. (2009). Discrimination and racial disparities in health: Evidence and needed research. *Journal of Behavioral Medicine, 32*(1), 20–47.

Woolf, S., & Braveman, P. (2012). The social and ecological determinants of health. In D. Scutchfield, J. W. Holsinger, et al. (Eds.), *Contemporary topics in public health*. Kentucky University Press.

Additional Resources

Carratala, S., & Maxwell, C. (2020). *Health disparities by race and ethnicity*. Downloaded from URL: https://www.americanprogress.org/issues/race/reports/2020/05/07/484742/health-disparities-race-ethnicity/

Galea, S. (2019). *Well: What we need to talk about when we talk about health*. Oxford University Press.

National Academies. (2017). The state of health disparities in the United States. In *Communities in action: Pathways to health equity* (Chapter 2). Downloaded from URL: https://www.ncbi.nlm.nih.gov/books/NBK425844/

National Center for Health Statistics. (2020). *Health United States, 2019*. National Center for Health Statistics.

Thomas, R. K. (2016). *In sickness and in health*. Springer.

Chapter 8
Population Health and Healthcare Delivery

In view of the developments that are driving the population health movement, this chapter addresses the practical implications for the delivery of healthcare. While it could be argued that "true" population health is not compatible with clinical medicine or personal healthcare, this chapter explores the ways in which the principles of population health can be applied in that arena. It describes the concept of "population health management," considers the role of the healthcare system in addressing social determinants and policy issues, and discusses the manner in which population health and personal health intersect.

In this chapter, the reader will be:

- Exposed to the application of population health principles within the healthcare system
- Learn about population health management and its attributes
- Find out the limitations of applying population health principles to healthcare delivery
- Understand the transformation required for the US healthcare system to adopt the population health model

Introduction

Population health purists would argue that it is not appropriate to apply the term "population health" to any activity that focuses on clinical care and/or individual patients. Any effort to do so, it is claimed, represents a perversion of the notion of population health and suggests a misunderstanding of the nature of this approach to community health improvement. This author would probably be included among those protesting the application of this concept to healthcare delivery.

This is not to say that a population health-based methodology can not be applied to patient management, but that some other term should be applied to the management of care for individual patients. While a case can be made that the term "population health" should be strictly reserved for initiatives involving geographically and/or demographically defined populations, the reality is that many in the field will continue to pursue efforts to apply the population health model to the management of individual patients in clinical settings.

Research by the Health Research and Education Trust found that as early as 2014 70% of hospital administrators indicated that existing patients/clients are an appropriate target for population health, 59% cited individuals experiencing a certain disease or condition, and 47% cited people who put the hospital at financial risk (Health Research and Educational Trust, 2015). Encouragingly, 69% of hospital representatives interviewed did consider a specified geographic population or community as an appropriate target for a population health initiative.

In actuality, virtually every aspect of care delivery can be impacted by the emerging population health paradigm—so much so that a serious rethinking of the way care is provided is required. The growing emphasis on outcomes, pay-for-performance, and the management of the health of defined populations requires different approaches to identifying and managing health problems. While a population health purist would contend that applying a population health approach to existing patients, plan members or employees represents a misapplication of the concept on the part of healthcare providers, the truth is that, for the healthcare delivery system to be successful in the future, it must incorporate population health principles. The sections that follow seek to clarify the distinction between population health in general and population health management as applied in healthcare delivery.

The Institute for Health Improvement (IHI) views the healthcare environment as including both clinical populations and geographically and demographically defined populations (Lewis, 2014). As the IHI describes them, *"discrete/defined populations* are enterprise-level populations that make business sense. Typically, they are a group of individuals receiving care within a health system, or whose care is financed through a specific health plan or entity. Examples of a discrete population include employees of an organization, members of a health plan, those within a practice's patient panel, or those enrolled within a particular accountable care organization. The members of a discrete population can be known with some certainty. On the other hand, *regional/community populations* are inclusive population segments, defined geographically or demographically. People within a community population are unified by a common set of needs or issues. However, these individuals may receive care from a variety of systems, may be unconnected to care, or may or may not be insured. It is often difficult to delineate community populations with certainty.

Micro-level assessments and interventions typically involve patients within a clinical setting. While the clinical management of patients might be thought of as the antithesis of population health, healthcare practitioners who are involved in the delivery of care are also being affected by a number of developments that are reflective of the population health movement. Increasingly, healthcare providers are being rewarded based on the quality of the care provided rather than on the quantity of care. This means that providers will have to demonstrate favorable clinical outcomes or face financial penalties.

The key here, and what moves it into the population health realm, is the emphasis on group rather than individual outcomes. This means that the health status of the entire patient pool will be taken into consideration over and above any individual patient outcomes. "Pay for performance" has become a buzzword in the healthcare arena as practitioners are increasingly being asked to contribute to higher quality care at lower costs. New Medicare regulations that limit reimbursement for hospital patients who are readmitted is the first of probably many such provisions in the future.

Although, in general, physicians treat individual patients and not populations, there are aspects of this process with relevance for population health. It is important that healthcare providers be aware of patterns of illness in the population being served. First, although a medical condition may result from the patient's lifestyle, the driving forces for this lifestyle may lie within the social environment. That is, the patient does not experience the impact of the social environment so much as an individual but as a member of a group. There is truth to the old adage that "common things are common"; in effect, a patient's condition is a symptom of population-wide health patterns. The underlying population prevalence should therefore affect the hierarchy involved in a physician's differential diagnosis.

Because of the social context in which patients live, efforts to help them alter health behaviors may be frustrated by social pressures. Indeed, the efforts by the Centers for Medicare and Medicaid Services to reduce hospital readmissions by limiting reimbursement has uncovered an important fact: The likelihood of hospital readmission has very little to do with the clinical circumstances and very much to do with the non-medical circumstances associated with patients (Hui et al., 2014). This means that it may prove more efficient to tackle a disease at the population level than by treating large numbers of individuals one at a time.

Interestingly, Kindig (1997) addressed this issue in the very early days of the evolution of the population health model. Foreshadowing the future pay-for-performance environment, he posited the following definition of population health: *the aggregate health outcome of health-adjusted life expectancy (quantity and quality) of a group of individuals, in an economic framework that balances the relative marginal returns from the multiple determinants of health*. This definition includes a specific measure of population health (health-adjusted life expectancy) as well as consideration of the relative cost-effectiveness of resource allocation.

These population-based factors are also important when it comes to the delivery of care in that the characteristics of patients may be as important in determining their clinical outcomes as the medical care they receive. To the extent that providers are going to be reimbursed based on their outcomes, it will be important for practitioners to understand the life circumstances, cultural contexts and social histories of their patients. As just one example, compliance on the part of patients has been documented to be heavily influenced by social factors and, to the extent that providers will be rewarded based on outcomes, it is important to be aware of the attributes of patients that will encourage or discourage their adherence to medical regimen.

Population Health Principles and Healthcare Delivery

At this juncture it might be important to revisit portions of Chap. 1 where the population health concept was originally introduced. It should be recalled that the application of this methodology was considered at two levels: (1) a micro-level whereby population health principles are applied at the point of care delivery; and (2) a macro-level wherein population health principles are applied at a more societal level independent for the most part of the healthcare system. While the contention here is that the latter represents a more appropriate application of population health, some consideration must be given to the application of these principles at the micro-level.

The following developments have encouraged healthcare providers to apply what they consider a population health approach to the delivery of care:

Emphasis on Group Outcomes There has been a major shift away from evaluating (and rewarding) providers for the successful management of individual patients. While the successful treatment of serious conditions is important, CMS and other third-party payers are more concerned about how a clinic's 100 patients or a health plan's 1000 enrollees are faring—and not just in terms of a specific health issue but in terms of their overall health status. Thus, the significance of clinical outliers is minimized, with those evaluating effectiveness or paying for services looking for across-the-board improvement rather than individual successes. Hospital executives' efforts at improving the overall health of a "managed" population, in fact, are increasingly being considered in their evaluations (Conn, 2016).

Emphasis on Quality Rather Quantity There has been a shift away from rewarding providers based on the *number* of cases treated, diagnostic tests run and procedures performed toward rewards for the *quality* of these services provided and their subsequent impact on the health of patient populations. "Quality" is notoriously hard to define and measure, but as imperfect as the measures might be providers will increasingly be judged in this regard. Quality measures, while perhaps considered an aggregate of individual measures, can be thought to provide a global indicator of the effectiveness of the care provided to a group of patients, plan members or employees.

Deficiencies in Disease Management Initiatives For two decades health plans and employers have attempted to control costs through the implementation of initiatives such as "disease management" and "patient management". The intent was to micromanage the care for a select number of high-cost patients. Diabetics have been a common target for such programs with some going so far as to assign case managers to assure timely access to services and patient adherence. Such programs have resulted in limited financial benefits and have failed to contribute to the overall health of the targeted population. Micromanaging a small number of patients has been found to have little impact on overall health, while focusing on at-risk populations, for example, has tended to yield better results. Ultimately, any initiative that attempts to improve population health one patient at time is not going to be effective in today's healthcare environment.

Emphasis on "Community Benefits" There is growing concern that healthcare providers (often with tax-exempt status) are focusing on their existing patients to the detriment of the health of the community. There is pressure on not-for-profit hospitals in particular to generate "community benefits" beyond the services they provide to their patients. Indeed, the Patient Protection and Affordable Care Act of 2010 mandated that not-for-profit hospitals conduct a comprehensive community health needs assessment at least every 3 years. The legislation made it clear that the emphasis was on the extent to which these providers served the total community and not just their own patients. In fact, existing regulations require that a plan be developed for addressing any identified gaps in services within the community whether or not the provider is involved in the delivery those services.

Emphasis on Non-clinical Factors A major contribution of the population health movement has been the spotlight placed on non-clinical factors and their impact on health status and health behavior. It has become increasingly clear that the demographic, socioeconomic, and psychographic attributes of populations play an important role in the health problems they exhibit and the subsequent health behavior of their members. These non-clinical factors often override the impact of the healthcare delivery system. These attributes determine who gets sick and with what disease, the likelihood of seeking treatment and/or complying with doctor's orders, and what happens to them after they leave the doctor's office or hospital. Indeed, it is now realized that one's ZIP Code of residence is a prime predictor of health status (Roeder, 2014) and that hospital readmissions are more a function of non-clinical factors than of anything that transpires in the healthcare system (Hui et al., 2014).

Emphasis on Patient/Plan Member/Employee Engagement Much of the ineffectiveness that has been documented related to the delivery of care has been traced to the failure to engage patients, plan members, employees and consumers in positive health behaviors. Social marketing efforts have been primarily geared to mass audiences, and interventions typically involve one-size-fits-all initiatives. A population health approach would involve the identification of subpopulations and their attributes, allowing for engagement efforts customized to the needs of targeted populations. Population health emphasizes the segmentation and profiling of defined populations in terms of their salient characteristics, thereby allowing for more informed intervention efforts.

Attributes of Population Health Management

To distinguish between the population health approach that is the focus of much of this text and the version that is applied within the context of healthcare delivery the term "population health management" is increasingly being used. Efforts at improving the individual experience of care, reducing the per capita cost of care, and improving the health of defined populations can all benefit from a population health approach. Many clinicians and medical managers, in fact, have begun to use the term *population health management* to describe "the iterative process of strategically and proactively managing clinical and financial opportunities to improve health outcomes and patient engagement, while also reducing costs" (Kindig, 2015).

Alternatively, the Agency for Healthcare Research and Quality (AHRQ) uses the term "practice-based population health" to describe the application of population health principles to patient populations (Cusack et al., 2010). The AHRQ definition reads: "an approach to care that uses information on a group of patients within a primary care practice or group of practices to improve the care and clinical outcomes of patients within that practice."

Some efforts geared toward improving the effectiveness of care continue to emphasize (perhaps inappropriately) the care of individual patients. As indicated below, there are ways in which to apply population health principles to the healthcare delivery system.

Segmenting and Profiling Populations and Subpopulations Rather than focusing on the characteristics of individual patients, population health emphasizes the attributes of groups—whether they be patients, employees, plan members or consumers. The need to develop an in-depth understanding of the characteristics of targeted populations has never been greater, and a first step is the identification of meaningful segments within any targeted population. Segmentation could be based on demographic or psychographic characteristics, levels of utilization, at-risk status or a variety of other attributes. Once meaningful segments have been identified they can be profiled in terms of their salient characteristics. This information can then be used as a basis for developing clinical intervention programs, education initiatives, patient engagement plans and any number of other activities supporting healthcare delivery.

Implementing "Group Therapy" While traditional clinical medicine is designed to manage one patient at a time, population health emphasizes the management of groups of patients (however the group may be defined). This may involve something as simple as group diabetes education management efforts or something as complex as developing an advanced treatment strategy for a defined set of patients. With subgroups of patients identified and profiled (see above) programs and initiatives can be developed on an informed basis. All plan members at-risk of diabetes, for example, could be aggregated for particular attention. Efforts to introduce interventions, educational programs, or marketing initiatives can take the characteristics of various population segments into consideration in a more targeted fashion.

Implementing Patient Education One existing activity at most health care organizations that could be considered a candidate for population health management is health education. Various providers have attempted to implement patient education activities for groups of patients who exhibit similar characteristics. Patients, plan members and employees may be at various stages in the process of health improvement and exhibit different levels of health literacy. Some may be only at the point of realizing they have health issues, and others may be informed but unmotivated, and others may actively be involved in positive health behavior and require on-going support. Having identified and profiled meaningful segments of the target population it is possible to tailor educational programs to the needs of the respective segments and develop engagement plans that take these differences into consideration.

Accounting for Life Circumstances One thing that should be clear from previous sections is the importance of non-clinical factors for both health status and health behavior. Life circumstances can perhaps be thought of as the everyday manifestations of the social determinants of health. These are the factors such as health literacy, joblessness, food insecurity, housing insecurity and unsafe neighborhoods that affect both the health status and health behavior of defined populations. We now realize that what has happened to a patient before they enter treatment and what happens to them after they leave treatment often have more of an impact on their clinical outcomes than the actual clinical care provided. Forewarned is forearmed and providers who have prior knowledge of the characteristics of the patients for which they have responsibility should be able to provide better care. Box 8.1 describes how "life circumstances" have relevance for population health management.

Box 8.1: Life Circumstance Intelligence and Patient Care

There is growing concern among healthcare providers, third-party payers and policy makers over the poor outcomes that are being generated by our healthcare system. Further, there are significant disparities in the outcomes for different groups with similar conditions. Members of different racial groups, for example, with similar health conditions, the same level of acuity, and the same treatment in the same health facilities, may record different outcomes suggesting that there are factors other than the quality of medical treatment that contribute to differential outcomes. Increasingly, characteristics attributable to patients before and after medical treatment are being analyzed for their effect on clinical outcomes.

Understandably, physicians exhibit a biomedical bias and place high priority on observed symptoms and diagnostic tests. Little attention is paid to information about a patient's context. Yet, factors like living arrangements may be as significant for the efficacy of treatment as the type of bacteria infecting the patient.

(continued)

Box 8.1 (continued)

A school of thought has developed that the "life circumstances" of patients are important drivers of healthcare outcomes. While there is no consensus with regard to what should be considered as life circumstances at this time, it is clear that certain attributes and conditions affect individual patients and consumers as well as families and households. Important conditions identified include: unemployment, household structure, substandard housing, a lack of health insurance, and low educational attainment. In addition, ethnic group membership, language proficiency and even religious affiliation can represent aspects of life circumstances. These might be thought of as the manifestation of the social determinants of health at the micro-level. These attributes are frequently incorporated into assessments of health disparities within communities and can become deep-rooted attributes that provide an on-going negative backdrop for the lives of affected patients and consumers.

Additional life circumstances attributes likely to affect households include family stability, housing stability (as opposed to housing quality), the safety of the living environment and surrounding community, the quality of the physical environment, and access to affordable healthy food. Other specific factors include access to transportation, personal assistance and access to social support, and information that informs individual health and well-being.

Quantifying the life circumstances of patient and consumer populations is an on-going challenge for healthcare providers, researchers and policy analysts. Much of the data necessary to create life circumstance metrics is not available. Household-level indicators are necessary in order to profile patients in terms of their life circumstances, and this information is often not available to providers.

One health data vendor has attempted to address this issue by developing a Life Circumstance Intelligence (LCI) model that analyzes data on the demographic, psychographic, socioeconomic, and other important characteristics of patients and their households. Developed by Health and Performance Resources, the LCI model compiles data on: household structure, household size, household income, home ownership/rental status, and length of residence. In addition, information is obtained at the household level on communication patterns, communication preferences and personal interests. Insights into the ethnicity, religious affiliation and language preferences are also included.

Access to life circumstances intelligence allows healthcare providers to anticipate social and cultural issues that may be relevant for patient management. To the extent that this type of information can be made available to clinicians prior to treatment, LCI has the potential to improve the effectiveness of patient care. For example, knowing that a scheduled patient lives alone, has a poverty-level income, and limited English proficiency not only makes the clinician aware of potential health challenges but suggests a need for careful discharge planning and aggressive follow-up care.

For additional information on life circumstance intelligence, visit: www.hpranalytics.com.

Predictive Modeling A critical aspect of population health management is the ability to predict the behavior of individual patients—particularly those who are heavy utilizers of services. A major tenet of population health is that we can predict future morbidity patterns with a reasonable level of certainty and, in turn, project the demand for health services of various types. For patient management purposes providers need to be aware of the future characteristics not only of their existing patient pool but those of prospective patients. After all, most of their future patients are not in their patient pool today. Box 8.2 describes the use of predictive modeling at the practice level.

> **Box 8.2: Using Predictive Modeling in Care Delivery**
> The growing popularity of personalized, predictive medicine, and its transformation into predictive modeling has raised the prospect of improved patient care (Saxena, 2015). By combining patient and community data with evidence-based healthcare practices, predictive modeling can make a significant contribution to population health management. Predictive medicine replaces the traditional paper-and-pen approach to collecting patient data by simplifying and personalizing the process. Combining previously stored data about the patient, mass amounts of evidence-based medical information and a user-friendly data infrastructure, predictive medicine can estimate when patients will become ill or when they'll be at risk for various health conditions. Including information on patients' life circumstances brings an additional dimension to this effort.
>
> In addition, predictive modeling allows physicians to catch conditions *before* they turn into medical emergencies or cause lasting damage. Patient alerts allow primary care physicians to handle preventive care in the office, freeing up emergency department doctors' time and workloads. It also cuts down on the amount of care needed to improve the health of individual patients. Patients are also empowered to be more proactive through knowledge of which symptoms qualify as actual medical emergencies, thus preventing unnecessary trips to the emergency department (ED) and avoiding further congesting the ED.
>
> When care providers are armed with information before patients are in the office, they can anticipate possible diagnoses. While this information may not always lead to a final diagnosis, it does allow providers to narrow down possible ailments. This capability not only can cut down patient wait time, but also free up more time for providers to help other waiting patients.
>
> While predictive modeling concerns individual patients, this technique can combine individual patients' data to give a picture of the health system's entire patient population. Expanding the principles of personalized medicine to hospitals and clinics, predictive modeling allows healthcare administrators to transform collected data into insightful guidelines for managing the future demands on the healthcare system. For example, predictive modeling could help administrators

(continued)

> **Box 8.2** (continued)
> more accurately forecast the number of patients who will arrive at the ED on a given day. This insight can aid administrators in making more informed decisions concerning everything from staff scheduling to supply ordering.
>
> Predictive modeling already has been used to lower wait times in certain healthcare facilities. Administrators at Johns Hopkins Hospital used predictive modeling and interactive software to lower patient wait times in their ED from an average of 10 hours to 4 hours in just one year. At Massachusetts Institute of Technology applying predictive parameters to hospital waiting rooms has been proven to lower ED wait times by 10% (or approximately 40 minutes).

Community Health Needs Assessment Progressive healthcare organizations have historically conducted community health needs assessments of various types—typically for the own strategic planning purposes. Now—at least for certain hospitals—this is not an option as the Affordable Care Act requires not-for-profit hospitals to conduct a comprehensive community health needs assessment at least every 3 years. Tax-exempt hospitals must demonstrate an understanding of the healthcare needs of the total community (even those segments that it does not serve), identify gaps in services (even those that it does not provide), and formulate a plan for addressing the gaps that have been identified. A key factor here is that the emphasis is on *consumers* and not just existing patients. Thus, a major hospital has to look beyond its walls into the community to identify issues that it must address even if they are not related to a service it provides. For example, Hospital ABC does not provide behavioral health services but finds through the community assessment process that there is a serious gap between the needs of the community and the behavioral health services that are available. Theoretically, at least, this hospital must quantify these gaps, demonstrate to the federal government that it has a plan to address them, and be able to document through subsequent assessments its effectiveness in helping to close the identified gap. Box 8.3 presents an example of the use of a CHNA for population health management.

Geospatial Analysis of Health Problems The healthcare industry has been slow to adopt the use of geographic information systems (GIS). Yet, this technology can be invaluable for population health management. Health problems are not randomly distributed within the population but exhibit spatially dependent patterns, and today the importance of the spatial dimension of health problems is finally being recognized. A growing body of evidence has linked health status to geographic location, and as noted one's ZIP Code of residence has been recognized as an important predictor of health status (Roeder, 2014). In applying population health management, it should be noted that existing patients all have a geographic identifier, and there is going to be a wide range of attributes associated with the location of residence. Patients for a particular provider often cluster in certain locations, and the health conditions that are likely to affect a given patient population can be linked to specific geographic areas. Box 8.4 presents a case study of the use of spatial analysis in the tracking of burn patients.

Box 8.3: Using a Community Health Needs Assessment to Improve Patient Care

A major hospital system in a medium-sized Southern city conducted a comprehensive community health needs assessment in compliance with the Affordable Care Act. In conducting the assessment, the analysts discovered a particular ZIP Code whose residents were responsible for a large proportion of the hospital's uncompensated care. Additional research was conducted to determine the nature of the issues surrounding the high use of healthcare resources by residents of this particular community.

The research uncovered a significant number of residents with co-morbid chronic conditions who were frequent users of the hospital's emergency department and regularly admitted as inpatients. It was also found that these high utilizers were clustered in certain locations suggesting that the local environment had an impact on health status and that there was a culture of ill-health characterisitic of these patients that led them to use similar health services.

The research also found that there was a significant portion of the population, as yet undiagnosed, at high risk for chronic conditions, particularly diabetes. The remainder of the population was only at moderate risk but, given the illness-inducing attributes of the community, there was concern over their future health status. Each of the three populations—high utilizers, high-risk and low-risk—were profiled in terms of their demographic, socioeconomic and psychographic characteristics. This information was used to inform the development of customized programs for each of these groups.

As a result of this exercise the hospital developed a three-tiered approach for addressing the health issues facing this community. For the 100 chronically ill high utilizers a case management program was established that involved the micromanagement of the care for each of these patients. Efforts were made to assure they received timely treatment, adhered to their medical regimen, and to the extent possible maintained a healthy lifestyle. For the estimated 4000 at-risk residents, an intensive patient education effort was developed that targeted their areas of residence. Like the high utilizers, the at-risk populations also tended to cluster together. For the relatively healthy low-risk population a social marketing program was developed that provided general information on healthy lifestyles and prevention.

Although the impact of such programs is difficult to quantify, the case management efforts vis-à-vis the high utilizers paid significant dividends in terms of reduced emergency department utilization and inpatient admissions. Many of the 4000 at-risk patients who received screening and prevention materials actually entered treatment programs for chronic conditions, although it is difficult to determine how much impact the hospital initiative had in this regard. Follow-up surveys by hospital analysts found that members of the general population (low-risk segment) had been exposed to health education materials, and many had actually participated in health fairs located in areas with concentrations of high-risk residents.

(continued)

Marketing Services to Patients and Consumers While some marketing efforts by healthcare providers might be considered "internal" in that they seek to develop relationships with existing customers in order to retain their business and cross-sell other products and services, the majority of marketing efforts are directed toward external markets. There is clearly a role here for the application of population health principles (as reflected in the section above on segmenting and profiling target populations). After years of mass marketing efforts on the part of healthcare providers, it was finally realized that the demand for healthcare does not represent a mass market. At any given time only some segment of the population is in need of health services (particularly complex services) and different segments of the population have different needs and respond to different types of marketing appeals. With the need for patients, plan members, employees and consumers to become engaged in positive health behavior, well-crafted marketing efforts are required. Box 8.5 discusses the role of marketing in promoting the population health approach.

Creating Financial Efficiencies and Maximizing Revenue The financial welfare of healthcare providers is never far from the surface and, not surprisingly, efforts toward population health management often focus on introducing financial efficiencies and maximizing revenue. Measures of success are increasingly focusing on the extent to which providers or health plans are providing cost-effective services. Providers that hope to survive the current environment must be able to control costs

---

Box 8.4: Using Spatial Analysis to Predict Pediatric Burn Care Needs
In an effect to understand the nature of pediatric burn injuries and the children that they affect, researchers in St. Louis, Missouri, examined data on pediatric burn cases from two children's hospitals. It was felt that a better understanding of the geographic distribution of burn cases would provide information for better anticipating future needs and hence providing more effective services to the affected population. Further, it was felt that this information would contribute to better prevention efforts.

Data were collected on over 300 children from the city of St. Louis who received burn treatment within a specified year. The patients were profiled in terms of their relevant characteristics and their place of residence. Patient addresses were matched to block groups using a geographic information system (GIS). Burn injury rates were calculated based on geography a propensity rating system developed for projecting future burn cases. Mapping software utilizing Bayesian analysis was utilized to create maps of burn rates and risk levels for the city of St. Louis.

(continued)

Box 8.4 (continued)

The researchers found that burn injuries were not randomly distributed across the city and were in fact <u>clustered</u> in certain sections. A wide range of injury rates was discovered with a particular concentration of burn injuries in North St. Louis. This high-risk geographic area was further disaggregated to reveal the highest risk areas within that community. The researchers were able to develop a hierarchy of risk linked to the various geographic subareas of the city. The map below illustrates the distribution of burn cases within the city of St. Louis.

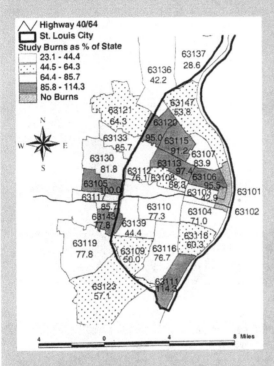

Burn Rates Reported by Study Hospitals

The researchers demonstrated the utility of using spatial analysis to analyze the distribution of burn injuries within a defined area. The combination of mapping injury rates and spatial analysis provided a detailed level of injury surveillance not available through any other means. Armed with this information, planning for prevention programs and the delivery of pediatric burn services could be carried out on an informed basis.

Source: Williams et al. (2003)

Box 8.5: Advancing Population Health: The Role of Marketing
Despite the apparent success of clinical medicine in the United States there is growing concern that the historical approach to care that emphasizes individual treatment has ceased to be effective at improving community health. This perspective is mostly foreign to healthcare providers who are unlikely to be cognizant of the social determinants of health contributing to their patients' pathology nor of the implications of life circumstances that affect their patients before they receive clinical care and after they leave treatment. It could be argued that the failure of the existing healthcare system to address population health issues is less a function of structural deficiencies—although these certainly play a part—and more a function of the manner in which resources are deployed.

This brings us to the issue of healthcare marketing and its role in promoting population health. It could be argued in fact that, from a population health perspective, the past efforts of marketers have been misdirected and have contributed to the problems inherent in the system. In the guise of "following orders" healthcare marketers could be accused of promoting the wrong services to the wrong populations, of marketing products that do not contribute to community health, and even of marketing services that may be detrimental to health.

The standard approach to marketing health services involves: marketing to individuals rather than groups, marketing to patients rather than consumers, marketing "downstream" rather than "upstream," marketing to sick people rather than well people, and promoting the "wrong" services. In view of historical incentives related to the healthcare system, this is exactly what marketers would be expected to do. At the end of the day, however, none of these actions can be considered to contribute to population health improvement. In some cases, it could be argued, they don't even contribute to personal health improvement and may, in fact, exert a negative pressure on health status.

In order to adapt to the changing demands of a population health approach, a major rethinking of healthcare marketing must occur. First, marketers must utilize their in-depth community knowledge as a foundation for population health initiatives. Marketers know more about the characteristics of patients and consumers than clinicians, yet this knowledge is often underutilized. Providers, of necessity, have a fractured perception of the characteristics of their patients. Even the most thorough assessment is not likely to reveal pertinent attributes that have implications for patient management. Even more important, marketers are likely to be familiar with the non-medical factors that contribute to health status—life circumstances, lifestyles and social contexts—factors now considered as important to patient outcomes as the

(continued)

> **Box 8.5** (continued)
>
> clinical treatment received. Marketers are also likely to be familiar with the motivations characteristic of various groups of consumers.
>
> Second, marketers are well acquainted with methods for influencing *groups* of consumers. Most marketing is geared toward the entire population or major subsets of the population, and this is an area where marketers have the expertise to profile populations and develop appropriately designed marketing initiatives. Third, marketers recognize the importance of the differentials that exist among subgroups within the population and have the capability to segment the population into meaningful subgroups. Different segments, for example, are likely to be at different stages in the continuum from awareness to action with regard to positive health behavior and, thus, require differing marketing approaches. Not only is this a necessary step in developing an informed marketing plan, but careful segmentation allows for efficient allocation of marketing resources.
>
> Finally, marketers have the skills necessary for engaging target populations in various behaviors. Most population health initiatives call for active participation of targeted populations. Indeed, the failure of many initiatives promoting improved health status reflect not flaws in the proposed intervention but an inability to engage members of the target audience in appropriate behaviors. Ultimately, providers are going to be evaluated (and rewarded), on the one hand, based on the extent to which their patient pool demonstrated more positive health behaviors and, on the other, on the extent to which the provider contributed to overall improvement in the health status of the community.
>
> Perhaps the most important role that the marketer of the future can play in promoting better community health status is as the "bridge" between the healthcare system and the community. Unlike all other parties, the marketer is in a position to view the situation from both sides of the street—from the perspective of the provider who is using his or her services and from the prospective of the consumers that the marketer is targeting. No one else is in a position to reconcile these perspectives and encourage the interface of personal health and population health.

and maximize revenue. CMS is increasingly offering financial incentives to Medicare providers who manage patients efficiently. To this end a number of vendors have developed methodologies (often under the label "population health") for assisting providers, health plans and accountable care organizations in improving their financial performance. CMS has encouraged such activity through its "shared savings" initiative. Box 8.6 provides an example of the shared savings approach.

Box 8.6: Using Population Health Management with Shared Savings Programs

The Integrated Health Association (IHA) is a statewide multi-stakeholder leadership group that promotes quality improvement, accountability and affordability of health care in California. Through its various partners it covers 875,000 Blue Shield members and is served by 135 physician groups. Its effort to align the pay-for-performance (P4P) programs of the largest commercial insurers in the state through consolidated measurement and the use of a common set of measures and methodology has attracted national attention.

The IHA P4P program was originally organized to develop statewide metrics and measurement activity because medical groups voiced concerned that their performance varied by health plan for the same measures. IHA added a Shared Savings, or "gainsharing", provision in order to augment its P4P program with efficiency incentives. Most of the California health plans faced deficits and needed to find new ways to effectively engage medical groups around efficiency.

To this end IHA developed initiatives designed to decrease variation in provider performance, improve quality, and lower the rate of spending growth. This effort centered on a series of resource use measures. Risk-adjusted rates were calculated using data from all of the IHA participating health plans, and the health plans then calculated savings using their own unit cost data. The initiative was hampered because health plans were hesitant to change the physician payment methods they had been using. Further, various plans addressed cost savings and pay-for-performance in different ways.

Despite the challenges, IHA was able to demonstrate considerable success. The largest savings were generated through the use of free-standing ambulatory surgical centers (ASCs). Blue Shield gave medical groups listings of contracted ASCs and made them aware of the services that were available in each. The medical groups were then able to move the percentage of patients receiving outpatient surgery in outpatient hospital surgical units to ASCs. Blue Shield focused on those members already receiving outpatient surgery and did not try to move inpatient surgeries to outpatient. The most pharmacy success was seen where Blue Shield could steer targeted messaging to practices (e.g., use of proton pump inhibitors, hypertension medications). Overall, two-thirds of the provider groups received some payout, and the groups have received the program positively.

The IHA initiative represents a useful example of population health management in that it utilizes actionable data to influence the behavior of groups of patients with the ultimate result of more effective care and subsequent cost savings for participating health plans.

Source: National Business Coalition on Health (2011)

Barriers to Population Health Management

Healthcare providers are naturally drawn to population health management since it involves activities with which they are already familiar. Despite this growing affinity for population health management, there are a number of factors that present challenges to applying this methodology within the context of healthcare delivery.

Limited Appreciation of Population Health and its Usefulness Despite the growing interest in population health, many if not most healthcare providers have a limited understanding of what it involves. Few in fact appreciate the macro-level application of population health while more are beginning to appreciate its application to the delivery of care. When health professionals consider challenges related to the delivery of care, they most frequently consider such things as the efficient processing of patients, utilization management and revenue maximization. These are pressing concerns for healthcare administrators, but the usefulness of population health management is not likely to be immediately obvious under the pressure of delivering care.

Lack of Appreciation for the Non-clinical Contributors to Health Status To the extent that the population health approach can be applied to the delivery of care, a major benefit is its emphasis on the non-clinical aspects of care. Few providers, however, are aware of the influence of poverty, inadequate housing, food insecurity and domestic violence on the health of their patient populations. Part of the failure to acknowledge the importance of social determinants is the notion that things that go on "out there" outside the walls of the institution are beyond the influence of healthcare providers. To a great extent, this is true (and will be discussed in a later section), yet better care can presumably be provided if providers are armed in advance with information on the life circumstances of their patients and the potential importance of social determinants on their patients' health status.

Lack of Incentives to Incorporate Population Health Management Historically there has been pressure on healthcare providers to process as many patients as possible as efficiently as possible. In fact, the pressure to do so has only increased as managed care arrangements have become widespread and increasing numbers of physicians are working under quotas as employees. This is not an environment that encourages the thoughtful introduction of population health management, and existing financial incentives typically do not encourage the activities that would be implemented through a population health approach. Not only do financial considerations influence consumer and patient behavior, they also influence the practice patterns of physicians. If there are financial incentives encouraging physicians to see more patients, conduct more tests, or provide more services, physicians will respond rationally by increasing volumes. Certainly, incentives are changing rapidly as the emphasis shifts to ensuring greater access, more effective outcomes and lower costs, but these new incentives have to be incorporated into the system before many providers embark on radical restructuring.

Discontinuity with Other Types of Non-medical Services It has become increasingly clear that medical care alone cannot advance population health. A comprehensive range of services is required to supplement the benefits of clinical medicine. Given the extent to which non-clinical factors contribute to health status, the system must be able to link healthcare providers with the providers of services existing independent of medical care. Obvious possibilities that come to mind are dentists, eyecare specialists, mental health counselors and social workers.

There is also a wide range of services thought to have an impact on clinical outcomes that are not typically considered by the system. These include services related to housing, food security, personal safety, environmental threats and the range of social determinants discussed in previous chapters. The lack of interface between providers of clinical services and these "external" service providers and the absence of financial incentives to establish such interfaces represent clear barriers to the implementation of population health management.

Lack of the Necessary Data to Support Population Health Management While significant advances have been made in accessing and analyzing the voluminous amount of clinical data available to healthcare providers, gaps remain with regard to the data required for population health management. Most data focus on historical utilization patterns for existing patients and do not provide much assistance to clinicians and administrators seeking to employ population health management. There is a lack of actionable data to allow practitioners to appreciate the factors that influence the health status and clinical outcomes for their patients, plan members or employees. Providers have limited information, for example, on the life circumstances that are likely to affect their patients' health status and their ability to benefit from treatment, information that is not likely to be obtained during history taking. For example, a clinician is not likely to know the economic circumstances of a patient (although these are of immense importance for the patient) and may not even know what type of insurance coverage (if any) a patient has. Similarly, a clinician is not likely to know the living arrangements of the patient, although these are likely to affect one's ability to adhere to a medical regimen.

Lack of Tools for Population Health Management There is no doubt that the amount of knowledge—and the expertise required of physicians—has increased exponentially in recent years. However, it is impossible for the best-informed physician to be knowledgeable concerning the range of factors that contribute to health status and health behavior. Further, within a population health framework providers need access to information—particularly of a non-medical nature—that would support their decision making. Not only are the requisite data not available but there are few tools available to the practitioner for applying population health management. To effectively apply this model practitioners need a toolkit that allows them to input the available data and generate "red flags" that would allow them to anticipate health problems and challenges to care on the part of their patients. These same needs exist with regard to insurance plan members and employees.

The Role of Healthcare in Population Health Improvement

As noted above, the application of the population health model at the macro-level is considered a more appropriate approach by most proponents of the population health concept. It is argued that the traditional *population health* definition should be reserved for geographically or demographically defined populations—populations that are the concern of public health officials, community organizations, and business leaders rather than the healthcare system. In this regard, Jacobson and Teutsch (2012) recommended to the National Quality Forum that "current use of the abbreviated phrase *population health* should be abandoned and replaced by the phrase *total population health*."

There are three components that come into play in efforts to improve population health: (1) clinical care; (2) social determinant modification; and (3) policy formulation. The clinical care component is the primary area in which the healthcare system is expected to have an impact. In thinking about improving population health one naturally thinks first of the healthcare delivery system and the tremendous resources at its disposal. Based on past successes it is not surprising that many—particularly health professionals—place unmerited faith in the system's ability to improve population health.

If the healthcare system is to have any relevance to this discussion of the three components, it has the most influence on the clinical care component. While the past accomplishments of medical science are unarguable, the question arises even here as to how effective the healthcare system is in this sphere. The deficiencies characterizing the system have been enumerated elsewhere, and except for the implementation of life-saving procedures, the current benefits of the healthcare system are thought to be limited. There are a number of reasons why the healthcare system is not in a position to lead the effort toward community health improvement and, in fact, may not be in a position to make a significant contribution to this effort.

Some population health purists would argue, in fact, that there is virtually no role for the healthcare system in population health improvement. Those taking that approach argue that even within the limited clinical care sphere the healthcare system is contributing more to the problem than to the solution and that any progress that is being made toward population health improvement is in spite of the healthcare system rather than because of it. In view of the uncertainty surrounding the contribution of the healthcare system to population health improvement, its role in this process needs to be carefully considered.

The healthcare delivery system has the potential to influence some factors related to social determinants, but this component can only be impacted by the health professionals actually looking beyond their own walls and thinking well outside the box. There is clearly not a very direct path for the healthcare system to affect poverty, housing insecurity, environmental threats, unsafe communities and so forth.

The final component—policy formulation—is essentially beyond the purview of the healthcare system. Health professionals are not in a position to influence policy at any level of government, and even the organizations that represent them (e.g., American Medical Association, American Public Health Association) have relatively less influence than policy-makers who are outside the healthcare arena.

There is now general agreement that medical care accounts for only about 10% of the variation in health status found in the US population. Yet 90% of our resources are devoted to clinical care at the expense of public health and to the exclusion of social concerns and policy matters. Further, as the situation has evolved, it is hard to imagine that even this figure can hold up, especially considering the extent of health problems actually caused by the healthcare system and the injuries and deaths resulting from inappropriate and/or unnecessary treatment.

A major limitation when it comes to the ability of the healthcare system to improve community health is its restricted range of vision. The healthcare system holds a fairly narrow view of health status and the factors considered in its assessment, yet the population health approach requires an expansive perspective. Healthcare providers are not trained for and often have little capacity to address the non-medical health issues of their own patients—much less those of the total population. While some engage in health promotion, health education and related prevention activities, the focus is usually on screening, detection and follow-up care for specific health conditions affecting a defined population.

Through no fault of individual practitioners, the primary barrier to a more comprehensive perspective is the existing structure of the healthcare delivery system and its supporting components (e.g., medical education, research). The premises underlying this structure are inimical to population health. It should be no surprise that practitioners (and this includes medical educators and researchers) are not sensitive to the significance of non-clinical factors; the structure of the healthcare system precludes it.

Medical science as it is taught and practiced retains a twentieth century mindset that focuses on treatment and cure (rather than prevention), on the importance of biological rather than social etiology, on "downstream" responses rather than proactive "upstream" actions, and on clinical care as the almost exclusive answer to observed health problems. Further, virtually all financial incentives and opportunities for professional recognition and advancement encourage practitioners to buy into premises that are no longer valid. Given this situation it is not surprising that physicians do not receive training in a variety of areas that are relevant to the implementation of even a population health management effort. Box 8.7 discusses topics that doctors should be familiar with but are not covered extensively in medical school.

With few exceptions, healthcare delivery systems have never had to deal with the social determinants of health and certainly not to the degree that public health

> **Box 8.7: What Every Doctor Should Know but Is Not Taught in Medical School**
>
> Research on patients visiting physician offices has found that a large portion of those presenting for care do not actually have physical health problems. While non-medical conditions may manifest themselves through physical symptoms, in a large proportion of the cases a non-medical condition has resulted in the office visit. Increasingly we find patients presenting with emotional or mental disturbances, nutritional, weight or metabolic problems, sexual disorders, addictive behaviors, and so forth. Yet, the medical school curriculum offers limited training in these areas and does not accord them the attention that their prevalence merits.
>
> Despite revisions of most medical school curricula in recent years, it is still the case that doctors-in-training receive limited exposure to information nutrition and diet, weight management and even eating disorders. Their advice on healthy lifestyles, in fact, is likely to be limited to "eat less and exercise more." Although there is typically a clinical rotation in psychiatry, there is limited exposure to psychological and emotional issues, behavioral health issues and addictive behaviors. Limited attention is paid to domestic violence and child abuse and the whole notion of family health (physical and mental) is honored more in concept than in practice. There is little exposure to sexuality and sexual dysfunction, and women's health issues, in particular, are given short shrift. Although chronic disease management is being increasingly emphasized, there is little emphasis on geriatric care even as the elderly population accounts for most chronic conditions. Despite the increased recognition given to oral health as a factor in physical health, this topic is also neglected. The importance of spirituality to health has been neglected for decades and is only now being revisited in medical school.
>
> Beyond these deficiencies related to the delivery of care, other factors that limit physicians' appreciation of population health issues is their lack of exposure to the social determinants of ill-health or to the influence of the physical and social environment on their patients' health. They even receive limited exposure to public health. Given the content of medical education it is not difficult to understand the lack of appreciation on the part of physicians of the significance of population health.

systems have. The American Hospital Association identified over 20 factors that influence health status but are outside the purview of the healthcare system (Hospital Research & Educational Trust, 2012). The narrow perspective of the healthcare system causes practitioners to focus on their patients to the exclusion of other populations. The recognition of these factors is an important first step in adopting a population health approach, but there is a long road from recognition to meaningful action.

By the same token, when solutions are proposed for ameliorating poor health status, they typically reflect the perspectives of the healthcare community and not those of affected population groups. An earlier chapter noted that the general public has a much different perception of community health problems than the medical establishment. To the extent that representatives of the healthcare system have proposed community-based solutions, these interventions have been imposed from the "outside" without consideration of the perspectives of the affected group. As a result, most such initiatives have not had a significant impact, nor have they contributed to sustained community health improvement. Most of these efforts involve imposing more of the same on populations that have not responded positively to similar initiatives in the past. Over the decades untold amounts of money, programs, personnel and effort have been applied toward the amelioration of persistent health problems and, yet, we find ourselves today with an increasingly sick population. The standard intervention involves a clinical medicine perspective that typically does not even reflect the paradigm shift from medical care to healthcare, much less the movement toward population health.

To the extent that a comprehensive approach is required for advancing population health that integrates a wide range of medical and non-medical services, healthcare providers are at a disadvantage. Providers often do not know the extent of the non-medical "treatment" that is required by their patients nor what resources are available within their communities. While evidence-based treatment for chronic conditions is constantly being advanced, the population continues to get "sicker" and little or no improvement in community health status is observed (Hagland, 2015). The system must be able to link healthcare providers with the providers of services existing independent of medical care. This includes the wide range of supportive clinical services and ancillary services that exist outside the healthcare arena. While some providers have established informal or formal relationships with other providers of health or social services, there is a wide range of services thought to have an impact on clinical outcomes that are typically not considered by the system.

Representatives of the healthcare system are at best vaguely aware of the role of the environment on the health of their patients and almost totally unaware of the environment's impact on the general population. It is not surprising that clinicians are not sensitive to the connection between social conditions and health status. They often do not understand that the environment—social and/or physical—has more influence on health status then the armamentarium that health professionals can bring to bear (Ellaway, 2014). For example, there is growing evidence that the best predictor of even clinical outcomes are non-medical factors—the patient's history, lifestyle, social circumstances and demographic traits.

Even for physicians who understand the role a patient's social context may play in their health status and the progression of a disease, this context is rarely taken into consideration in treatment planning and the provider's expectations of the patient. At the same time, it would be impossible for healthcare providers to not note the impact of life circumstances on some of their patients, to bemoan a lack of compliance with "doctor's orders", and to observe the frequent recidivism of their patients. Unfortunately, these fragmented and sporadic glimpses into the role of the environment on health status do not provide a basis for assessment much less action. Thus, patients with the same or similar treatment plans from the same institution often exhibit quite different outcomes as the result of disparities and barriers that have virtually nothing to do with the care received (Hopper, 2011).

Further, a local healthcare system faces a major drawback when it comes to population health that communities are not likely to face. There are parties within healthcare that are not enthusiastic about improving the overall health status of the population and may, in fact, create institutional barriers. These parties are doing quite well financially under the current system and may stand to lose influence and wealth should health status improve. While there may be those with vested interests in other spheres within the community that may be ambivalent with regard to efforts at population health improvement, few representatives of these entities are likely to publicly state that they are opposed to improving health status or to openly block these initiatives. However, there is every reason to believe that vested interests in healthcare would be willing to thwart efforts at improving health status if it preserved their financial position. (See, for example, the case of the Susan B. Komen Foundation as reported by Swissler [2015]).

In the third domain—public policy—the role of the healthcare system is very limited. Although there is certainly some concern among providers over national and/or state-level health policies, most providers remain uninformed and/or uninvolved with regard to the policy sphere. While they may have some understanding of public health policies and procedures from a system and community perspective (and strong opinions with regard to government regulations and programs), they are typically not aware of the implications of public policies and regulations as they affect patient health. This is especially the case with policies that are outside the sphere of healthcare and affect some seemingly unrelated aspect of the community (e.g., housing, employment, education).

This situation partly reflects the lack of interface between the healthcare system and the public health establishment. Public health officials are, by definition, more concerned with policy issues than private sector practitioners. They live in a world of government regulations and deal every day with policy issues if only implicitly. The fact that there is so little interface between the two sectors is emblematic of the lack of coordination inherent in our system. Indeed, in response the Affordable Care Act mandated that not-for-profit hospitals seek input from public health authorities in the development of the required comprehensive community health assessments.

This leaves most of the policy "space" unaffected by the healthcare system, except, for lobbying efforts on the part of those representing public and private health interests. The public health establishment is noteworthy for its efforts in this regard at the national and state levels. Yet, to the extent that APHA efforts have been successful, few of these advances have been adopted by private sector medicine. Representatives of the private sector focus almost entirely on the defense of their interests and not on behalf of patients or consumers. Even here it is found that the American Medical Association (AMA), the presumed "voice" of American physicians focuses its efforts almost entirely on the welfare of the organization, often to the detriment of both physicians and patients (Gorman, 2009).

While national-level policies (e.g., economic development, housing, nutrition, physical activity, education) may have some relevance for population health, most policy changes will have to take place at the state and/or local levels and are essentially beyond the control of the healthcare system. Next to education, state legislatures allocate more funds for healthcare than for any other function. Yet decisions concerning the allocation and disbursement of these funds are often driven more by political than health-related concerns. Since each state has a department of health the potential is there for input into health policy decision-making on the part of public health interests. The private health sector, on the other hand, is only likely to have input through lobbyists, making for very inconsistent state-by-state input. Indeed, recent state-level decisions concerning the expansion of Medicare under the Affordable Care Act have been essentially political decisions unaffected by the objections of representatives of both the public and private health sectors.

The Role of the Healthcare System in Population Health

Of the three areas of concern, the healthcare system only interfaces with the clinical care component—with limited ability to address social determinants or influence policy formulation. There are too many disincentives to reasonably expect the healthcare system to take a lead role in this process, and these barriers are presented above. Yet the system has an important role to play albeit a supporting one. A case is made later for the role of the community—however defined—in implementing a population health approach. Given the social determinants of ill-health, it could be argued that only through the collective impact of a variety of community forces can a population health approach be successful.

While it is essential to have healthcare providers as part of a "team" approach to patient care their role in population health should be limited to improving clinical decision-making and patient adherence, and only then if the patient's life circumstances are taken into consideration. Even this role should be informed by community data and patient information that is not normally available to practitioners. Ideally, the medical community will be turned to whenever there is a need for input related to the management (within the community) of a health issue. Even here, however, it is likely to be public health officials who have the most to offer.

One clear role for the healthcare system is in the area of partnership development. While virtually every hospital maintains partnerships within the community, the relationships are often limited to organizations that have direct bearing on the delivery of care or represent social causes in which the hospital may have an interest. However, the scope of these partnerships is likely to be limited leaving a wide swath of community organizations outside the circle.

In order to support the population health movement, a web of partnerships has to be established that encompasses all aspects of the community that have relevance for population health. There are examples across the nation of efforts to create health consortiums, often including non-healthcare entities. And certainly, there are community-based coalitions that attempt bring together the various interests within the community in order to create some level of collective impact. As yet, it seems there are no examples of community-wide coalitions that include all relevant healthcare entities and all of the various community-based organizations and government entities that could be expected to impact population health.

A population health approach is needed that is "systemic" but targeted to what can be changed in a limited amount of time and with limited resources—that is, an approach that emphasizes changes in services offered, the social context, and the physical infrastructure of communities. A focus on strategies to overcome current structural and functional barriers that negatively affect health status and access to care-seeking behavior is needed. Box 8.8 describes attempts to merge the management of personal health concerns with the population health model.

> **Box 8.8: Merging Personal Health and Population Health**
> In view of the seemingly mutually exclusive nature of population health and population health management, is there any potential for interfacing or perhaps merging these two perspectives? Despite the respective stances on population health, there do appear to be ways in which the two seemingly disparate perspectives can be seen to merge. The proponents of population health management must first come to appreciate the broader application of population health that exists primarily outside the walls of healthcare institutions. This is understandably a challenge for practitioners who are in the trenches. Further, it has been demonstrated that people are not likely to develop an understanding of a concept if their income depends on them *not* understanding it.
>
> That being said, those involved in healthcare delivery must come to appreciate the principles of population health and strive to apply them to the practice setting. A large part of this is shifting the emphasis from individuals to groups with the intention of advancing the health status of the entire patient pool rather than individual patients. This may mean something as simple as providing the same educational input to the total patient population rather than just those with existing diagnoses.
>
> Further, those in healthcare delivery need to look beyond their walls for three major reasons. First, most of the health problems today are originating "out there"—i.e., they are being driven by environmental factors, social conditions, life circumstances and so forth that are non-clinical in nature. The first principal of diagnosis is to determine the cause, and this will take a change in mindset among practitioners. Second, it is the social, cultural and economic attributes of patients that are driving much of their behavior. The facts that they were exposed to a health risk in the first place, that they chose to present themselves for treatment, and that they may or may not follow doctor's orders reflect the social context in which they live. Third, the focus needs to shift away from patients to consumers, on the assumption that health status can

(continued)

Box 8.8 (continued)

only be improved if the total population is included and not just existing patients.

Unless the non-medical attributes of patients are taken into consideration medical care will have limited effect. The facts that patients report recurrences of previously "cured" conditions and that non-medical factors are driving hospital readmissions indicates a need to better employ resources outside of the healthcare system to address these issues. Progressive health care organizations involved in *population health management* are working with other partners to advance *total population health* across geographic populations, with these efforts considered as *"population medicine expanding into total population health" (Health Catalyst, 2016)*. At the same time, clinicians are in a position to provide feedback to those taking a broader population health approach. For example, to the extent that the life circumstances of patients are taken into consideration, how helpful is this to clinicians for more efficient diagnosis and the development of care plans? What different information might be useful? What other resources might be brought to bear?

As we begin to understand populations, the lines between a population management/medicine focus on healthcare services and a population health focus on the broader determinants of health become blurry with certain population segments. The identification, understanding, and segmentation of a population; the redesign of services for that population; and the delivery of those services at scale require organizations to understand and address the broader social, environmental, and behavioral determinants of health in order to achieve better outcomes, improve the care experience, and control total cost (Lewis, 2014).

Proponents of population health must conceptualize ways in which population health principles can be applied within the healthcare delivery system. Substantial research is on-going related to the social determinants of health and how, ultimately, they may impact individual patients. Information gained and lessons learned should be channeled back into the healthcare system to support population health management efforts. Population health proponents should harness the private sector of the community to provide input into the care delivery process and to coordinate public/private efforts toward population health improvement.

The healthcare system is going to require more comprehensive data than in the past and the ability to access it. The system is essentially limited to the data that it generates internally and occasional market data. Yet, effective population health management is going to require external data on a variety of topics—topics only limited by the breadth of the social determinants involved. Agencies outside of healthcare can play a role in generating and disseminating data to healthcare providers that they would not otherwise have access to

(continued)

> **Box 8.8** (continued)
>
> (e.g., life circumstance intelligence) or even know they need. Bare facts are worthwhile but healthcare organizations need the ability to manipulate data in support of population health management. This means that tools must be made available to them that they can use to interface external and internal data and perform the analyses required. The community health needs assessment tool developed by the Healthy Communities Institute is an example (Healthy Communities Institute, 2014).
>
> Finally, the healthcare system is used to operating as an independent entity essentially isolated in terms of healthcare delivery from the other institutions of society. Guidance will be required with regard to the interface of healthcare with other institutions and the development of a working relationship with disparate organizations.

A New Mindset

The previous sections should make it clear that the population health approach requires an entirely different mindset on the part of healthcare professionals—whether operating at the micro- or macro-level. Progressive healthcare organizations that understand and implement a population health strategy will be positioned to not only respond to the demands of regulators, insurers, and government mandates but to proactively address the needs of their service area populations.

Adopting a population health approach, it must be conceded, is not an easy task. In effect, this approach sets the healthcare system on its head. Health professionals must forget much of what they know about health and healthcare delivery in order to adopt a perspective that supports a population health approach. This will require a different mindset that thinks in terms of populations not individuals, of consumers not patients, of prevention not cure, and of non-traditional approaches to improving community health. This type of outside-the-box thinking represents a challenge for health professionals but is a requirement for the adoption of a population health approach.

In keeping with a new mindset, healthcare entities must transform themselves into the type of organization that can operate within a population health model. This involves an even more radical conversion since we are advocating changing the direction of an "ocean liner" in a very short period of time. Organizational transformation is already underway at a number of healthcare organizations. Too often, however, this transformation is limited to trying to adapt existing processes to the new environment. Unfortunately, there can be no "business as usual" in the future. Healthcare organizations are going to have to recreate themselves to survive in the new environment—an environment that emphasizes outcomes over volume, quality over quantity, prevention over treatment, and keeping people out of treatment. These types of mandates can be expected to increase in the future as payers, government regulators and policy makers realize that the only way to improve community health status is through a population health approach.

According to Health Catalyst (2016), in order to have any significant impact on population health the healthcare system must make major changes. Healthcare delivery systems must add public health professionals and epidemiologists to their management and executive staff. They need to build the skills to interact with and develop health intervention strategies in concert with law enforcement; social support services in the community, including charitable and religious organizations; job growth and economic development in communities that ensures patients can afford care when they need it; adequate affordable housing in the community; and healthy options for eating in the community. They must assure access to adequate dental care; primary and secondary education programs that encourage healthy lifestyles; violent crime reduction; and environmental strategies to ensure that communities have clean air and water. These are traditional public health issues that health professionals need to apply in the healthcare arena in order to promote population health.

At the end of the day, health issues are not a health system problem, they are a societal problem. No longer can the issues facing our society be shunted off to be addressed within the walls of our healthcare institutions. They are not in a position to do this and we should not expect them. As demonstrated in the next chapter population health is increasingly becoming a community issue that will require collective impact for its management.

Summary

Population health purists would argue that it is not appropriate to apply the term "population health" to any activity that focuses on clinical care and/or individual patients, and a case can be made that the term "population health" should be strictly reserved for initiatives involving geographically and/or demographically defined populations. The reality is that virtually every aspect of care delivery can be impacted by the emerging population health paradigm, and many in the field will continue to pursue efforts to apply the population health model to the management of individual patients in clinical settings. The term "population health management" is increasingly being applied to these types of initiatives.

The developments that are encouraging the use of population health management include: an emphasis on group outcomes, deficiencies in existing disease management initiatives, growing emphasis on "community benefits," an appreciation of non-clinical contributors to health, and an emphasis on the engagement of targeted populations. These developments have encouraged healthcare providers to utilize population health management to segment and profile targeted populations, devise population-based diagnosis and treatment strategies, redouble patient education efforts, take life circumstances into consideration, rethink marketing strategies, conduct community health needs assessments, and adopt analytical methodologies such as predictive modeling and spatial analysis. Importantly, population health principles are being applied to utilization management and revenue maximization.

A number of barriers exist for healthcare providers seeking to employ population health management. Providers have a limited appreciation of population health and its usefulness, do not fully appreciate the importance of non-clinical contributors to health status, do not see incentives in place for immediate benefits, and do not interface with providers of non-medical services. Further, they typically lack the necessary data for applying population health principles and the tools with which to apply the data.

Despite the interest in population health management on the part of healthcare providers, there are limits to the role that the healthcare system can play in population health improvement. Of the three spheres that comprise population health—clinical care, social determinants and policy—the healthcare system can contribute only to the first of these. Even here there are concerns that the healthcare system as currently operating can have little impact. Its potential contributions to the reduction of social factors affecting health and to policy formulation are extremely limited.

To the extent that the healthcare system can participate in population health improvement it is in a supporting rather than a leadership role. Beyond providing the clinical services required for individual patients, the healthcare system can offer insights into the effectiveness of using population health management to meets its objectives while at the same time informing those operating at the macro-level of the usefulness of this approach for improving patient care and reaching financial goals.

Two developments that are required for the successful adaptation of population health to healthcare delivery are a new mindset and organizational transformation. Adopting a population health approach is not an easy task. Health professionals must forget much of what they know about healthcare and develop a perspective that thinks in terms of populations rather than individuals, consumers rather than patients, prevention rather than cure, and well people rather than sick people. Healthcare entities must also transform themselves into the type of organization that can operate within a population health model. They must restructure themselves to survive in the new environment—an environment that emphasizes outcomes over volume, quality over quantity, population health improvement over patient success stories. Mandates like those found in the Affordable Care Act can be expected to increase in the future as payers, government regulators and policy makers realize that the only way to improve community health status is through a population health approach.

Key Points

- While population health purists believe that the concept should only be applied at the macro-level, there are numerous ways in which population health principles can be applied within the healthcare delivery system.
- The term "population health management" is increasingly be used to describe these activities.
- A number of developments in healthcare are encouraging providers to employ a population health management approach, and incentives are increasingly being offered to providers that take this approach.
- Healthcare organizations are using population health management to segment and profile targeted populations, develop initiatives that affect their entire covered population, and consider the life circumstances of their target audience.
- Population health principles are being applied to community health needs assessments and methodologies such as predictive modeling, spatial analysis and revenue maximization are being employed.
- The adoption of population health management by healthcare providers is beset by a number of barriers including a lack of understanding of population health and the societal factors that are driving the movement, a lack of appreciation for the non-medical contributors to health, and limited interface with community-based organizations outside of healthcare.
- Healthcare providers typically lack access to the data necessary for population health management and to the tools necessary for manipulating what data are available.
- While the healthcare system cannot drive population health improvement it can play an important supporting role.
- There are numerous ways in which population health and population health management can be interfaced to the benefit of both.

References

Conn, J. (2016). Hospital executives earn bigger bonuses as value-based care takes hold. *Modern Healthcare*. Downloaded from URL: http://www.modernhealthcare.com/article/20160806/MAGAZINE/308069982

Cusack, C. M., Knudson, A. D., Kronstadt, J. L., et al. (2010). *Practice-based population health: Information technology to support transformation to proactive primary care*. Downloaded from URL: https://pcmh.ahrq.gov/citation/practice-based-population-health-information-technology-support-transformation-proactive

Ellaway, A. (2014). "The Impact of the Local Social and Physical Environment on Wellbeing," in Burton, E., and R. Cooper (editors) *Wellbeing and the Environment Vol. 2*. Oxford: Wiley-Blackwell.

Gorman, L. (2009). *Who does the AMA really represent*. Downloaded from URL: http://health-blog.ncpa.org/who-does-the-ama-really-represent/#sthash.dUOGhiaG.dpbs

Hagland, M. (2015). Chronic care world: What a new California report tells us about the future of U.S. healthcare. *Healthcare Informatics* at URL: http://www.healthcare-informatics.com/blogs/mark-hagland/chronic-care-world-what-new-california-report-tells-us-about-future-us-healthcare

Health Catalyst. (2016). *Population health management: Systems and success.* Downloaded from URL: https://www.healthcatalyst.com/population-health/

Health Research and Educational Trust. (2012). *Managing population health: The role of the hospital.* Downloaded from URL: http://www.hpoe.org/population-health.

Health Research and Educational Trust. (2015). Top of the pops. *Hospitals and Health Networks* October 13:25.

Healthy Communities Institute. (2014). *Interactive online tool streamlines the community health needs assessment process.* Downloaded from URL: http://www.healthycommunitiesinstitute.com/news-release-interactive-chna-guide/

Hopper, K. (2011). *Disparities in Cardiac Rehab.* Unpublished presentation. Downloaded from URL: http://www.aacvpr.org/Portals/0/events_edu/annualmeeting11/2011%20Online%20Syllabus%20PPT/BO31Hopper.pdf

Hui, J., Gonsahn, M. D., & Nerenz, D. R. (2014). Socioeconomic status and readmissions: Evidence from an urban teaching hospital. *Health Affairs, 33*(5), 778–785.

Jacobson, D. M., & Teutsch, S. (2012). *An environmental scan of integrated approaches for defining and measuring Total population health by the clinical care system, the government public health system, and stakeholder organizations.* National Quality Forum.

Kindig, D. A. (1997). *Purchasing population health: Paying for results.* University of Michigan Press.

Kindig, D. (2015). What are we talking about when we talk about population health. *Health Affairs Blog.* Downloaded from URL: http://healthaffairs.org/blog/2015/04/06/what-are-we-talking-about-when-we-talk-about-population-health/

Lewis, N. (2014). *Populations, population health, and the evolution of population management: Making sense of the terminology in U.S. Health Care Today.* Downloaded from URL: http://www.ihi.org/communities/blogs/_layouts/ihi/community/blog/itemview.aspx?List=81ca4a47-4ccd-4e9e-89d9-14d88ec59e8d&ID=50

National Business Coalition on Health. (2011). *Shared savings case study: Integrated healthcare association.* Downloaded from URL: http://www.nbch.org/PPR-Case-Study%2D%2D-Integrated-Health-Association

Roeder, A. (2014). *Zip code better predictor of health than genetic code.* Downloaded from URL: http://www.hsph.harvard.edu/news/features/zip-code-better-predictor-of-health-than-genetic-code/

Saxena, A. (2015). Improving medicine with predictive modeling. *Hospitals and Health Networks.* Downloaded from URL: http://www.hhnmag.com/articles/6662-improving-medicine-with-predictive-modeling

Swissler, M. A. (2015). *Running from the truth: How the Susan G. Komen Foundation Fights Health Care Reforms and Fails Breast Cancer Patients.* Downloaded from URL: http://www.southernstudies.org/2012/02/flashback-how-the-komen-foundation-fights-health-reform-and-fails-cancer-patients.html

Williams, K. G., Schootman, M., Quayle, K. S., et al. (2003). Geographic variation of pediatric burn injuries in a metropolitan area. *Academy of Emergency Medicine, 10*(7), 743–752.

Additional Resources

Begley, C. E., Lairson, D. R., Morgan, R. O., et al. (2013). *Evaluating the healthcare system: Effectiveness, efficiency, and equity.* Health Administration Press.

Evashwick, C. J. (2013). *Hospitals and community benefit: New demands, new approaches.* Health Administration Press.

Health & Performance Resources website for information on life circumstances: www.HPRAnalytics.com.

Ozdenerol, E. (2017). *Spatial health inequalities.* CRC Press.

Prochaska, J. O., & Velicer, W. F. (1997). The Transtheoretical model of health behavior change. *American Journal of Health Promotion, 12*(1), 38–48.

Chapter 9
Population Health and Public Policy

> *There are a number of levels at which a population health approach can be applied and the highest is at the policy level. More so than clinical medicine, population health requires a policy environment that is conducive to the implementation of initiatives geared to the health of populations rather than the health of individuals. To date, it could be argued that existing policy at various levels of government (and particularly at the federal level) hinder rather than help the application of population health to our nation's health problems. This chapter underscores the critical role of policy in community health improvement.*
>
> In this chapter the reader will:
>
> - Be exposed to the various types of public policies that exist and the different levels at which they operate
> - Learn about the history of public policy as it relates to health and healthcare in the US
> - Understand the various forces that influence the promulgation of public policy
> - Find out about the "health in all policies" approach and the use of health impact assessments
> - Explore how policies that exist in non-health-related sectors have implications for the health of the population

Defining Public Policy

The impact of public policy on the health status of the population is often overlooked. The enactment of policies in not only the healthcare sphere but in the education, criminal justice and economic arenas, among others, will inevitably have implications for the health of the population. Some policies may have a direct impact on health status and health behavior, as in previous policies prohibiting the immigration of people infected by AIDS, or they may be more indirect in their impact, as in the case of efforts to defund Planned Parenthood.

We might begin by defining "public policy" based on a definition offered by Longest (2010) and modified to read:

> *Public policies are authoritative decisions that are made in the legislative, executive or judicial branches of government. These decisions are intended to direct or influence the actions, behaviors or decisions of others with regard to the accomplishment of some goal.*

While much of this chapter will deal with public policies (particularly those promulgated by governments at various levels), other arenas will be discussed in which policies might be implemented that, in some cases at least, may have more influence on behavior than overarching public policies. Box 9.1 discusses the issue of who should benefit from public policy.

The United States is noteworthy for its lack of broad-reaching societal policies, and there are a variety of reasons why policy setting does not occur at the national level. For one thing, there is no formal mechanism for setting national goals and priorities, and the fragmentation of power leaves no entity in a position to formulate an overaching policy. In addition, the federalist system under which the society operates mitigates against a strong influence on the part of the central government.

It should be recalled that the federal government has a "residual" role in that it only can exhibit its prerogatives in areas not considered under the auspices of the states. While policy can be enacted through promulgation of federal legislation, the most effective option available to the federal government is through the control of federal expenditures. However, strong vested interests make it difficult to establish consensus on the acceptable degree of government involvement, much less on the nature of that involvement. Lobbyists representing many special interest groups provide millions of dollars in campaign contributions in an effort to shape or undermine the establishment of a broad-reaching policies.

Box 9.1: Policies for Whom?
The United States is faced with a number of issues in a variety of arenas, but only some of these issues rise to the level where they become matters of public policy. Most problems start out as "private" problems, affecting only the individuals involved. Many health-related decisions are made at the individual level (e.g., unhealthy dietary practices), and there are policies that directly affect said individuals (e.g., "sin taxes"). There are situations when an individual problem becomes widespread enough to have societal implications. If these individual decisions result in consequences for society (e.g., an

(continued)

Box 9.1 (continued)

"epidemic" of obesity), they may rise to the level of public interest and call for a broad-based policy approach. Any number of similar situations can be cited.

The acquisition of health insurance by individuals has historically been a personal matter mediated in some cases through the role of employers or government-sponsored health plans. Since the 1980s, however, individuals have faced increasing barriers to the acquisition of health insurance at a time when healthcare costs were skyrocketing. At the end of the twentieth century, tens of millions of Americans were not covered by health insurance. A lack of insurance resulting in medical debt has been found to be a major contributor to the soaring bankruptcy rate in the United States Further, tens of thousands of Americans are dying unnecessarily every year simply because they do not have a means to pay for their healthcare. Thus, what was once considered a personal issue rose to the point of a public policy issue and ultimately led to the incorporation of numerous provisions into the Patient Protection and Affordable Care Act of 2010.

This raises the question of for whom or what are public policies enacted. Kindig and his colleagues (2008) proposed using a population health approach as a framework for planning and implementating goals, policies and interventions aimed at improving health outcomes. This approach would downplay policies that target individual behaviors in favor of policies that focus on organizations and communities.

To the extent that policies can target organizations there is an unlimited number of options. Obviously, government agencies at every level represent potential entities to which policies can be targeted. Outside of government, the entities run the gamut from healthcare organizations, schools (where school health programs are being implemented), private industry, social service organizations, and various other entities in a position to promote population health.

A third option is to target entire communities with policy initiatives. There is in fact a growing movement, discussed in a later chapter, toward funding the efforts of communities to bring about collective impact with regard to community health status. These initiatives have been funded by the federal government, foundations and professional organizations. Most of these programs reflect the fact that the healthcare system is unable to contribute significantly to community health improvement. It must be a community-wide effort that marshals the resources across a wide range of community sectors.

Ultimately, all three categories of entities must be brought into the process. A community cannot not effect population health improvement if its component organizations are not on board. Similarly, policies that are implemented that do not engage the population they are meant to serve are not likely to be very effective.

The United States stands apart from other comparable societies in regard to its health policy development. Although there have been brief periods during which health *planning* was emphasized, these initiatives were short-lived and were strongly opposed by various interest groups. The primary influence of the federal government on health policy has been through the provision (or withdrawal) of funding for various health-related programs. The size and nature of the physician manpower pool (for example) has been affected by subsidies for medical school training. Healthy lifestyles have been encouraged through financial support for health education programs. The thrust of the healthcare system has been influenced by the selective allocation of research funding. Examples of broad-ranging policies related to cost containment include efforts to control the operation of the Medicare and Medicaid programs. By controlling the financing mechanism (and virtually no other aspect of the process), the federal government has set "policy" with regard to the provision of care. A very different example involves the prohibition introduced through federal legislation against research on gun violence. This "policy" has had the effect of limiting our ability to address gun violence as a public health issue. More often than not failure to establish a policy represents a policy statement in its own right.

Spheres for Policy Development

There are a number of spheres in which policies may be implemented, with policies classified in terms of their emphasis. These would include macro-level policies with broad social impact (e.g., national 5-year economic development plan), public policies meant to address a specific issue (e.g., access to green space and parks), organizational policies (e.g., provider policies with regard to the acceptance of insurance), and professional policies (e.g., restricting "kickbacks" to referring physicians).

At the same time, policies can be classified based on the level of government at which they are promulgated. Policies developed in the United States at the federal level are typically designed to be applied society wide based on the assumption that the policies can be expected to affect everyone in the society. At the state level, policies are promulgated with the notion that their impact will be restricted to residents of the state or those otherwise having dealings with state entities. At the local (city and county) level, policies are enacted that are expected to primarily affect residents governed by the local political entity, those who have reason to be physically in the political jurisdiction or those doing business with the political entity. Because policy-setting processes operate relatively independent at the different levels there is often a lack of coordination between the various levels of government and even some measure of conflict.

Macro-level Policies

Macro-level policies are overarching policies typically enacted at the societal level that may affect many areas of public concern. Macro policies are uncommon in the United States given its antipathy toward centralized government planning. Among the few examples from our own history are the national public works programs implemented in response to the Great Depression. While some federal agencies and others at state and local levels may have responsibility for policies related to healthcare, none of these rises to the macro level.

It could be argued that the 2010 Patient Protection and Affordable Care Act (ACA) represents a form of macro policy because of its wide-reaching provisions. The fact that the purchase of health insurance was mandated for all individuals represents an unprecedented use of federal legislation to encourage a specific behavior. Even within the healthcare arena the scope of the legislation is restricted (with most of the impact on insurance practices) with limited impact on such critical issues as healthcare personnel shortages, the maldistribution of services, and the increasing cost of healthcare.

Although there is no formally enacted national health policy for the country, certain policies are implicit in the goals of various health agencies. These policies are reflected in the regulations that are enacted and in the manner in which funds are allocated. Although there is no omnibus healthcare policy, the overriding concerns gleaned from disparate sources include: (a) improving the quality of life through disease and death prevention, (b) improving the quality of life by improving disease treatment, (c) fostering a set of behavior patterns conducive to better health, and (d) improving the understanding of the causes and prevention of disease through medical research. None of these stated concerns, however, have resulted in the promulgation of macro-level policies (although the Medicare and Medicaid programs can be thought to contain elements of macro-level policy making). Box 9.2 discusses national health insurance as a public policy issue.

The one clear effort in this direction during the last century was the wide-reaching health planning regulations enacted by the federal government during the Johnson administration. Formal healthcare planning in the United States can be traced back to the Comprehensive Health Planning act of 1966. This planning initiative was in response to the discovery in the 1960s that large segments of the population did not have access to mainstream healthcare, along with concerns over perceived inequities in the provision of services to different segments of the population. This act called for the establishment of a federally funded and coordinated planning initiative for assuring access to adequate healthcare for every American.

The Act established statewide and area-wide (i.e., sub-state) planning agencies for the implementation of the planning process. These agencies were charged with the development of state plans and were assigned responsibility for coordinating healthcare activities within the geographic areas under their jurisdiction. Planning agencies established guidelines for the development of facilities and programs based on a state plan. The primary means of control was through the review of projects that were proposed. However, these agencies could only make recommendations with regard to proposed projects and had limited power to affect change.

> **Box 9.2: National Health Insurance as Public Policy**
>
> In 1990, the Congressional Health Care Commission (the Pepper Commission) issued a document that probably comes closer to being a national healthcare policy statement than anything that preceded it. The proposed policy would have expanded private health insurance to most of the 37 million Americans (including more than 12 million children) who at that time were without coverage, and it would have developed a system that would have guaranteed long-term healthcare for persons in need regardless of their financial status. Components of the plan included: (a) mandatory health insurance coverage for businesses with 100 or more employees, (b) tax credits and subsidies to smaller companies to encourage them to offer an insurance plan, (c) free coverage for uninsured pregnant women, as well as children under age 6 in families below 185% of the federal poverty level, and (d) no out-of-pocket expenses for patients for the first three months spent in a nursing home. A similar proposal was offered by the American Medical Association (AMA) in 1990. That plan would have created state risk pools to provide group insurance for the medically uninsurable, as well as small businesses and others unable to afford coverage.
>
> In late 1990, Senator Bob Kerrey (D-Nebraska) introduced "The Health USA Act of 1991." The key to the bill was that healthcare coverage would no longer be tied to the workplace. It would have also subsumed the Medicare and Medicaid programs. The legislation was designed to provide care for all US citizens and permanent residents. Among the services covered were: primary care, inpatient and outpatient hospital care, hospice care, dental care for children to age 18, and preventive services. A combination of federal income, corporate, and state taxes were expected to fund the program. No such sweeping bill was ever authorized.
>
> An absence of health insurance coverage, at the very least, denies a large segment of the population ready access to healthcare. Besides the lack of treatment for certain types of less serious maladies, early diagnosis for more serious illnesses does not occur, resulting in more pain and suffering along with more expensive treatments at a later point in time. In fact, it can be argued that the provision of subsidized health insurance (and therefore care) is in the long run much less expensive than the current system, which places relatively little emphasis on prevention and early diagnosis.
>
> A national health insurance program did not become policy at that time and has not since then. While the feasibility of such an approach could be debated, the failure to establish any national health policy reflected ideological opposition to federal involvement in healthcare and pushback from vested interests who benefit from the existing system.

A primary tool for use in health planning is the certificate of need (CON) process. Although the details of the process differ from state to state the intent of CON programs is to establish a basis for evaluating the appropriateness of the development, expansion, or significant change in health facilities. The facilities that are covered vary from state to state. CON regulations are theoretically synced up with state health plans (for states that operate a CON program) and must comply with standards and restrictions embedded in the state plan or in other state legislation.

The Regional Medical Program (RMP) was another federal initiative established in the mid-1960s with responsibility for coordinating and promoting health services within a defined geographic area. These programs were established nationwide and were charged with facilitating the diffusion of medical technology and other breakthroughs from major medical centers to surrounding areas. While planning was not a stated responsibility of these programs, a certain level of planning was required in order for the RMPs to successfully disseminate medical knowledge throughout their regions.

Planning activities were revitalized nationwide in 1974 with the enactment of the National Health Planning and Resources Development Act. This act was prompted by growing concern over the lack of uniformly effective methods of healthcare delivery, the maldistribution of healthcare facilities and personnel, and the increasing cost of care. With a better financial footing than the 1966 planning initiative, this act called for the creation of statewide health coordinating councils and the establishment of local health systems agencies.

This "experiment" in health planning came to an end under the Reagan administration in the early 1980s. Despite some successes, comprehensive health planning had not created many political allies and essentially had few constituents. As a result, the demise of these programs represented the end of any formal federal health planning initiatives. Some vestigial remains of federal health planning policy implementation exist through initiatives like Healthy People 2020 and agencies like the Health Resources and Services Administration (HRSA). A few states and local governments have retained limited health planning functions.

Public Policies

Public policies are promulgated by governments at various levels and typically focus on a particular issue. Although the lines are blurred between macro-level policy and public policy as defined here, examples of the latter are typically more narrow in their scope. The most broad-reaching public policies are enacted at the federal level, although states and local governments may also enact such policies. Major federal policies are manifested through the Social Security, Medicare and Medicaid programs.

These programs represent policy statements endorsed at some time or another with regard to an identified need. While the focus of this discussion is health-related policies, a major contention of this book is that policies outside the healthcare arena have as much impact on community health status as those within healthcare. Those policy areas are considered below as are policies enacted at other levels of government. Box 9.3 discusses how competing perspectives hamper the development of effective public policy.

Box 9.3: Competing Perspectives and Public Policy

One factor that complicates the promulgation of public policy in the U.S., particularly in the healthcare arena, is the competing perspectives that exist within American society. When there is no consensus with regard to important societal issues, it is difficult to enact policies to address them. In many cases, there are outright value conflicts as in the case of the abortion issue, thereby creating a situation where there may be no broadly accepted policy solution. Some of these competing perspectives may be based on utilitarian viewpoints wherein it is argued that funding is not available for implementation even if the policy itself is considered beneficial. Increasingly, it appears, these competing perspectives reflect deep-seated ideological stances that often are not rooted in fact but in partisan opinions.

An example of a competing perspective involves the question of whether healthcare is a privilege or a right. Although the preponderance of opinion appears to have shifted over time toward the notion of healthcare as a right, there are still those—many in key political positions—who maintain that healthcare should not be considered a right but is a resource that should be purchased like any other commodity. Obviously, the stance that one takes in this regard is critical for the policy-making process.

A related issue centers on what the acceptable role of government in the operation of the healthcare system should be. If, for example, one considers healthcare as a right of all citizens, it could be argued that government has an important role in assuring this right. On the other hand, if healthcare is viewed as a commodity, then the role of government should be limited to assuring that a fair and equitable market exists for the purchase of health services. Here, too, ideology may play a role in that conservative elements of the political system oppose virtually any role for government related to healthcare to the point of decrying Michelle Obama's initiative for healthier school lunches as an effort on the part of the government to tell Americans what they should and should not eat.

One final example among many possibilities that is also related to the two examples above involves the question of whether healthcare is an individual responsibility or an amenity that society has a responsibility to provide. Historically, it was held that individuals were responsible for their own health. They should make decisions with regard to healthy or unhealthy lifestyles, are responsible for obtaining health insurance, and are ultimately responsible for their health status. Here, too, there has been a shift in orientation over time, with the growing recognition that individuals have limited ability to control the factors that contribute to positive health. To the extent that unhealthy physical and social environments, limited access to food, housing and green space, and structural barriers prevent individual progress toward good health, it could be argued that the onus shifts to society to assure the potential for a healthy life for all citizens. A premise of the population health model is that unless society assures that an opportunity to pursue good health is in place, individuals are powerless to accomplish this.

Public policies like most policies can be addressed in terms of their direct and indirect effects. Direct policies refer to those legislative efforts designed purposefully to affect the delivery and quality of healthcare or the health status of the population. For example, funding for federally qualified health centers represents direct involvement in the provision of care, while federal funding for public health activities involves a more indirect approach. Indirect policies are those whose basic intent is to affect some non-healthcare outcome, although in the process the provision of healthcare or the health status of the population is impacted. In the federal budgetary process, appropriations for healthcare and non-healthcare programs alike are negotiated in order to meet overall dollar limits. Therefore, direct, indirect, and non-healthcare policy issues are sometimes closely linked. Past efforts to cut federal spending through "sequestration" indirectly affected healthcare policy to the extent that at least some service agency budgets shrank as all "social services" funding was trimmed. Direct effects would be realized as specific programs (e.g., Medicare and Social Security) were targeted for reductions.

At the state level a number of policy areas are evident. This reflects the role accorded to states under the Constitution whereby the federal government in effect has residual responsibility for those functions *not* assigned to the states. States, thus, often enact policies independent of federal policies and, in some cases, in direct opposition to federal priorities. With regard to healthcare states have licensing and oversight responsibilities for health professions and health facilities. States have almost total responsibility for certain behavioral health problems, and primary responsibility for public health, environmental protection and highway safety. With regard to public health, each state health department sets its priorities and, although significant funding flows to the states from the Department of Health and Human Services, federal agencies have limited control over how the funding is spent within a budgeted category.

State governments also play a pivotal role when it comes to health insurance and the policies that govern health plans. Insurance is regulated at the state level and different states have different requirements that govern the actions of insurers. These requirements typically determine the rate-setting process and the types of services that must be provided. A state agency typically manages the state's Medicaid program and has considerable latitude in terms of the provisions governing the operation of this joint federal-state program. The threshold for eligibility can be set by the state as well as the services that can be covered. As a result, these provisions vary from state to state, even to the point of encouraging low-income families to move across state lines to access insurance. The ACA was an unprecedented step with regard to federal involvement as it created a national health insurance exchange and standardized insurance provisions across all states.

One area for which states have primary policy responsibility is health planning—to the extent that any states participate in this endeavor. A number of states develop state-wide health plans in an effort to manage the development of health resources within the state. These "state plans" vary in scope and frequency of preparation as well as in the "teeth" they have for enforcement. Further, there is little consistency in the structure and operation of certificate of need programs (CON) across the various states that maintain them. Implicitly or explicitly these plans reflect policy decisions reached at the state level. Like the state health plans, CON guidelines presumably reflect policies that individual states have enacted.

Local government has less latitude in terms of policy development than states and the federal government. Their responsibilities are limited to the city or county over which they have jurisdiction. Their role may include oversight of public health functions and, in some cases, management, oversight, funding or other involvement with public health facilities. In some rare cases, local government may be directly or indirectly involved with health planning activities. There are some aspects related to health that local authorities may be directly or indirectly involved with. Local governments may provide direct services to the community by virtue of the health department, with local priorities influencing the nature of the public health services provided. They also have oversight with regard to environmental issues. Local authorities also establish policies with indirect implications for health such as housing policies, transportation policies, and the regulation of farmers markets. Box 9.4 addresses the different levels of society at which policy may be introduced.

Organizational Policies

Organizational policies are developed at the organizational level and affect the actions that organizations take with regard to both internal and external constituencies. Typically codified in operational protocols and policies and procedures manuals, these policies are intended to encourage the achievement of organizational goals on the one hand and to prohibit actions that would be considered detrimental to the organization or deter goal achievement on the other. While these internal policies certainly do not have the broad sweep of federal or state policies, they often are established in response to governmental regulations. In some cases, these policies have the effect of law while in others they are in response to regulatory mandates. Unlike sweeping federal regulations these policies directly affect those on the front lines of healthcare delivery.

A key issue related to healthcare involves organizational policies for the management of personal health information (PHI). Federal regulations require that patient confidentiality be maintained and that patient records are secured against inappropriate access. Strict policies are enacted at the organizational level to assure the integrity of personal health information.

An aspect of organizational policies that attracts controversy involves policies related to accepting patients for care. While discrimination with regard to race, ethnicity, sex and other attributes has long been outlawed, some providers still subtly discourage patronage by certain categories of patients. While such discrimination is seldom blatantly pursued, it most often takes the form today of selective acceptance of payment. Providers may require payment at the time of (or even before) service is provided or may refuse service to individuals who are not covered by health insurance. Even among the insured, some providers may reject Medicare patients

Box 9.4: An Approach to Policy Formulation and Implementation

Level of attack	Areas of emphasis	Thrust	Sample task	Objective	Change agents
Societal (nation, state)	Government policies	Advocate for public health	Encourage politicians to fund health disparities research	Reduce health disparities	Government/public health officials; politicians/policy setters
	Laws	Advocate for health education	Encourage policy setters to enact legislation	Encourage healthy eating by students	Government officials; politicians/policy setters; educational administrators
	Regulations	Advocate for prevention coverage	Require insurance plans to cover preventive care	Prevent/delay the onset of diabetes	Government officials; politicians/policy setters; insurance regulators; employers
	Taxation	Influence tax policy	Tax unhealthy foods; tax benefits to healthy companies	Encourage healthy behavior	Government officials; politicians/policy setters; employers
	Budget formulation	Influence budgetary process	Lobby for fund allocations that support healthy lifestyles	Use government funds to improve lifestyles	Government officials; politicians/policy setters
Community (city, neighborhood)	Government policies	Advocate for adequate government services	Encourage use of city facilities for health improvement	Facilitate improved citizen health	Government officials; politicians/policy setters
	Laws	Use local laws to reduce unhealthy activities	Regulate sales of unhealthy foods	Limit or tax distribution of unhealthy foods	Government officials; politicians/policy setters
	Regulations	Advocate for regulations supportive of food access	Remove prohibitions against farmer's marketers	Improve diets through access to fresh foods	Government officials; politicians/policy setters
	Community priorities	Leverage existing community resources for good health	Establish coalitions to support access to fresh foods	Increase access to fresh foods in underserved areas	Local government, community organizations, religious leaders
	School policies	Schools as a vehicle for health education	Enact policies that support physical activity, access to healthy food and treatment compliance	Improve health knowledge of students; provide access to healthy food	School board; educators; PTAs; local government

(continued)

Box 9.4 (continued)

Level of attack	Areas of emphasis	Thrust	Sample task	Objective	Change agents
Organization (business, church)	Policies	Encourage workplace health	Provide employee incentives	Healthier, more productive workforce	Employers; business coalitions; health professionals; health plans
	Regulations	Advocate for organization-friendly regulations	Incentives for not-for-profit-supported farmers markets	More flexible programming by community organizations	Employers; business coalitions; health professionals; NFP staff
	Relationships	Encourage coalition development	Coordinate activities of like-minded community organizations	Leverage existing resources for better health	Community activists/organizations; local government
Group (family, social group)	Family "policies"	Support family structure	Establish family-friendly fitness facilities	Use family to encourage health of members	Families; community organizations; churches; local government
	Group activities/priorities	Discourage unhealthy behaviors	Educate families/groups on healthy foods	Eliminate unhealthy foods from the household	Families; community organizations; churches; local government
Individual	Personal lifestyles	Encourage healthy diet	Educate individuals on healthy foods	Improve dietary habits	Individuals; families; social groups; churches
	Spiritual involvement	Encourage support of faith-based organizations	Church-based health education/wellness	Leverage church influence to improve dietary habits	Families; churches
	Community service	Encourage volunteerism	Volunteer for health education/wellness programs	Incentivize citizens to volunteer	Local government, community organizations, religious leaders

(although this has become rare) or Medicaid patients (and this has become more common). There is anecdotal evidence that some providers have rejected patients covered under the healthcare exchange established through the ACA legislation. If anything, the existence of such practices underscores the fact that the healthcare system cannot effectively contribute to community health improvement and may, in fact, be part of the problem.

Professional Policies

Professional policies are implemented to guide the behavior of those operating within professional settings. These are particularly relevant to healthcare given the potential ethical issues within the healthcare arena. Other professions such as law, accounting and architecture establish ethical frameworks but the significance is much greater for healthcare given the potential for harm to a large segment of the population. While most professional ethics do not take the form of law, some of them reflect existing legal statutes (e.g., inappropriate dispensing of regulated drugs).

Within healthcare the range of ethical issues is quite broad. Many of the proscriptions relate to physician behavior (and in some cases to other health professions). There are ethical considerations related to physician referral practices, physician ownership of related businesses, kickbacks for prescribing drugs and products, and the receipt of gifts or other perquisites from parties seeking to influence practice patterns.

There is a whole range of issues unique to healthcare that have clinical dimensions but may fall into a grey area. The manner in which providers should deal with abortions, assisted suicide, and child abuse involves ethical issues that cannot always be codified in ethics guidelines.

Health in all Policies

One attempt to bring attention to the impact of policy decisions on health involves the "Health in All Policies" movement. According to the American Public Association (Rudolph et al., 2013) Health in All Policies (HiAP) represents a collaborative approach to population health improvement that incorporates health considerations into decision-making across sectors and policy areas. The goal of Health in All Policies is to ensure that decision-makers are informed about the health, equity, and sustainability consequences of various options during the policy development process.

This approach engages diverse stakeholders in an effort to directly improve health while simultaneously advancing other societal goals that indirectly contribute to community health improvement. Health in All Policies builds on a long public health tradition of successful multisectoral collaboration. This approach encompasses a wide spectrum of activities but particularly benefit from on-going collaboration across many agencies. Ultimately the Health in All Policies approach seeks to institutionalize considerations of health, equity, and sustainability as a standard part of decision-making processes across a broad array of sectors.

Since health is influenced by the social determinants previously noted, Health in All Policies incorporates health considerations into decision-making across sectors and policy areas. At its core this approach supports improved health outcomes and health equity through collaboration between public health practitioners and those non-traditional partners who have influence over the social determinants of health. These partners would include representatives from education, healthcare, housing, criminal justice, community development and other sectors.

According to the American Public Health Association, Health in All Policies includes five key elements:

- Promoting health and equity
- Supporting intersectoral collaboration
- Creating co-benefits for multiple partners
- Engaging stakeholders
- Creating structural or process change

Health in All Policies thus encompasses a wide spectrum of activities and can be implemented in many different ways. The Health in all Policies approach has been adopted by individual communities, state governments, and federal initiatives, including the interagency health promotion council established under the Affordable Care Act of 2010. Case Study 9.1 describes a health-in-all-policies approach to obesity.

One of the tools available to support a health-in-all-policies approach is the Health Impact Assessment (HIA). Increasingly, governments and businesses are being encouraged to consider the consequences for health, and for health disparities, of proposed policies in transportation, housing, education, taxation, land use, and so forth. Health impact assessments have been commissioned to study the potential health consequences of policies concerning such diverse topics as minimum wage laws and freeway widening. Health impact assessments can help communities, decision makers, and practitioners make choices that improve population health through community design.

HIA is a process that helps evaluate the potential health effects of a plan, project, or policy before it is built or implemented. HIA brings potential positive and negative public health impacts and considerations to the decision-making process for plans, projects, and policies that fall outside traditional public health arenas, such as transportation and land use. The steps involved in conducting an HIA are:

- ***Screening*** During screening, practitioners (who may include staff from health departments, foundations, private organizations, or others with training in HIA methodology) briefly describe potential connections between the proposed policy,

> **Case Study 9.1: Health in all Policies and the Obesity "Epidemic"**
>
> The causes of the obesity epidemic are complex, including the food, physical activity, social, and economic environments that shape individuals' opportunities to make healthy food and beverage choices and incorporate exercise into daily routines. More than one-third of adults and almost one-fifth of children in the United States are obese, and obesity rates have more than doubled for adults and tripled for children since 1980. Obesity increases the risk of many health conditions including coronary heart disease, stroke, high blood pressure, Type 2 diabetes, some cancers, osteoarthritis, and infertility. It may also shorten population life expectancies for future generations.
>
> The increased prevalence of sedentary lifestyles, which contributes to rising obesity rates, is related to changes in patterns of land use and transportation, increased distances from homes to school and work, parental fears about children's safety, shifts in the nature of work, and cultural changes. These factors suggest that personal actions can have limited impact on obesity patterns within the population.
>
> The standard prescription of "eat less, exercise more", even if faithfully followed, cannot overcome the influence of "fast food nation" and the power of the food industry. Increased consumption of foods and beverages with high caloric density and little nutritional value is encouraged by the proliferation of time-saving processed convenience foods, pressures on working parents, intensive marketing, and government subsidies for commodity products such as corn and soy.
>
> Reducing the prevalence of obesity and chronic disease will require that public health practitioners address people's environments, which will in turn require working across multiple sectors. Those representing transportation, agriculture, economic development, education, recreation, and housing all need to be involved in order to advance a comprehensive approach to obesity and chronic disease prevention. It will also require exploring the links between these sectors and environmental sustainability, as well as addressing inequities in how communities are impacted.
>
> Source: Rudolph et al. (2013)

program, plan, or project and the health of affected communities and individuals. If the proposed undertaking is likely to have significant health impacts—either positive or negative—and an HIA would provide additional information for the decision-making process, proceeding with the HIA process is recommended.

Scoping This step identifies primary health outcomes of interest, affected and vulnerable populations, and issues identified by stakeholders. Practitioners also outline the research methodology, including data sources and analysis plans. Scoping determines the nature of community involvement and the depth of the assessment.

Assessment This stage follows through on plans set during scoping and compiles relevant data and information for analysis. Data may be qualitative or quantitative and from a broad range of fields. Analyses should also incorporate stakeholder perspectives. Throughout the process, practitioners must be clear about the limitations of available data and findings.

Recommendations HIA does not prescribe a decision. Rather, it presents actions to maximize health benefits and minimize harm, especially to vulnerable groups, for the decision alternatives. Recommendations specify the parties or stakeholders that should be responsible for implementation.

Reporting The HIA report describes in detail the first four steps, including the proposed policy, plan, or program; stakeholders and their involvement; data sources and analysis; findings; recommendations; and a plan for monitoring and evaluation. The report must be clear and easily accessible to all stakeholders. For maximum utility, the report format and timeline should align with economic, political, and social considerations and decision points.

Monitoring and Evaluation The HIA process, impact of the HIA recommendations, and health outcomes after implementation should be evaluated. This stage is especially important given that HIA is a new and rapidly developing field. A HIA is usually voluntary, although several local and state laws support the examination of health impacts in decision making and a few explicitly require the use of HIA.

The health impact assessment is a useful tool to assess how a proposed decision will disproportionately affect the health of a vulnerable population. The goal of HIA is to provide recommendations during the decision-making process that will protect health and reduce health inequities. The Centers for Disease Control and Prevention (2016) considers it a promising tool for supporting community health improvement because of its:

- Applicability to a broad array of policies, programs, plans, and projects.
- Consideration of adverse and beneficial health effects.
- Ability to consider and incorporate various types of evidence.
- Engagement of communities and stakeholders in a deliberative process.

Case Study 9.2 provides an example of a health impact assessment.

This holistic approach to public policy has been endorsed by the World Health Organization and numerous prestigious foundations. Major initiatives of the MacArthur Foundation, the Robert Wood Johnson Foundation and the W.K. Kellogg Foundation have reinforced the message that "place matters." Armed with a new field of research that collects data at the neighborhood level, communities are beginning to use HIAs to document and rectify local social and environmental conditions through influencing the policy-making process. Box 9.5 describes how misplaced priorities can influence the course of policy development.

Case Study 9.2: Health Impact Assessment of Three Growth Scenarios
Humboldt County, California, famed for its redwoods, is home to the tallest tree on earth—the 379-foot-tall hyperion in Redwood National Park. When this rural county began to update its general plan in 2008 it recognized the importance of its decisions for the health of the county's population. Land use planning decisions are often made based on population projections, economic considerations, political realities, and community input, yet a substantial body of evidence suggests that these policies have significant impacts on population health. Planning impacts health by affecting the community determinants of health—the social, economic and environmental factors that influence well-being including for example: access to housing, fresh produce, educational opportunities, parks, and transportation among other amenities. Other factors that affect health include economic inequality, residential segregation, substandard housing, lack of supermarkets, poor schools, insufficient public transit, and disruptions to family and social networks.

When the county decided to update its General Plan, it conducted a health impact assessment (HIA) to determine how the health of its approximately 125,000 residents would be affected. The local health department and the Humboldt Partnership for Active Living (a coalition of local organizations) teamed up with Human Impact Partners and community members to identify 35 indicators of community health. Through the HIA it was possible to evaluate how these factors would be impacted by each of the three alternative growth scenarios being considered in the General Plan update.

The three options under consideration were: Alternative A (focused growth emphasizing development within established areas already served by amenities); Alternative B (emphasizes in-filling within established boundaries but allows for expansion of boundaries and some exurban development); and Alternative C (allows for unlimited growth that would support population increase at twice the rate of the first two alternatives).

Ultimately, the analysis pointed strongly toward "focused growth"- new development in areas already served by existing infrastructure such as public sewage and utilities - as better for the county than unrestricted growth, or a mix of the two. The HIA indicated that one outcome from focused growth would be fewer miles driven. That, in turn, could lead to fewer traffic injuries and more walking and biking (and therefore less risk of cardiovascular disease, diabetes and obesity). Having families live closer to schools should likewise encourage walking and biking, which could further improve health and reduce pollution.

The county health and planning departments endorsed the HIA recommendations, and the planning department followed HIA guidelines, in developing their proposals for the final General Plan.

Source: Pew Charitable Trust (2008)

Box 9.5: Public Policy and Misplaced Priorities
One premise of this book is that a major reason the healthcare system cannot contribute to population health improvement is that it is beset by various misplaced priorities. Perhaps the one that underlies many of the other misplaced priorities is our system's emphasis on "sickness" rather than "health". Our present healthcare model requires people to be sick in order for vested interests to generate a profit, and there are three trillion reasons why established players support the current priorities. Unfortunately, the "preservatives" (i.e., those trying to protect status quo/revenue) often cling to old models. Despite the fact that many health systems are not for profit, they reflexively view revenue growth as their objective. This may be due to the fact that non-profit boards are typically made up of business leaders from environments where revenue growth is the goal.

Related to this discussion is the fact that financial incentives within the healthcare system are misplaced. Although significant changes are underway—some of which are paving the way for a population health approach—the incentives in place continue to favor: more care rather than less care; more expensive care rather than less expensive care; more specialty care rather than primary care; and treatment rather than prevention. Despite the fact that some physicians have begun to take a more enlightened approach to patient management, the default response continues to be to do more diagnostics and treatment rather than less.

There is continued emphasis on treatment rather than prevention—despite the proven benefits of the latter. The aforementioned financial incentives continue to favor the provision of services and, even when incentives are modified, old habits are hard to break. Despite the emphasis on prevention under the Affordable Care Act, the financial incentives are still limited. The fact that physicians are not well trained in preventive techniques is also a consideration.

Tied into the above discussion is the emphasis placed on technology. The United States has the most technological healthcare system of any country but what it has to show for this is: (1) over-utilization of high-end diagnostic tests; (2) overly expensive healthcare; (3) unnecessary treatments (and deaths) as a result of misdiagnosis, false positives, and the consequences of testing/treatment; and (4) worse clinical outcomes than other similar countries. There are financial incentives, of course, that encourage the use of advanced technology and certainly circumstances that warrant it. However, when the question comes down to whether or not to employ advanced technology, for most practitioners more is better than less.

One final area where policy priorities are misplaced involves medical research. Despite the proven benefits of prevention, virtually all federal research dollars are dedicated to advancing reatment modalities. This is perhaps no more obvious than in the case of cancer where it is widely recognized that prevention provides the best hope for reducing cancer morbidity and

(continued)

Box 9.5 (continued)

mortality. Yet, billions of research dollars are devoted to testing the effect of various "poisons" on the treatment of cancer. Further, research on conditions where there are clearly "epidemics" underway (e.g., obesity, mental illness) is limited in deference to "sexier" research foci. The fact that support for disparities research by minority researchers on the part of the federal government is limited offers further evidence of misplaced priorities (Weller et al., 2020).

Social Domains and Public Policy

The gravitational pull of healthcare in the past has kept the policy focus on reorganizing care, implementing information technology, and reforming the payment system, with less consideration of issues outside of medicine. This approach has been rooted in the belief that bringing efficiency to the existing system would contribute to community health improvement. In actuality, expanding health insurance coverage, improving the quality of care and other "tweaks" to the system contribute little to saving lives and controlling medical spending. Alternatively, a population health approach focuses on policies to improve environmental conditions, reduce health disparities and promote healthier behavior. A number of policy areas outside of healthcare are described below along with examples of policy-related efforts to address the challenges to health improvement presented by those areas.

Education

In the United States education has generally been a function carried out at the local level, with policies set by individual school districts. Over time, however, state governments became increasingly involved in education, supporting state institutions of higher learning as well as certain secondary school programs at the local level. The U.S. Department of Education has also played an increasingly important role in public education. Federal monies are transferred to the respective states (and then to the local school districts) for general support as well as for support of specific programs. In the first decade of the twenty-first century the No Child Left Behind initiative was established at the federal level and imposed upon the various states. This represented an attempt (although considered misguided by some) to promulgate a national policy related to academic standards in response to the growing concern over lagging academic achievement. This initiative, however, did not address the health issues facing students.

The US Department of Education has responded to concerns over inequitable access to educational opportunities, recognizing the role of education as a social determinant of health. These concerns have been exacerbated by virtue of the COVID pandemic. The Department is leveraging funding from the American Rescue Plan to address these issues in an effort to equitably serve all students. The Department sponsored an Equity Summit in 2021 and has carried out extensive research on the extent to which health disparities have influenced the impact of the pandemic (US Department of Education, 2021).

Promise Neighborhoods is part of the White House's Neighborhood Revitalization initiative (U.S. Department of Education, 2016). This collaboration between the White House Domestic Policy Council, the White House Office of Urban Affairs, and the Departments of Education (DOE), Health and Human Services (HHS), Housing and Urban Development (HUD), Justice (DOJ), and the Department of the Treasury aimed to transform high-poverty neighborhoods into more functional communities. Led by DOE, Promise Neighborhoods were intended to address the significant challenges faced by students and families living in distressed communities. This was done by providing resources to plan and implement a continuum of services from early childhood education to college and career with the goal of improving educational and developmental outcomes for children and youth. Services range from improving neighborhood health, safety, and stability to expanding access to learning technology and Internet connectivity. By building capacity to revitalize underserved neighborhoods, the Promise Neighborhoods program has helped eliminate health and educational disparities.

An example of an effort toward a policy-oriented solution to poor dietary habits have been efforts on the part of some public school systems to increase healthy food options while decreasing access to unhealthy options. While implemented at the local level (with state support in some cases), this issue was elevated to the federal level due to the commitment of Michelle Obama to improving the dietary habits of school children. Although it is difficult to determine what role the First Lady's support played, improvement has been noted in the case of many school systems as a result of food service "reforms". This has included the inclusion of healthy cafeteria items and the removal of unhealthy foods from vending machines and cafeteria menus. In many school districts clear results have been demonstrated (U.S. Department of Agriculture, 2015), with students eating healthier meals, avoiding unhealthy options, and otherwise experiencing health benefits. Despite these successes there continues to be ideologically based pushback from some quarters (Confessore, 2014).

Housing and Community Development

Housing and community development are functions generally carried out at the local level and, for the most part, by private sector organizations. The U.S. Department of Housing and Urban Development (HUD) does play a role in initiating federal programs to be administered at the local level and in the allocation of funds for specific needs (e.g., housing for the homeless and people living with AIDS). The federal government has also historically played a role in the development of public and subsidized housing. By providing funding to localities, HUD has supported the establishment of public housing projects and subsidized the cost of so-called "Section 8" housing for the indigent. The availability of affordable housing continues to be a national issue as does the rise in homelessness, and the resolution of this issue has been left primarily to local government which has to depend on private sector entities to address this issue. However, HUD has become increasingly involved in neighborhood redevelopment and provides funds to localities with an emphasis on preserving existing communities rather than abandoning them.

There are at least two aspects related to housing with implications for population health. One has to do with housing stability and the other with housing adequacy. With regard to the former, the inability to maintain stable housing—primarily due to its unaffordability—represents a major threat to the health of those affected by instability. Affordable and safe housing is important to the well-being and health of families. Without adequate housing, families have trouble managing their daily lives. When this happens, their health suffers.

Research has shown that affordable housing may help individuals living with chronic diseases to better maintain their treatment regimens and seek medical care more frequently (Johns Hopkins, 2016). For patients who are homeless, properly storing medication, maintaining a healthy diet and consistently going to the doctor are difficult to do when they are spending a good deal of time trying to find a place to sleep. When families cannot afford adequate housing, they may be forced to live in homes that are too small for their needs or to live with family or friends in a crowded situation. This makes it difficult for them to maintain healthy relationships and to handle personal stress. High levels of stress can lead to or exacerbate a number of health issues Stable housing provides a foundation for individuals with chronic illness to improve their health outcomes.

One effort toward reducing the health impact of housing insecurity is Jubilee Housing (Jubilee), a non-profit affordable housing organization operating 280 housing units in Washington, D.C. These organizations provide an array of supportive services, such as housing stability, health services, youth services and family programming. Jubilee is currently launching a model that will report rental payments to the credit bureaus to help residents build their credit. Jubilee is also working to provide families access to financial education, and access to a low-cost credit building loan that reports on-time rent payments to the credit bureaus. Jubilee Housing is collaborating with local partners to provide this suite of key services leading more families to financial stability.

Inadequate housing also represents a serious health threat. Nationwide there are more than six million substandard housing units. Residents of these units are at increased risk for childhood lead poisoning, asthma, fire and electrical injuries, falls, rodent bites, exposure to indoor toxicants, and other illnesses and injuries. HUD has developed a Healthy Homes initiative to addresses health-related issues associated with inadequate housing (U.S. Department of Housing and Urban

Development, 2021). This initiative reflects concerns raised over the disproportionate impact of inadequate housing on disadvantaged populations. The Healthy Homes strategic plan addresses these issues through a number of strategies. Short-term strategies include: creating a mechanism for coordinating federal healthy homes activities, conducting research to characterize the potential indoor air quality benefits of green construction, collaborating with other HUD offices to promote healthy housing principles in areas where there is a critical public health need (e.g., smoke-free housing, injury prevention, post-disaster environments), and enhancing lead hazard control programs' capability to address broader housing issues that impact occupant health.

In the long term, HUD will assess the effectiveness of healthy homes training and public outreach/education efforts, support the creation and adoption of health-protective housing codes and enforcement strategies, identify and pursue opportunities to promote healthy homes concepts to private and public sector entities, and continue to act as a convener of national, state and local partners through national healthy homes conferences and workshops. This work will be done in coordination with the Office's ongoing efforts in lead poisoning prevention, as the need to create and maintain lead-safe housing for low income families remains substantial.

The Healthy Homes Initiative seeks to:

- Broaden the scope of single-issue public health programs, such as childhood lead poisoning prevention and asthma programs, to address multiple housing deficiencies that affect health and safety.
- Build capacity and competency among public health, environmental health, and housing professionals, and others who work in the community, to develop and manage comprehensive and effective healthy homes programs.
- Promote, develop, and implement cross-disciplinary activities at the federal, state, tribal, and community levels to address the problem of unhealthy and unsafe housing through surveillance, research, and comprehensive prevention programs.
- Facilitate the collection of local data and monitor progress toward reducing or eliminating housing deficiencies and hazards.
- Develop guidelines to assess, reduce, and eliminate health and safety risks.
- Promote research to determine causal relations between substandard housing and adverse health effects.
- Expand collaborations with national associations and organizations, academia, community-based organizations, and others.
- Identify and implement low-cost, reliable, and practical methods to reduce health and safety risks in substandard housing.

Transportation

The predominant types of communities and the distribution of the US population today are a reflection of past transportation policies. Decisions were made, primarily at the federal level, with regard to allocation of funds for infrastructure development. These decisions directed federal funding away from railroads and toward airports and highways. These policies resulted in the United States becoming an automobile-centric society, to the detriment of other forms of transportation.

There are at least two major implications of these past decisions. One relates to the impact of the built transportation environment on health. A second quite different implication relates to the availability of public transportation (or the lack thereof) with its implications for direct access to health-promoting resources (e.g., medical care) and for indirect access to health-promoting resources (e.g., healthy food).

Public health, transportation, and planning professionals increasingly recognize how the built environment affects the physical, social, and mental health of communities. Transportation is an important part of the built environment and significantly influences physical activity and well-being, safety, and the ability of community members to access destinations that are essential to a healthy lifestyle. The U.S. Department of Transportation (DOT) has aggressively supported efforts to ameliorate the negative health consequences of transportation policies.

The second implication relates to the cost of and access to transportation. The Center for Housing Policy (2016) estimates that for every dollar that incomes have increased in the largest metro areas since 2000, combined housing and transportation costs have risen $1.75, making it all the more critical to preserve or create affordable housing near public transit. Nationally, working families face a trade-off between paying a larger share of their incomes toward housing or facing longer commutes and increased transit costs by living in lower-cost housing further from their jobs. The Center for Housing Policy found that for every dollar a working family saves on housing, 77 cents more of its income must go for transportation. Furthermore, when housing and transit costs are considered together, 44.3% of working families put more than half of their household expenditures into these two categories. Most US cities lack well-planned transit access that strategically links low-income communities and affordable housing with the jobs that residents need to support their families.

Living in communities with high quality public transportation or in well-designed and walkable transit-oriented developments can lead to a range of health benefits. These include: reduced vehicle crash injuries, reduced exposure to pollution, increased physical activity, improved mental health, reduced financial burdens and increased access to essential goods and services. Transit access can be a particularly critical issue for low-income older adults who no longer drive and rely on public transportation to reach necessary services, including medical and dental offices. Seniors can more easily and safely "age in place" in communities that are walkable and well-served by transportation.

The U.S. Department of Transportation (DOT) recognizes the role of transportation as a social determinant of health and has developed initiatives to ameliorate the impact of transportation-related issues on disadvantaged populations. The stated goals of the Department in this regard (US Department of Transportation, 2013) are:

1. Improving pedestrian infrastructure or increasing public transportation service in low-income and minority communities to improve connectivity.
2. Using roadside barriers, vegetation, or bottleneck removal to reduce the impacts of pollution on communities located near high-volume roads.
3. Offering reduced public transportation fares for students or youth and working with employers to extend public transportation benefits to employees.
4. Targeting demand response service toward communities with high concentrations of older adults and poor access to shops and services.
5. Addressing housing affordability through a regional strategy for promoting a variety of housing options at different price points for people of all stages and walks of life.

The Department's Complete Streets program provides guidance and support (particularly for rural areas and small towns) for making streets safe and exercise friendly (Smart Growth America, 2021). In view of the transportation challenges facing rural residents, the Department has developed the Rural Transportation Toolkit, an application that offers information, resources, and best practices for rural communities seeking to implement transportation programs that can help improve access to needed services and opportunities (Rural Transportation Information Hub, 2021).

Economic Development

The economy is the most important sector of US society, and an inordinate amount of energy and resources at the federal level are devoted to monitoring economic trends, encouraging economic development, and regulating interstate commerce. Federal policies have long encouraged private sector development, and the amount of "corporate welfare" that exists continues to be a controversial topic. The U.S. Department of Commerce uses monetary policy to attempt to steer the economy in the "right" direction, encouraging growth and discouraging inflationary practices. Numerous agencies like the Small Business Administration have been established to support business development, and job training and workforce development are activities supported by the federal government through grants to states and localities.

Of historical significance is the "war on poverty" initiated in the 1960s as it was realized that a shocking proportion of Americans lived in poverty situations that were generally invisible to the rest of an increasingly affluent society. Policies were promulgated related to poverty amelioration including an expanded welfare program and the introduction of "food stamps" to provide an adequate diet for those living under the poverty level. The Medicaid program was introduced to help address the healthcare issues of impoverished Americans. These policies, accompanied by economic growth, served to moderate the level of poverty in the United States for two or three decades. However, in the 1980s the nation experienced an upward trend in the number of Americans living in poverty, and this peaked at historic levels during the economic downtown beginning in 2008. Current policies, it could be argued, are not adequate to address the growing number of impoverished Americans and, indeed, it is suggested that the current generation of young Americans will be worse off economically than previous generations.

Much has been made of the negative health effects of unemployment, but limited research has been conducted on the link between *employment* and health. At least one study (van der Noordt et al., 2014) found that gaining employment had benefits for mental health status but did not have enough cases to assess the impact on physical health. A large body of research has established that employed individuals are healthier than those who are not employed (Yelin & Trupin, 2003). This association cuts across many demographics, including sex, age, and disability status (Goodman, 2015). Thus, some analysts hypothesize that enhancing employment opportunities for working-age people with disabilities may improve health status and thus decrease healthcare costs.

The National Prevention Strategy (U.S. Department of Health and Human Services, 2017a) highlights how the federal government and community leaders can expand access to jobs and economic opportunity to better promote healthy living. The National Prevention Strategy, outlines specific policies that elected officials and community leaders can implement to prevent disease, promote health, and control costs. A subsequent action plan showcases more than 200 specific prevention and wellness actions federal departments and agencies are currently undertaking toward these ends. The action plan highlights strategies designed to promote good jobs and better health. The Departments of Labor and Agriculture, for example, are providing grants to advance approximately 40 high-growth industries in economically disadvantaged regions to promote jobs that provide access to health insurance coverage and prevention services.

Food Access and Security

The most influential change agents in efforts to help Americans eat well and stay active may be the agencies and business interests that determine advertising messages, supermarket locations, school lunch menus, after-school and summer sports programs, food labels, and the built environment. Key actors include city planners, state officials, federal agencies, legislatures at both the state and federal levels, employers, school boards, zoning commissions, developers, supermarket chains, restaurants, and industries ranging from soda bottlers to transit companies. Initiatives by hospitals, medical societies, and insurers to reduce health care disparities remain vital, but the front line in narrowing health disparities lies beyond health-care (Woolf & Braveman, 2012).

In recognition of the implications of access to food for health, PolicyLink and The Food Trust have been working together for several years to advance policies to help entrepreneurs and food retailers build or expand stores in underserved communities (Policy Link, 2013). Bringing grocery stores to low-income underserved areas creates a healthier food environment that supports making healthier choices: having easy, regular access to grocery stores or other food markets that sell fruits, vegetables, produce, and other staples at affordable prices is necessary for the well-rounded, nutritious diet essential for good health. Supermarkets and other retail outlets that sell healthy foods are also major contributors to strong, local economies. Supermarkets, for example, are often "economic anchors" that draw in foot traffic to support additional stores. They not only create many local jobs, but also foster other commercial development and breathe new life into neighborhoods that have experienced disinvestment for decades. Successful advocacy by hundreds of organizations working to promote equity, health, entrepreneurship, and community development has helped bring over $1 billion in resources to healthy food access projects across the country through the federal Healthy Food Financing Initiative (U.S. Department of Health and Human Services, 2017b) and similar efforts in more than 10 states and localities.

The presence of so many new and diverse innovations in healthy food retailing has provided researchers with more opportunities to examine the relationship between the "food environments" in which people live and their diets, as well as the relationship between food retailing and community economic development. The recent material also reflects researchers' growing intentions and capacities to measure change over time in terms of better access to healthy food. While much progress is being made in developing new models of food retailing, the evidence continues to suggest that many families are underserved and that the problem is most pronounced for residents of low-income communities and communities of color. Leaders in many communities are crafting sustainable and authentic solutions to the grocery gap, creating healthier communities, and contributing to the nation's health and well-being. Policy Link and its partners have also seen how supportive policy can generate solutions in communities with the impetus coming sometimes from local policymakers and other times from the state or federal level.

Criminal Justice

Policing has historically been a local function in the US, and the founding fathers discouraged the establishment of a national police force. Indeed, except in unusual circumstances, the military cannot be deployed within the United States. At the same time, the federal government has over time become much more involved with criminal justice at state and local levels. Criminal justice "policies" have been promulgated primarily through the allocation of federal funds through the

U.S. Department of Justice. There are a variety of programs that support police staffing, training and equipping. After the attacks on the World Trade Center on 9/11 the Department of Homeland Security was established, and this agency has aggressively funded equipment for local police agencies.

The "policies" in place with regard to criminal justice can be determined by the focus of enforcement activities. A prime example of this is the so-called "war on drugs" initiated under President Ronald Reagan in the 1980s. In response to a perceived increase in illegal drug use, the Drug Enforcement Agency was established to prosecute drug suppliers and drug users. Despite the mind-boggling amount of money and resources devoted to the war on drugs, most experts agree that the war has been lost. Indeed, this is probably a case study in the emergence of unintended consequences, in that rather than reducing the volume of illegal drug use in the U.S., these efforts have contributed to continued high use by making the drug "industry" so lucrative.

It has further been argued that the war on drugs was a smokescreen for a "war on minorities" since it was believed, rightly or wrongly, that minorities were more likely to be drug users than whites. This represented a way to counter the civil rights legislation of the 1960s and 1970s. In this regard, the policy has been effective in that our prisons are filled with African-Americans and Hispanics who have been convicted of minor drug crimes.

The state of California has taken a broad view of the impact of sentencing on the condition of those involved including their health status. On the belief that reforming California's sentences for low-level crimes would alleviate prison and jail overcrowding, make communities safer, strengthen families, and shift resources from imprisoning people to treating them for addictions and mental health problems a Health Impact Assessment was carried out to determine how changes in sentencing policies would reduce crime, recidivism, racial inequities in sentencing, and save the state and its counties hundreds of millions of dollars. Human Impact Partners (2014) conducted an in-depth assessment of the public health and equity impacts of reclassifying six non-serious offenses–crimes of drug possession and petty theft–as misdemeanors.

Many people are convicted of crimes that pose no serious threat to others but can be traced to their own substance abuse and mental health problems. They need treatment, not punishment. And treatment is much less costly than punishment, returning $3.77 in benefits for every dollar spent. A shift in how we charge and sentence people who have committed non-serious, non-violent, and non-sexual crimes has far-reaching implications for the health and well-being not only of those who commit these offenses, but for their families, their communities, and the public.

The key to achieving the full benefits of sentencing reform is funding and implementation of the treatment, prevention, and recovery services called for in the initiative. Evidence is overwhelming that providing treatment to offenders who have substance abuse problems or mental illnesses reduces crime and recidivism. Treatment instead of punishment not only benefits their health and well-being, but that of their families and the entire community.

Summary

Policy implementation is expected to play a key role in any efforts to improve community health. Policy can take a number of forms including macro-level policies (affecting the entire society), public policies (affecting specific aspects of society), organizational policies (affecting the operation of organization inside and outside of healthcare), and professional policies (affecting the behavior of those within the healthcare system). Policies can be formulated at various levels of government, with the federal government, individual state governments and various local governments (city and county) addressing their respective issues through policy formulation.

It is felt that many of the deficiencies in the US healthcare system are a result of either a lack of well-thought out policies or policies that are dictated by misplaced priorities. There has been significant movement toward a health-in-all-policies approach to addressing community health improvement. The HiAP model contends that virtually every decision made in terms of policy or legislation has implications for health and well-being. Thus, programs being planned for educational services, transportation projects, housing expansion and various other endeavors should take the implications of decisions being made on the health of the population into consideration. The health impact assessment (HIA) is a tool that has come into widespread use in support of the health-in-all-policies approach. Specific steps are followed in evaluating the direct and indirect, intended and unintended impact a project will have on the health of the community and populations that are directly affected.

While policies related to healthcare might be thought of as the ones most relevant for community health, it is increasingly felt that policies that affect societal spheres outside of healthcare perhaps warrant more consideration. The implications of policies promulgated in the areas of housing, transportation, economic development, criminal justice, education and other spheres that reflect the social determinants of health and illness need to be considered. Policy implementation in these areas, it could be argued, have more potential for contributing positively to community health improvement than health-related policies.

Key Points

- "Public policies" are authoritative decisions made by the legislative, executive and judicial branches of government that are intended to direct or influence the actions, behaviors or decisions of others with regard to the accomplishment of some goal.
- Policies can be formulated in a number of different spheres:

    Macro-level policies
    Public policies
    Organizational policies
    Professional policies

- The United States is noteworthy for its lack of macro-level (society-wide) policies and "policy" often being established by default
- Many of the deficiencies of our healthcare system can be attributed to policies that reflect misplaced priorities
- There is a national movement supported by the public health profession as well as other interests for a health-in-all-policies approach
- The health impact assessment (HIA) is a tool that is increasingly being utilized in order to assess the impact of any decision being made and, as such, is useful to those pursing a health-in-all-policies approach
- Policy analysis should be undertaken in all of the social domains that relate to the social determinants of health and illness
- Policies formulated within the domains of housing, education, economic development, food security, criminal justice, transportation, and other domains should be examined for their impact on community health
- Ultimately, the manner in which policies are implemented vis-à-vis areas that affect health and illness may be more important than any efforts by the healthcare system toward improved population health

References

Center for Housing Policy. (2016). *Paycheck to paycheck*. Downloaded from URL: http://www2.nhc.org/chp/p2p/

Confessore, N. (2014). How School lunch became the lastest political battleground. *The New York Times Magazine*. Downloaded from URL: https://www.nytimes.com/2014/10/12/magazine/how-school-lunch-became-the-latest-political-battleground.html?_r=0

Goodman, N. (2015). *The impact of employment on the health status and health care costs of working-age people with disabilities*. Downloaded from URL: http://www.leadcenter.org/system/files/resource/downloadable_version/impact_of_employment_health_status_health_care_costs_0.pdf

Human Impact Partners. (2014). *Rehabilitating corrections in California: The health impacts of proposition 47: Executive summary*. Downloaded from URL: http://prop47impacts.org/docs/SR_HIP_execsum_091514.pdf

Johns Hopkins (Center to Reduce Cardiovascular Health Disparities). (2016). *Stable housing*. Downloaded from URL: http://www.jhsph.edu/research/centers-and-institutes/johns-hopkins-center-to-eliminate-cardiovascular-health-disparities/about/influences_on_health/stable_housing.html

Kindig, D., Asada, Y., & Booske, B. (2008). A population health framework for setting national and state health goals. *Journal of the American Medical Association, 299*, 2081–2083.

Longest, B. B. (2010). *Healthcare policy making in the United States* (5th ed.). Health Administration Press.

Pew Charitable Trust. (2008). *Humboldt County, California*. Downloaded from URL: http://www.pewtrusts.org/en/research-and-analysis/analysis/hip/hip-case-study-humboldt-county-ca

Policy Link. (2013). *Access to healthy food and why it matters: A review of the research*. Downloaded from URL: http://thefoodtrust.org/uploads/media_items/access-to-healthy-food.original.pdf

Rudolph, L., Caplan, J., Ben-Moshe, K., & Dillon, L. (2013). *Health in all policies: A guide for state and local governments*. American Public Health Association and Public Health Institute.

Rural Transportation Info Hub. (2021). *Rural transportation toolkit.* Downloaded from URL: https://www.ruralhealthinfo.org/toolkits/transportation

Smart Growth America. (2021). *Complete streets: Rural areas and small towns.* Downloaded from URL:https://smartgrowthamerica.org/resources/complete-streets-rural-areas-and-small-towns/

U.S. Department of Agriculture. (2015). *Fact sheet: Schools serving, kids eating healthier school meals thanks to healthy, hunger-free kids act.* Downloaded from URL: https://www.usda.gov/media/press-releases/2015/09/01/fact-sheet-schools-serving-kids-eating-healthier-school-meals

U.S. Department of Education. (2016). *Promise neighborhoods.* Downloaded from URL: http://www2.ed.gov/programs/promiseneighborhoods/index.html

U.S. Department of Education. (2021). *Department of Education announces actions to advance equity in education.* Downloaded from URL: https://www.ed.gov/news/press-releases/department-education-announces-actions-advance-equity-education

U.S. Department of Health and Human Services. (2017a). *National Prevention Strategy.* Downloaded from URL: https://www.surgeongeneral.gov/priorities/prevention/strategy/index.html

U.S. Department of Health and Human Services. (2017b). *Healthy Food Financing Initiative.* Downloaded from URL: https://www.acf.hhs.gov/ocs/programs/community-economic-development/healthy-food-financing

U.S. Department of Housing and Urban Development (2021). *Leading our nation to healthier homes: The healthy homes strategic plan.* Downloaded from URL: https://www.hud.gov/sites/documents/DOC_13701.PDF

U.S. Department of Transportation. (2013). *Health and equity.* Downloaded from URL: https://www.transportation.gov/transportation-health-tool

van der Noordt, M., Ijzelenberg, H., Droomers, M., et al. (2014). Health effects of employment: A systematic review of prospective studies. *Occupational and Environmental Medicine, 71*(10), 730–736.

Weller, C. E., Sharpe, R. V., Solomon, D., et al. 2020). *Redesigning federal funding of research and development.* Downloaded from URL: https://www.americanprogress.org/issues/race/reports/2020/08/18/489609/redesigning-federal-funding-research-development/

Woolf, S., & Braveman, P. (2012). The social and ecological determinants of health. In D. Scutchfield, J. W. Holsinger, et al. (Eds.), *Contemporary topics in public health.* Kentucky University Press.

Yelin, E. H., & Trupin, L. (2003). Disability and the characteristics of employment. *Monthly Labor Review May,* 20–31.

Additional Resources

American Public Health Association. (2012). *Promoting health impact assessment to achieve health in all policies.* Downloaded from URL: https://www.apha.org/policies-and-advocacy/public-health-policy-statements/policy-database/2014/07/11/16/51/promoting-health-impact-assessment-to-achieve-health-in-all-policies

Centers for Disease Control and Prevention. (2016). *Healthy housing reference manual.* Downloaded from URL: https://www.cdc.gov/nceh/publications/books/housing/housing_ref_manual_2012.pdf

Collins, J., & Koplan, J. P. (2009). *Health impact assessment: A step toward health in all policies.* Downloaded from URL: https://pubmed.ncbi.nlm.nih.gov/19602691/

Health and Resource Services Administration: www.hrsa.gov.

Health in All Policies Task Force Report to the Strategic Growth Council Executive Summary. (2010). Sacramento (CA): Health in All Policies Task Force.

References

Healthy Community Design Initiative (Federally funded health impact assessments.
National Association of County and City Health Officials. *Health in All Policies*. Downloaded from URL: http://archived.naccho.org/topics/environmental/hiap/.
National Conference of State Legislators (certificate-of-need reference): https://www.ncsl.org/research/health/con-certificate-of-need-state-laws.aspx.
Thomas, R. K. (2021). *Health service planning* (3rd ed.). Springer.
U.S. Department of Transportation. (2015). *Transportation and health tool*. Downloaded from URL: https://www.transportation.gov/transportation-health-tool

Chapter 10
Traditional Approaches to Community Health Data

The traditional approach to conducting a community health needs assessment reflects the historical orientation of the healthcare system. This approach was developed primarily by epidemiologists, so it is not surprising that these assessments rely heavily on epidemiological data. These assessments also place a great deal of emphasis on the availability of healthcare resources and observed utilization patterns. Traditional data categories are reviewed, along with some neglected categories that should be included in an assessment. The drawbacks of these data types for a health needs assessment are reviewed.

In this chapter the reader will:

- Review the types of data traditionally used for assessing health status and conducting community health needs assessment
- Be exposed to the drawbacks of traditional data and the need for a different approach
- Find out about the importance of non-traditional health data and non-health-related data
- Learn about sources of data useful for traditional community health analyses

Introduction

Community health needs assessments have long been carried out in the US, and some standard approaches have been established. Part of the process involves accessing data that are thought to provide insight into the health status of the targeted population. The sections that follow describe the categories of data that are typically accessed for a health needs assessment and the sources where relevant metrics can be found. This is followed by a critique of the traditional data categories that leads into the next chapter's discussion of population health assessments.

Traditional Categories of Data for Health Needs Assessment

The sections below describe the types of data that have traditionally been collected and analyzed in the implementation of a community health needs assessment.

Demographic Data

Demographic data serve as the foundation for most needs assessment activities. Not only are demographic data important for profiling the community, but they serve as the basis for the calculation of a number of statistics relevant to the analysis. While an understanding of the demographic composition of the target population is important in its own right, this information is also essential for identifying the prevalence of health conditions and determining utilization patterns within the community. Importantly, certain demographic attributes have historically been considered proxies for health status metrics.

From an analytical perspective, it is useful to categorize demographic variables into *biosocial* variables and *sociocultural* variables. Biosocial characteristics are clearly distinguished as demographic variables by their link to biological traits. The demographic variables included in this category are: *age*, *sex* and *race*. (*Ethnicity* is sometimes included because of its close relationship to race). The sociocultural variables reflect one's position within the social structure and include income, education, marital status, occupation and other socially assigned attributes.

Age is probably the best single predictor of the utilization of health services. Age is related not only to levels of service utilization but to the type of services utilized and the circumstances under which they are received.

The *sex* distribution of community members is another factor influencing both health status and health behavior. Females are more active than males in terms of health behavior and are heavier users of the healthcare system. They tend to visit physicians more often, take more prescription drugs, and, in general, use other facilities and personnel more often.

Racial and ethnic characteristics influence the demand for health services and tend to be associated with extreme health disparities. Detailed information on the racial and ethnic characteristics of the population should be compiled, including qualitative data on attitudes and preferences. While differences in utilization may be traced to differences in the types of health problems experienced by these populations, many of the distinctions reflect variations in lifestyle patterns and cultural preferences. The language spoken by the community population or sub-populations may also be a factor influencing healthcare communications and the efficient delivery of services

Sociocultural traits are important in profiling the population because of their correlation with health status and health behavior. The sociocultural variables discussed below include: marital status and related attributes, education, income, occupation/industry, and other sociocultural factors. Additional information on insurance coverage, psychographic categories, and community attitudes is included.

Marital status, household structure and, to a degree, *living arrangements* are all of interest to health analysts. Marital status refers to one's current legal status with regard to marriage. Household structure refers to involvement in the physical household–i.e., where one actually lives. Living arrangements refer to the relationship between those sharing a household–i.e., roommates, married with children, unmarried relatives. For community health planners, marital status and household structure may have implications for the types of health problems that exist and the patterns of health services utilization.

Education is an important factor to consider during an assessment, since the educational level of the population is closely correlated with both health status and health behavior. This information is often important for the development of services that are compatible with the level of sophistication of the target audience.

Income and related variables, such as poverty status, are obviously critical for any analysis at the community level. Income, measured in terms of annual household income or per capita income, is an important predictor of both the level of morbidity within the community and likely patterns of health services utilization. The overall level of community affluence will influence both the healthcare "wants" of the population and the level of resources available.

Occupation and *industry* are important variables in profiling a community. Not only do individuals in different occupations and industries have differing consumer behavior habits, but the occupational or industrial profile of an area is an excellent indicator of the mix of healthcare services and products required by the target population. Distinctive patterns of healthy and unhealthy behavior have been correlated with different occupations and industries. Further, the occupational structure is likely to determine the extent to which employer-sponsored health insurance is available.

There are other sociocultural characteristics that might be important in different communities. *Religion* is a characteristic of the population that is difficult to measure and has, in fact, played a limited role in a health needs assessment. However, there are occasions when knowledge of a community's religious preferences may be appropriate for health services planning. For example, there may be segments of the population that have strong ties to church-affiliated health facilities within the community or sects that may have an aversion to medical care.

Epidemiological Data

Epidemiological data have historically represented the primary basis for assessing health status and identifying health service needs. Traditional community health assessments have focused on the "five Ds": death, disease, disability, discomfort, and distress, and most early attempts at measuring health status took this approach. The five Ds form a hierarchy, from objective, numerical measures to more subjective, qualitative indicators, and also from those that are routinely collected (e.g., death certificates) to those that are not routinely tracked by epidemiologists. The sections below provide an overview of various examples of epidemiological data.

Morbidity Measures

Morbidity refers to the level of sickness and disability characterizing a population. Morbidity may be used to refer to a person or a group, with the former referring to the health status of an individual and the latter to the health status of a population. Traditional health needs assessments have tended to think of a community's health status as the sum of individual characteristics. Proponents of a population health approach are, on the other hand, almost exclusively interested in morbidity as associated with populations and seldom with the morbidity of individuals—reflecting the distinction between individual (clinical) morbidity and group (epidemiological) morbidity. Box 10.1 addresses the subjective nature of morbidity.

Most classification systems used for assessing a population's level of morbidity focus on physical illness rather than mental illness (although there is some overlap between the two types of systems). The most widely recognized and utilized disease classification system is the *International Classification of Diseases*. The ICD system is the official classificatory scheme developed by the World Health Organization within the United Nations. The version currently utilized in the United States is ICD-10-CM. The ICD system is designed for the classification of morbidity and mortality information and for the indexing of diseases and procedures that occur within a clinical setting. The present classification system includes two components: diagnoses and procedures. Other classification systems are used to categorize other types of conditions (e.g., mental illness, disability).

"Reportable" conditions, or notifiable diseases, represent another system of disease classification. Reportable diseases are singled out by public health authorities primarily because of their communicable nature. Public health officials are particularly interested in conditions that have the potential to spread to epidemic proportions. It should be noted that notifiable diseases are virtually all acute conditions, at a time when chronic conditions represent the dominant health threat. For this reason, notifiable morbid conditions have become less useful over time as indicators of health status.

Box 10.1: The Subjective Nature of Morbidity
While we typically think of illness being determined based on clinical measures, this objective depiction of ill-health is not the only manner in which illness is conceptualized. It is, in fact, a "modern" notion of the nature of illness. Societies (and even individuals) are likely to develop notions of health and illness that are particular to the situation and the social context. For that reason, it would not be unusual to find a disparity between the clinically identified conditions within a population and the conditions members of that population identify. While biologically based health conditions are concrete and finite, socially defined conditions are more abstract and elastic. To understand the true level of morbidity within a population, both the objective and subjective dimensions need to be considered.

All things being equal, the absolute level of need should not vary much from population to population. Researchers working independently should draw the same conclusions with regard to the level and types of health conditions characterizing a specific population. This notion of an absolute level of morbidity relates more closely to the concept of biologically based "illness" than societally defined "sickness."

While epidemiologists are likely to find similar levels of morbidity from society to society, the subjectively defined levels of morbidity levels will typically be quite different. Anthropologists tell us of societies where certain clearly identifiable diseases exist but society members assure them that it is not a disease but something "normal" among this population. Malnutrition that might be identified by a scientist within a population may be considered normal by that population. In our own society, we have individuals who deny the existence of disease even though it may be clinically identifiable. While the detrimental effects of obesity have long been known, there are still segments of the US population that consider extreme overweight as a positive and even desirable state. Certainly, many Americans who could be diagnosed with a mental disorder would deny that any such condition exists.

There are plenty of examples of the subjective nature of illness that could be cited. Classic examples include the military induction center, where most prospective inductees are deemed disease free when there is high demand for servicemen, but a "normal" amount of morbidity is discovered when there is no pressure on recruitment. Similarly, during the time of the Soviet Union, if a factory was not meeting its quota, the on-site physician might diagnose few cases of illness that would merit time off from work. On the other hand, if quotas were being met, a "normal" amount of morbidity was revealed.

Mortality Measures

Mortality refers to the level of death characterizing a population, and the study of mortality involves research on the who, how, why, and when issues related to dying. The most basic way to measure mortality is simply to count the number of deaths that occur within a population during a specific period of time. Such counts are usually based on a one-year period and may be reported for the nation as a whole, states, metropolitan areas or smaller geographic areas. Virtually every death in the United States is recorded and as a result mortality data are of very high quality. Compiling death counts over a period of years allows demographers to identify trends with regard to increases or decreases in mortality. Insights into mortality can be gained by cross-classifying deaths by the medical, social, and economic characteristics of the deceased.

The *causes of death* affecting a population are a major factor in determining the level of mortality. Populations in different times and places are subject to different causes of death. Knowing the number of people who died is one thing but knowing what they died from provides valuable insights into the overall health status of the population and the types of health conditions that afflict it. With a preponderance of chronic diseases, it is often the case that death can and should be attributed to a factor other than the underlying cause of death. For example, patients with AIDS do not typically die as a direct result of AIDS but due to system failure as a result of AIDS. This situation has led to a growing lack of confidence in the ability of cause-of-death data to accurately reflect health status.

One other frequently utilized mortality indicator is the infant mortality rate, and this is sometimes considered a proxy for a population's overall health status. Although this measure only applies to a limited segment of the population (i.e., those under 1 year of age), it is considered by many as more useful than the overall mortality rate. The premise is that the infant mortality rate reflects environmental safety, diet, prenatal care, the educational and economic status of the parents, the age of the mother, the occurrence of neglect and abuse, and a number of other factors. As with the overall mortality rate, however, infant deaths occur rarely enough that measures of infant mortality have less salience as indicators of a population's health than they did historically.

Health Behavior

Health behavior can be defined as any action aimed at restoring, preserving, and/or enhancing health status. Both formal activities such as physician visits, hospital admissions, and prescription drug consumption and informal actions on the part of individuals such as diet, exercise, and risk-taking should be considered. (It should be noted that utilization rates represent a dimension of health behavior, and these are discussed in some detail in the section below.)

One set of models of health behavior focuses on the individual level and considers how individuals make decisions with regard to their health. Studies of behavioral intentions suggest that the likelihood of intended audiences' adopting a desired behavior can be predicted by assessing (and subsequently trying to change or influence) their attitudes toward and perceptions of the benefits of the behavior, along with how they think that their peers will view their behavior.

Traditional health needs assessments are likely to view health behavior at the individual level. This assumes that individuals are making health behavior choices of their own volition and that their actions should be viewed in isolation. This conventional perspective flies in the face of the population health model, which would contend that decisions related to health behavior are not made in a vacuum but are influenced by the social context. It could be argued that health behavior—like health status—arises out of the social and cultural environment and reflects the operation of the social determinants of health.

Lifestyles affect health behavior in several direct and indirect ways. A clear example relates to food preferences. Youth and many adults adopt a "fast-food lifestyle" and seldom eat any other type of food. To do so would risk ridicule from their peers. Healthy foods once promoted by certain subcultures (e.g., the greens and vegetables associated with African-American culture) are eschewed in favor of inexpensive but unhealthy processed foods. The churches patronized by members of certain subcultures, for example, are notorious for their unhealthy church supper fare. Many observers consider lifestyles to be a major determinant of health behavior.

Healthcare Resources

A key component of the typical health needs assessment is an inventory of the health-related resources available to the community. "Resources" are viewed in the broadest sense here, ranging from facilities to personnel to sources of funding for healthcare. The focus here is on facilities involved in the direct provision of care. The most important types of community resources are described below.

Facilities

A major component of resource identification involves the inventory of the facilities available for meeting the healthcare needs of the population. These include all types of facilities devoted to the treatment of physical or mental illnesses. The following are representative of the types of facilities that must be inventoried:

Hospitals The central role of the hospital in the provision of care warrants a careful inventory of the area's inpatient facilities. This includes not only general hospitals but any specialty hospitals that might serve the population. Some categories of hospitals may ultimately be eliminated from the analysis (such as military hospitals or others that serve small, selected populations), but all should initially be included. Hospitals should be categorized in terms of the auspices under which they operate (e.g., governmental, private for profit, faith-based not-for-profit). The number of available hospital beds should be determined, with careful attention paid to operational versus licensed beds.

The range of services offered by area hospitals should be determined since not all services are offered by all facilities. For example, all general hospitals must offer emergency services, but the quality and level of specialization can vary greatly. Another example would be maternity services. Not all hospitals deliver babies, and, among those that do, their capabilities for dealing with premature and low-weight births will vary.

Area hospitals should be profiled in terms of admissions, occupancy rates, specialty areas and any other relevant characteristics. The market share controlled by the hospitals within the community should be calculated to the extent possible. Trends in relevant indicators should be identified and the physical location of hospitals and other facilities with regard to population concentrations needs to be considered. Any identifiable trends in the characteristics of local health facilities should be noted.

Clinics The number of clinics providing health services should be determined, particularly since this is the setting in which most clinical encounters occur. ("Clinic" here refers to any freestanding outpatient facility that dispenses medical care.) The key category, of course, is the physician-based clinic, and these clinics should be inventoried in terms of size, specialty, and any other relevant characteristics. Most of these will be private practices, but community-based clinics (such as federally qualified health centers) should be included and counted toward the overall resource base. Other types of clinics (non-physician) that should be considered include: eye care clinics, chiropractic clinics and podiatric clinics. The type of reimbursement accepted by various physician clinics is likely to affect access to care for community residents. Given the observed level of maldistribution of clinical services the distribution of clinics in relation to population concentrations should be noted.

Nursing Homes The other major institutional facility besides hospitals is nursing homes, with nursing home access becoming a growing issue as the number of elderly Americans increases. The number of nursing homes should be determined, along with the number of beds, occupancy rates, and the categories of clients served. The type of reimbursement accepted is also an important consideration with regard to nursing home access.

Residential Treatment Facilities Another form of institutional care involves residential treatment centers. Typically reserved for behavioral health and substance abuse patients, residential treatment centers represent "inpatient" facilities in the sense that their clients remain overnight at the facility. They do not typically have the around-the-clock intensive clinical support that a hospital would provide. The types of clients that these facilities cater to is an important consideration for the resource inventory, as well as the type of reimbursement that is accepted. The opioid abuse epidemic has highlighted the need for—and serious lack of—substance abuse treatment centers.

Home Health Agencies/Hospices Home health agencies have come to play a major role in the delivery of health services, particularly as the emphasis has shifted from inpatient care to outpatient care. These are technically not facilities since they actually provide care in the client's home. The range of services provided in a home setting has steadily grown and, in communities that suffer a shortage of physicians, home health agencies may represent an important source of care. The inventory should identify home health agencies in terms of the services they provide and the type of reimbursement they accept.

Hospices typically do not involve physical facilities but constitute a program of care that is implemented in the patient's home (although some hospice services may be provided in a hospital or some other setting). Although hospice services will not be a major factor in the overall operation of the delivery system, they are necessary to assure a comprehensive ranges of services.

Mental Health Centers Mental health services (increasingly referred to as behavioral health services) have often been overlooked in inventories of healthcare facilities due to the bias toward physical medicine. However, a growing proportion of the US population receives some type of behavioral health service, and the demand is expected to grow as lifestyle- and stress-related conditions proliferate. Mental health centers should be identified in terms of their volumes, the types of clients they serve, and their sources of reimbursement.

Diagnostic Centers As a result of the effort to move care out of the inpatient setting, a number of freestanding facility types have emerged, including outpatient diagnostic centers. These may be multipurpose diagnostic centers or they may focus on a particular diagnostic category such as radiology. The number and types of freestanding diagnostic centers should be determined as well as their organizational affiliation.

Surgery Centers Freestanding outpatient surgery centers have been another product of the shift from inpatient to outpatient care. As various specialties have shifted their surgical load from the inpatient setting to the outpatient setting, outpatient surgery centers have been the primary beneficiaries. As with other facilities, the type of patients, volume of services, reimbursement arrangements, and organizational affiliation should be determined as part of the inventory.

Urgent Care Centers Urgent care centers (called by a variety of names) have become increasingly common sources of basic health services. Initially developed as an alternative to emergency room care and as an option for off-hours care, urgent care centers have become a mainstay for segments of the population that do not have a regular source of care. They are, however, designed for episodic care and technically do not serve as true primary care centers. The number of centers, their volumes, and their acceptable reimbursement should be determined, along with their organizational affiliation.

Recent years have seen the emergence of "retail" clinics in drug stores, grocery stores and "big box" chain establishments. While these mini-clinics offer limited services, they do represent an alternative for those seeking convenience or lacking personal physicians. A more specialized version of this has emerged in the form of "shot nurses" who administer both required vaccinations (e.g., for school) and discretionary vaccinations (e.g., for overseas travel).

Programs and Services

A distinction is often made between "programs" and "services", with the former typically referring to a multipurpose operation that integrates a number of functions. The latter typically refers to a specific treatment modality that might be offered in a stand-alone fashion or as part of a program. Thus, an agency that provides personal assistants for the home might be considered to offer a service, while a home health agency that offers a full-range of nursing services, rehabilitation services, and home infusion, in addition to personal assistance aides, would be considered to have a program.

The identification of programs and services separate from health facilities and personnel is perhaps more important than it seems on the surface. This is primarily because services define the facility more than the facility defines the services in many cases. Further, healthcare consumers and referral agents are more likely to be seeking a particular service and may not care what type of facility provides it. For example, someone seeking treatment for an eating disorder will be searching for that type of service and it probably does not matter whether it is located at a hospital, a residential facility, or an outpatient facility. It would be rare for a consumer to select a hospital and *then* determine if it had the required service. (An exception would be cases where one's insurance restricted the use of facilities.)

Personnel

It could be argued that the availability of health professionals within a community is the most important indicator of resource adequacy. The treatment capabilities available to the population are more a reflection of the personnel available than the facilities available. Personnel should be identified in terms of type, number, characteristics and distribution.

Physicians The physician remains the pivotal player in the healthcare system, despite the shifts in control that have occurred in recent years. For this reason, as precise an inventory of physician resources as possible should be carried out. Physicians should be inventoried as a group and in terms of their distribution by specialty. To the extent possible, other characteristics should be identified as part of the profile. These include subspecialty areas, ages, type of practice (e.g., office-based, hospital), level of effort, hospital affiliation, and so forth. Of particular importance is the distribution of physician practices vis-a-vis the distribution of the population. Health professional shortage areas (for primary care physicians) are designated by the Health Resources and Services Administration (HRSA) and are useful for assessing the adequacy of physician resources.

Of particular importance is an assessment of the sources of reimbursement accepted by physician practices. To the extent that physicians to not accept patients who are uninsured or are covered through Medicaid, a significant barrier to care may exist.

A basic distinction that should be made is between primary care physicians and specialty physicians. The primary care physician is responsible for basic services and, as such, family practitioners, obstetricians, pediatricians, and general internists are considered the backbone of the system. Increasingly, they serve as the "gate-keepers" who channel patients into the system.

Nursing Personnel Nurses have historically served as the backbone of the healthcare delivery system, while constituting the largest category of health personnel. While the number of nurses practicing in a community may be more a function of demand than supply, the existing nurse staffing patterns provide an important perspective on the delivery system. Increasingly, nurse practitioners, nurse clinicians, and other highly trained nursing personnel are practicing independently. In fact, such personnel, usually practicing under a physician's supervision, may provide the bulk of the primary care in certain underserved areas. The longstanding–and growing–nurse shortage has implications for the ability of a community to provide certain services.

Other Independent Practitioners Several categories of independent practitioners should be inventoried as part of this process. These include dentists, pharmacists, optometrists, chiropractors, and podiatrists. These practitioners typically occupy specific niches within the delivery system, usually supplementing but sometimes competing with the services of physicians. In fact, in an era of managed care, it has become common to substitute "lower" level services from optometrists, chiropractors, and podiatrists for the more expensive physician services of ophthalmologists, neurosurgeons and orthopedic surgeons.

Mental Health Personnel Mental health personnel are frequently overlooked when community assessments are conducted. Their position at the fringes of mainstream healthcare has historically prevented them from being effectively inventoried in such projects. The community assessment should identify and inventory the variety of practitioners that provide psychological, behavioral health, and psychiatric services to the community. These practitioners are likely to be especially important when the needs of the community's vulnerable populations are considered, with the increasing prevalence of behavioral health problems drawing them more into the mainstream of health services delivery.

Alternative Therapy Providers A growing category of practitioners that requires inclusion is the variety of alternative therapy providers within a community. Until recently, such practitioners where considered outside the mainstream of conventional medical care. Today, however, it is realized that consumers spend as much of their healthcare dollar on alternative therapies as they do on conventional medical care. Alternative therapists are used both as adjuncts to conventional care and as substitutes. Thus, the community's complement of acupuncturists, herbalists, homeopaths, nutritional therapists, and so on should be identified along with the more conventional practitioners. This is especially the case in communities with large ethnic populations that are likely to maintain certain forms of traditional medical practices.

Health Insurance

An increasingly important health-related resource is health insurance. The US healthcare system is unlike any other system in the world in that it: (1) operates primarily on a fee-for-service basis; (2) includes a significant for-profit component; (3) covers costs on a "reimbursement" basis after services are provided; and, importantly, (4) places health insurance at a pivotal point between healthcare consumers and the system. Increasing portions of the population are covered under the Medicare and Medicaid programs, making the federal government the major purchaser of health services. Around one-third of the population is covered through private insurance with most of this offered through their place of employment. Another 25 million or more Americans are uninsured for health problems. Because of the limitations on available insurance coverage, medical bills are the major contributor to the high rate of bankruptcy in the US.

It is increasingly recognized that access to health insurance is a major consideration with regard to community health status and, indeed, an estimated 45,000 Americans die each year simply because they have no health insurance coverage. Even many with coverage would be considered "under-insured" due to substandard policies or the limited coverage provided under most state-run Medicaid programs. Although access to health insurance does not assure access to health services nor guarantee health maintenance or improvement, it is recognized as such a critical aspect that it is discussed in the chapter on the social determinants of health. Box 10.2 discusses the relationship between health insurance and health status.

Networks and Relationships

A thorough inventory of community health services should include a review of existing networks and relationships within the delivery system. This has become an increasingly important consideration with the emergence of the population health model. Some of these relationships may be formal and totally overt; others may take the form of "gentlemen's agreements" and be not widely appreciated by the general

> **Box 10.2: Health Insurance Coverage and Health Status**
>
> The United States is unique among modern, industrialized nations with regard to the financing of health services for its citizens. Most similar countries have national healthcare systems with a single mechanism (usually taxes) through which individuals pay for the healthcare they receive. Although in the US the government does play a role in the financing of healthcare, this is primarily through the Medicare and Medicaid programs (for the elderly and the indigent, respectively). For those not qualifying for Medicare or Medicaid, their primary option is commercial insurance (either through group or individual plans), often provided through one's place of employment. In recent years the proportion of US residents covered by employer-sponsored insurance has declined, while the proportion covered under government programs has increased.
>
> A significant portion of the population is uninsured and, although addressed somewhat by the passage in 2010 of the Affordable Care Act, tens of millions of Americans still lack health insurance. Of those who do have insurance, almost one in five has two or more different types. The extent to which an individual or family has health insurance varies with the situation and is liable to change over time. It is not unusual for a patient to have his medical costs covered through some combination of sources (e.g., Medicare, Medicaid and out-of-pocket payments).
>
> Data generated through the National Health Interview Survey indicate a correlation between type of insurance coverage and health status. All Americans over age 65 are eligible for Medicare insurance coverage, and their health status is not generally associated with their insurance status. For those under 65 years of age, however, the health status of those with private insurance was reported to be much higher. Similarly, people covered through private insurance are less likely than those covered under Medicaid or those lacking insurance to report chronic diseases or conditions limiting their daily activities.
>
> The relationship between presence of and type of health insurance and morbidity is a complicated one, and the nature of the relationship is not always clear. However, for our purposes it can be argued that type of insurance coverage is a reasonable predictor of health status in general and the prevalence of certain health problems in particular.

public. It could be argued that the presence or absence of certain relationships has been a major barrier to efforts at community health improvement.

The assessment of community facilities should consider the relationships that exist among various organizations. The extent to which hospitals have diversified into other areas such as home health and hospice, urgent care centers, or fitness centers, for example, needs to be determined. A similar process should be utilized with personnel to determine the relationships that exist. In most communities provider networks have been established by hospitals, health plans or some other entity.

In some communities, business coalitions have been established by major employers to negotiate directly with healthcare providers and/or insurance plans. These relationships may involve exclusive contracts between major purchasers of care and local health systems that must be taken into consideration.

An important aspect of this analysis involves referral relationships. "Referral patterns" is used broadly here to include actions that channel consumers toward the use of a service or the purchase of a product. In many communities the utilization of services is significantly influenced by existing referral networks. Referral patterns within the population health context are probably most important in relation to public health services and community clinics. The analyst needs to develop a clear understanding of the processes by which consumers come to access publicly supported services and the extent to which the safety net protects the medically indigent.

Health Services Utilization

The extent to which available health services are utilized by the population is an important factor, and a number of indicators that are commonly used to measure utilization. Each of the key utilization indicators is discussed in turn below, although the various aspects of these indicators cannot be discussed in detail in the limited space available here.

Hospital admissions is one of the most frequently used indicators of health services utilization, since the hospital represents the focal point for treatment in the system. The terms "admissions" and "discharges" are used to refer to episodes of inpatient hospital utilization. The hospital admissions rate serves as a proxy for a variety of other indicators, since hospital admissions are correlated with tests conducted, surgeries performed, and allocation of other resources. Since hospital care is both labor and capital intensive, one admission carries a great deal of weight in terms of significance in overall healthcare expenditures. Admissions may be measured for the entire community or for a particular facility or be decomposed into components of utilization. This could involve the calculation of admission rates by clinical specialty, demographic attribute, geographic origin, payor category, and so on.

Patient days refers to the number of hospital days generated by a particular population. The total number of patient days is calculated and they are converted to a rate calculated in terms of the number of patient days generated per 1000 residents. This indicator refines hospital admissions as an indicator by reflecting the total utilization of resources, since measuring patient days serves to adjust for variations in length of stay for various conditions. Like admission rates, patient days may be calculated by diagnosis, type of hospital, patient origin, and payer category. Over time, patient days have become more of a standard unit for the measurement of resource utilization than hospital admissions.

Another indicator used to measure hospitalization is the *average length of stay*. This is typically reported in terms of the average number of days patients remain in the facility during a specified time period. This metric is also based on the patient day indicator and involves dividing the total patient days generated for a time period (usually a year) and then dividing the total by, in this case, 365 days. This indicator provides a useful measure of resource utilization as well. In fact, Medicare and many health care plans reimburse hospitals on a per diem rate.

Emergency department visits represent an increasingly important indicator of health services utilization. There are many more emergency episodes than there are hospital admissions, and the frequent use of hospital emergency departments for primary care services makes the tracking of emergency service use an important indicator. The emergency department visit rate is calculated in terms of the number of visits per 1000 population per year. There is typically a correlation between the use of emergency services and the availability of insurance. The long-term increase in the emergency department visit rate is often considered a reflection of issues with access to health insurance.

There are several *other facility indicators* that might also be mentioned. While not all of them carry the significance of hospital admissions, each is important in its own way. Utilization rates may be calculated for hospital outpatient facilities, freestanding emergency centers, freestanding minor medical centers, freestanding surgery centers, and freestanding diagnostic centers, among others.

The most useful indicator of health services utilization is probably the volume of physician encounters. This is typically measured in terms of *physician office visits* although telephone contact, physician visits to hospitalized patients, and telehealth "visits" are sometimes considered. Since the physician is the "gatekeeper" for most types of health services, and, since virtually everyone uses a physician's services at some time, physician utilization is a more direct measure of utilization levels than hospital admissions. Physician utilization rates are often broken down by specialty, since the level of utilization for different specialties varies dramatically.

There are *other types of personnel* for whom utilization rates might be calculated. Most of these, like physicians and dentists, are independent practitioners who practice without the supervision of other medical personnel. Examples include optometrists, podiatrists, chiropractors, nurse practitioners, and physician's assistants, as well as various mental health counselors and therapists. Other health care personnel, who generally cannot operate independently, but for whom utilization rates might be calculated, include home health nurses and various technical personnel. Physical therapists and speech therapists are other categories of healthcare personnel for whom utilization rates might be developed if, for example, the analyst was involved in planning for rehabilitation services.

Another indicator of the use of health services is the level of *drug utilization* exhibited by the target population. Analysts of drug use typically focus on the consumption of prescription drugs, since these (rather than over-the-counter medicine) are thought to more closely reflect actual utilization of the formal healthcare system. Rates of prescription drug utilization are typically calculated in two different ways. First, the number of prescriptions *written* by physicians and other clinicians is tracked, and this can be converted to the number of prescriptions within a given year per 1000 population. Alternatively, the average number of prescriptions written annually per person may be calculated. Second, the number of prescriptions *filled* might be determined and the average number and rate per 1000 residents calculated. The former information is obtained from surveys of consumers or physician offices and the latter from pharmacy records. There is inevitably a discrepancy between the number of prescriptions written and the number filled. The question of the ultimate disposition of prescribed drugs also arises as some drugs are never consumed and others may be diverted for inappropriate and even illegal use.

Non-Traditional Health Data Metrics

Proponents of a population health approach have argued that analysts often rely on data that do not offer a true picture of health status. Indeed, the metrics often cited by epidemiologists reflect the perceptions of health professionals and not those of the community under study. Community respondents are not likely to cite death rates as their main health problems but conditions more likely to affect their everyday lives. They are more likely to describe a lack of food, poor housing, or other non-medical factors as the health problems they are facing, along with often-neglected measures of health status as obesity, substance abuse and domestic violence. The following section describe health conditions that are often neglected when assessing a community's health.

Obesity

Obesity is a "disease of civilization" and reflects the lifestyles of populations in modern society. The terms "overweight" and "obesity" refer to body weight that is greater than what is considered healthy for a certain height. People classified as obese have an abnormally high and unhealthy proportion of body fat. Obesity is considered a morbid condition in its own right and is associated with a wide range of other health conditions. Among the disorders considered to be caused, triggered or exacerbated by obesity are: coronary heart disease, hypertension, stroke and diabetes. Although obesity has traditionally been considered a contributing factor in the onset of other chronic diseases, its importance is elevated within the population health framework on the contention that obesity is not an individual problem but a societal one, one that is more reflective of the environment that American society has fostered than of individual behavior. Box 10.3 describes the use of the BMI metric as a health status indicator.

Mental Illness

Modern Western thinking recognizes a clear distinction between the physical and the mental domains. This perspective was reinforced by the deep entrenchment of germ theory in the medical model paradigm. The biomedical model's emphasis on

Box 10.3: BMI as a Measure of Morbidity
The steady increase in the collection of healthcare data via disease reports, administrative data, and surveys has made it possible to create a variety of morbidity and comorbidity indices. These indices are subsequently used in a host of analyses designed to provide insights into the changes in the levels of sickness and illness. In addition, the indices are linked to mortality data in order to better understand shifts in death rates (Chaudhry et al., 2005).

One index receiving significant attention in recent years is a simple one, the body mass index (BMI). The BMI is generated through a simple calculation:

$$\text{BMI} = \frac{\text{mass (Kg or pounds)}}{(\text{height (m or inches)})^2}$$

The BMI is not a direct measure of morbidity, but an indicator of risk for morbid conditions such as high blood pressure and diabetes. BMI scores are classified into seven categories ranging from severely underweight, index score less than 16.5 (e.g., a person who is 5'5" and weighs less than 118 pounds) to Obese Class 111 (e.g., a 5'5" person weighing 290 pounds or more). BMI scores can be calculated by age, thus allowing for the objective identification of persons who are overweight for their age.

It should be noted that the BMI has several shortcomings. The BMI sometimes overestimates adiposity in those who have more lean body mass and underestimates adiposity in those who have less lean body mass. For example, those with intermediate BMI scores are sometimes found to have a higher risk of death from diseases such as coronary artery disease than those with higher BMI scores (Romero-Corral et al., 2008).

However, the BMI is relatively easy to calculate and comparing scores over time provides a good summary of the growing problem of obesity in the United States and other developed countries. By examining shifts over time in the distribution of BMI scores among children, researchers have been able to document the growing epidemic of childhood obesity. The importance of obesity as a precursor to a variety of health conditions makes this simple index invaluable.

biological causes led to the separation of conditions that demonstrated clear biological pathology (physical illnesses) from those that did not (mental illnesses). This distinction is reflected in what is essentially a separate sector within the healthcare system for the treatment of mental disorders, with distinct facilities and practitioners. A clear demarcation is maintained today between mental hospitals and general hospitals and, in medical practice, between psychiatrists and other physicians.

Physical illness and mental illness do differ from each other in a number of ways. Physical illness is generally characterized by clear-cut, clinically identifiable symptoms, while mental illness is not. The symptoms of physical illness reflect biological pathology while those of mental illness reflect disorders of mood, behavior, and/or thought. Clearly, the diagnosis of most mental disorders is more subjective than that of physical disorders because of the lack of clinical diagnostic tests. Although a small portion of mental disorders can be attributed to some underlying biological pathology (e.g., nervous system damage), most mental conditions are thought to reflect either internal psychological pathology or the influence of external stressors. Neither of these lends itself to traditional clinical diagnostic techniques.

The definitions of mental health and illness reflect the same models or perspectives associated with physical health and illness. The medical model remains important, primarily due to the pivotal role of the psychiatrist in diagnosis and treatment. However, the functional model is particularly relevant in that mental pathology is more likely to be identified based on some functional impairment rather than a biological impairment. Indeed, most cases of mental disorder go undetected until social relationships are so disrupted that a response is required. It should also be remembered that mental health or illness is sometimes defined from a legal perspective. The courts may be placed in the position of determining the mental capacity of the effected individual.

The classification of morbidity related to mental problems is conceptualized somewhat differently from physical illness, and this is reflected in a classification system specific to mental disorders. The definitive reference on the classification of mental disorder is the *Diagnostic and Statistical Manual of Mental Disorders.* Now in its fifth edition, it is commonly referred to as DSM-V. Its 16 major categories of mental illness and over 300 identified mental conditions represent an exhaustive review of observed conditions.

Disability Data

"Disability" refers to any short- or long-term reduction of a person's activity as a result of an acute or chronic condition. While it would appear a simple operation to enumerate the blind, deaf, or otherwise handicapped, the situation is actually quite complex. Quite often a "diagnosis" of disability is a subjective process, and there are many hearing-impaired individuals and amputees, for example, who would take exception to being classified as disabled.

Despite their widespread use each of the classification systems suffers from limitations of one kind or another. From a research perspective, the use of self-reported measures raises questions concerning the standardization of the participant's answers. Disability measures have also been problematic as public policy-making tools. The nation's social security insurance programs rely on the narrowly defined criteria of the disease model to determine disability. They do not adequately address psychological difficulties nor do they provide insight into certain social contributions to disability. Systems measuring limitations in major activities, on the other hand, may indicate the presence of some social contribution to disability but do not provide sufficient information to inform health interventions. These limitations have been recognized, but there has been no consensus on a system that could provide a sufficiently broad understanding of disability.

The inclusion of disability data raises the issue of quality of life. Many observers would argue that data on morbidity and mortality are of little use if the quality of life is not taken into consideration. Indeed, while we find that more Americans are living to old age, this increase in longevity carries an increased chronic disease burden. Any improvement in life expectancy should be viewed against a quality-of-life backdrop if a meaningful assessment of health status is to occur. Box 10.4. discusses the importance of including a quality-of-life component in any health status assessment.

Box 10.4: Quality of Life as a Health Status Metric
"Quality of life" (QOL) reflects the degree to which an individual is healthy, comfortable, and able to participate in or enjoy life events. The World Health Organization (WHO) defines QOL as "an individual's perception of their position in life in the context of the culture and value system in which they live and in relation to their goals, expectations, standards and concern." Standard indicators of quality of life include wealth, employment, physical and mental health, education, and recreation, among others.

Quality of life (QOL) is a broad multidimensional concept that usually includes subjective evaluations of both positive and negative aspects of life. Although the term "quality of life" has meaning for nearly everyone and every academic discipline, individuals and groups can define it differently. While health is one of the important domains of overall quality of life, other domains to consider include jobs, housing, schools, and neighborhoods. The impact of social determinants on health at one level can be considered along with the impact of life circumstances at another level should be considered.

Today, increasing numbers of Americans are living to advanced ages. However, there is growing concern that people are living longer but are in poorer health. A poor quality of life, it is contended, negates the benefits of increased longevity. Health-related quality of life (HRQoL) is a multi-dimensional concept that includes domains related to physical, mental, emotional and social functioning. It goes beyond direct measures of population health such as life expectancy and causes of death and focuses on the impact health status has on quality of life. The CDC has defined HRQoL as "an individual's or group's perceived physical and mental health over time." Health-related quality of life is viewed as an outcome of the health factors included in the *County Health Rankings*. Being healthy incorporates length of life and also the quality of those years.

Health-related quality of life has traditionally been concerned with those factors which fall under the influence of healthcare providers and healthcare systems. However, as the population health model has emerged, the quality of life related to other domains has come to be seen as important as health-related quality of life. HRQOL considers community-level resources, conditions, policies, and practices that influence a population's health perceptions and functional status. As the population health model is refined greater attention is likely to be paid to not only health-related quality of life but to the quality aspects related other spheres of existence.

Dental Health Data

Another neglected indicator of health status is the dental health of the population. Part of the reason for this neglect is the lack of understanding of the relationship between dental health and other health problems. A "silent epidemic" of dental and oral diseases is affecting some population groups—a burden of disease that restricts activities in school, work, and home and often significantly diminishes the quality of life. Untreated tooth decay is more than twice as prevalent among children with family incomes below the federal poverty guidelines (FPG) than among children with family incomes above 200% of the FPG. The disparity in oral health care between income groups is even more marked among adults. Low-income adults are much less likely to have had a dental visit in the past 12 months and have higher rates of dental disease compared to those with higher incomes. Approximately 15% of the population live in a dental health professional shortage area (HPSA) where available providers are able to only meet less than half of the need for dental services. Despite these unsettling facts, the state of the population's oral health continues to be neglected in community needs analyses.

Sources of Data for Health Needs Assessment

The variety of data typically included in a community health needs assessment would suggest that a wide variety of sources must be tapped in order to harness the range of data required. The sections below provide an introduction to the sources of data utilized for health needs assessments.

Sources of Demographic Data

The federal government—primarily through the Census Bureau—is the world's largest generator of demographic data. The value of the census to health planners clearly rests with its demographic data. These data have direct application to the performance of market analyses and indirect applications as input into models for generating prevalence and demand estimates. Although the census is only conducted every 10 years, the Bureau maintains the capacity for generating population estimates and projections on an on-going basis. These figures may not be as detailed as some commercially produced ones—e.g., they are only calculated down to the county level—but they are broken down in terms of age, race, income, and other important variables.

Census data are made available by the Census Bureau for virtually every formally designated geographic unit in the United States, and this is a clear advantage of census data over some other type of data. Statistics generated by the census are disseminated for states, counties, ZIP Codes, metropolitan areas, and cities. Data are also published for specially designated areas created by the Census Bureau, including census tracts, block groups, and blocks

The Census Bureau produces 30 different series of projections for each year. The Bureau provides relatively detailed population estimates for the current year and projections as far as 50 years into the future down to the county level. Most states also generate population estimates and projections that are available through state agencies.

A number of commercial data vendors have emerged in recent years to supplement the efforts of government agencies. Data generated by these vendors have the advantage of being available down to small units of geography (e.g., the census block group) and they are often provided in greater detail (e.g., sex and age breakdowns) than government-produced figures. They also offer the flexibility to generate estimates and projections for "custom" geographies (e.g., a market area) that government statistics do not have the ability to do. The drawback, of course, is that some precision is lost as one develops calculations for lower levels of geography and for population components. However, the ease of accessibility and timeliness of these vendor-generated figures have made them a mainstay for health services planners.

Sources of Epidemiological Data

The tracking of vital statistics in the United States involves data collection on births, deaths, marriages and divorces and, in some jurisdictions, induced abortions. The collection of data on vital events is initially the responsibility of the local health authority. Health departments at the county (or county equivalent) level are charged with filing certificates for births and deaths. These data are forwarded to the vital statistics registry within the respective state governments. The appropriate state agency compiles the data for use by the state and transmits the files to the National Center for Health Statistics (NCHS). NCHS has responsibility for compiling and publishing vital statistics for the nation and its various political subdivisions.

The compiled statistics are typically presented based on both the place of occurrence of the event (e.g., the location of the hospital) and the place of residence of the affected individual. Considerable detail is provided in the reports for a wide range of geographic units including states, metropolitan statistical areas, counties, and urban places. Data for other geographic areas may be available through state and local government agencies. Yearly summary reports are produced and published by the National Center for Health Statistics, though monthly summaries are also available through the monthly vital statistics reports.

Vital statistics reports are also made available by most state governments and most local health departments. Although basic data will always be reported by these agencies, the format, detail and coverage vary from state to state and county to county.

Surveillance activities at the Centers for Disease Control and Prevention generate weekly data on the occurrence of diseases defined as "notifiable" by the Council of State and Territorial Epidemiologists (CSTE). Notifiable disease reports are received by the CDC from 52 US jurisdictions (Washington, D.C., and New York City report separately) and five territories. The number of diseases and conditions reported is quite large. The list of monitored diseases includes, among others, anthrax, botulism, cholera, diphtheria, food-borne disease, leprosy, mumps, and toxic shock. Statistics on notifiable diseases are published weekly by the CDC in *Morbidity and Mortality Weekly Report* (MMWR) and compiled in an annual report published by the agency. Box 10.5 describes the nature and operation of the National Center for Health Statistics.

Much of what we know about morbidity within the US population is based on data drawn from various registries of patients with health conditions. The CDC maintains a number of registries that track certain types of health problems. The National Notifiable Diseases Surveillance System (NNDSS), tracks the conditions that must be reported to public health authorities. By 1990, all 50 states were using CDC's National Electronic Telecommunications System for Surveillance (NETSS) to report individual case data that included demographic information (without personal identifiers) for most nationally notifiable diseases. These data are important for evaluating the demographic correlates of the occurrence of infectious diseases, monitoring infectious disease morbidity trends, and determining the relative disease burden among demographically diverse subpopulations (Centers for Disease Control and Prevention, 2013).

Box 10.5: The National Center for Health Statistics

The National Center for Health Statistics (NCHS) is considered by many to be the Census Bureau of healthcare. As a division of the Centers for Disease Control and Prevention (CDC), the NCHS performs a number of invaluable functions related to data on health and health care. Since 1960, the Center has carried out the tasks of data collection and analysis, data dissemination, and the development of methodologies for research on health issues. The NCHS also coordinates the various state centers for health statistics.

The compilation and analysis of data on morbidity is an important function, and the Center has been responsible for the development of much of the epidemiologic data available. To this end, a variety of registries are maintained on health-related topics, some in conjunction with the CDC. A major responsibility is the compilation, analysis, and publication of vital statistics for the United States and each relevant subarea. This massive task of compiling and analyzing births and deaths provides the basis for the calculation of fertility and mortality rates. These statistics, in turn, provide the basis for various health-related estimates and projections made by other organizations.

Potential (suspect) cases of notifiable diseases are reported to local, regional, or state public health authorities. These reports might be based on a positive laboratory test, clinical symptoms, or epidemiologic criteria. When a suspect case is determined to meet the national case definition, de-identified data are sent to the CDC. This can include information reported to public health by laboratories and healthcare providers, along with other information collected during public health investigations.

Currently, there are 52 infectious diseases designated as notifiable at the national level. Infectious disease data are also available for all 50 states, the District of Columbia, and 122 selected cities. The data are available on a monthly basis in *Morbidity and Mortality Weekly Report,* a CDC publication, and at http://www2.cdc.gov:81/mmwr/mmwr.htm. Additional information on notifiable diseases can be found at http://www.cdc.gov.

The CDC also maintains specialized registries focusing on specific diseases. One example would be the Outpatient Influenza-like Illness Surveillance Network (ILINet) consisting of about 2400 healthcare providers in 50 states reporting approximately 16 million patient visits each year. Each week, approximately 1300 outpatient care sites around the country report data to CDC on the total number of patients seen and the number of those patients with influenza-like illness (ILI). The percentage of patient visits to healthcare providers for ILI reported each week is weighted on the basis of state population and compared each week with the national baseline. Box 10.6 describes the survey research carried out by the National Center for Health Statistics.

Box 10.6: Survey Research Conducted by the National Center for Health Statistics

The National Center for Health Statistics (NCHS) is the foremost administrator of healthcare surveys in the nation. Its sample surveys are generally large scale and fall into two categories: community-based surveys and facility-based surveys. The National Health Interview Survey (NHIS), in which data are collected annually from approximately 50,000 households, is perhaps the center's most important survey. The NHIS is the nation's primary source of data on the incidence/prevalence of health conditions, health status, the injuries and disabilities characterizing the population, health services utilization, and a variety of other health-related topics. Other surveys that involve a sample from the community are the National Medical Care Utilization and Expenditures Survey (NMCUES), the National Health and Nutrition Examination Survey (NHANES), and the National Survey of Family Growth (NSFG). Another survey, the National Maternal and Infant Health Survey (NMIHS), involves a sampling of certificates of birth, fetal death, and infant death.

(continued)

Box 10.6 (continued)

The NCHS also surveys a variety of healthcare institutions in its efforts to identify morbidity levels (among other objectives). Data are abstracted from the records of physician offices, hospitals and nursing homes. Healthcare providers are randomly selected for participation in the data collection process. The National Ambulatory Medical Care Survey (NAMCS) samples the patient records of 2500 office-based physicians to obtain data on diagnoses, treatment, and medications prescribed, along with information on the characteristics of both physicians and patients. Important facility-based surveys include the National Hospital Discharge Survey and the National Nursing Home Survey.

The National Hospital Ambulatory Medical Care Survey (NHAMCS) was established through combining previous surveys and collects data on inpatient care, emergency services, hospital outpatient services and hospital-provided ambulatory care surgery. Data are abstracted from a sample of medical records for patients who are hospitalized or using hospital outpatient services. The NHCS reports include personal health data to allow for tracking patients across the various services.

Additional surveys conducted by the Center include the National Survey of Ambulatory Surgery (NSAS), the National Nursing Home Survey (NNHS), the National Home and Hospice Care Survey (NHHCS), the National Study of Long-Term Care Providers (NSLTCP), the National Survey of Residential Care Facilities (NSRCF), and the National Health and Nutrition Examination Survey (NHANES). These surveys vary in their frequency of administration.

The data collected through NCHS programs are disseminated in a variety of ways. The center's publications include annual "books" such as *Health, United States* (the "official" government compendium of statistics on the nation's health) and series of publications such as *Vital and Health Statistics*. These data are available today primary via the Internet at the NCHS website. Much of the data collected—including raw data from NCHS surveys—is also available on-line from the NCHS website. The NCHS sponsors conferences and workshops offering not only the findings from center's research but training in its research methodologies.

From the perspective of a health data user, there are other resources that the Center can offer. By contacting the appropriate NCHS division it is possible to obtain detailed statistics, many unpublished, on the topics for which the Center compiles data. Center staff members are also available to help with methodological issues and provide that "one number" that the health data analyst may require. In short, the NCHS is a service-oriented agency that performs a number of invaluable functions for those who require data on health and healthcare. Additional information is available on the National Center for Health Statistics at www.cdc.gov/nchs.

Sources of Healthcare Resources Data

The federal government is the major source of nationwide data on health facilities. The Directory of Health and Human Services (DHHS) Data Resources is a comprehensive file of inpatient facilities maintained by the federal government. The institutions included in this data collection effort are hospitals, nursing homes and related facilities, and other custodial or remedial care facilities. The data resources file is kept current by periodically adding the names and addresses of newly established facilities licensed by state boards and other agencies. Annual surveys are used to update information concerning existing facilities.

The facilities databases established by DHHS include data on facility size, personnel, admissions, discharges, services offered, type of ownership, and type of certification. These data are available through various published reports and much of this information is obtained initially from professional associations and processed by the NCHS or some other federal agency. The Center for Medicare and Medicare Services (CMS) is now making available a set of data files on health facilities and other providers of care. Its "Provider of Services" files include every provider that has filed claims with Medicare.

Arguably, the nation's most complete hospital registry is maintained by the American Hospital Association (AHA). Data are compiled annually on the availability of services, utilization patterns, financial information, hospital management, and personnel (American Hospital Association, 2003). The database is continuously updated through an on-going survey of the nation's hospitals. These data are available for a variety of geographic units (including regions, divisions, states, counties, and cities). Some of the information is reprinted in secondary sources such as the *County and City Data Book* and *Health, United States*. Certain commercial data vendors have also established hospital databases.

Since most health facilities are licensed by the state, information is usually available from the state agency charged with that responsibility. Increasingly, local organizations such as planning and regulatory agencies and business coalitions maintain facilities databases. For facilities other than hospitals, some private data vendors have begun collecting and disseminating data. There are now vendors selling data on health maintenance organizations, urgent care centers, freestanding surgery centers, and a variety of other types of facilities.

An inventory of mental health organizations is maintained by the Center for Mental Health Services (within the U.S. Department of Health and Human Services) and is updated every two years. The agency publishes periodic reports on the status of mental health services in the U.S., although the format varies from edition to edition. The Substance Abuse and Mental Health Services Administration (SAMHSA) also provides information on mental health conditions, services and facilities.

Since many mental health services are administered by state governments, the respective state agencies represent a source of mental health statistics, although the data provided vary in terms of accessibility, content, and format. While rather detailed statistics have become available on ambulatory care services for physical illness, this is not the case for mental illness. Some limited data on mental health outpatient activity may be available through reports filed by comprehensive community mental health centers.

The federal government is the primary source data on *health personnel* at the national level. The Department of Health and Human Services is responsible for collecting and disseminating data on the status of health personnel in the United States. These requirements have led to the establishment of registries for various categories of health professionals. The Department also generates projections of the future personnel pool for selected categories of professionals. In addition, the listing of health professional shortage areas maintained by the Health Resources and Services Administration within DHHS is often of use to health planners. This database tracks the counties, communities, and special populations (e.g., Indian reservations) that report less then the recommended number of primary care physicians. In addition, the Center for Medicare and Medicaid Services maintains detailed registries of many types of health professionals that receive reimbursement under federally sponsored health programs.

The Bureau of Labor Statistics maintains data on all occupational categories within the economy, including healthcare occupations. As part of the Bureau's responsibilities, it produces projections on the size of various occupational categories in the United States for 10 to 15 years into the future. Six projection models are generated, each containing a number of variables reflecting different scenarios reflecting changes in the total labor force, the aggregate economy, industry demand, and industry employment, among other factors. Three sets of employment projections are created based upon differing sets of assumptions. Of interest here are the various categories of health-related occupations (e.g., dentists, physicians and surgeons, and therapists by specialty) and supportive occupations (e.g., dental and medical assistants, nurse's aides). In recent years, health professions have been prominent among the occupations with the greatest projected growth. Data on occupational categories are available from the Department of Labor through regularly published reports and, increasingly, via the Internet.

State governments often represent more direct sources of information on health personnel than federal agencies, since the various states have the primary responsibility for the licensing and monitoring of virtually all health professions. As part of their administrative activities, they necessarily establish registries for specific categories of health personnel. The databases created at the state level for physicians, nurses, physician assistants and other categories of health personnel are typically up to date. However, the detail provided and the usefulness of the data collected for planning, marketing, and business development purposes varies widely from state to state.

Other major sources of health personnel data include the AMA physician master file; medical, osteopathic, dental, and nursing school enrollment data; the American Academy of Physician Assistants master file; the American Dental Association dental practice survey; the Inventory of Pharmacists; and licensure information from the National Council of State Boards of Nursing and various accrediting bodies and professional associations serving the allied health profession (e.g., laboratory technicians, dietitians, physical therapists).

State licensure agencies also maintain databases on health professionals registered in the respective states. While this information is often available to the public, mere registration in a jurisdiction does not necessarily indicate an active practice. Further, these databases are likely to include only the barest of data required to carry out the mandated functions of the licensing agency. Specialty boards and other organizations also maintain registries on their members or certification recipients. While this information is often available in printed directories, the availability of the actual databases varies.

Many local organizations have begun to develop and maintain personnel databases for their particular service areas. Since most healthcare markets are local, national databases are of limited usefulness. Business coalitions have led the way in support of database development in many local markets.

Commercial data vendors maintain databases of physicians and other personnel, and some of these are comparable to the more traditional databases maintained by the professional organizations and government agencies. Data vendors may identify emerging professions or "marginal" practitioners that do not have an association base or are not tracked by the government. Other vendors repackage data from government organizations or association sources, and resell the data in modified form.

The federal government does provide some data related to *health insurance*, but, since insurance plans are regulated at the state level, the information available will vary from state to state. The American Community Survey does provide data on health insurance coverage down to the census block group level. It breaks out the population in terms of the type of insurance coverage and can provide considerable detail by demographic category. The ACS also profiles the uninsured population. The Centers for Medicare and Medicaid Services (CMS) provides some data on Medicare enrollees and beneficiaries and on Medicaid enrollees. Since the Medicaid program is administered at the state level, some agency of state government may be able to provide geographically based data on the Medicaid population.

It should be noted that there is limited systematic information available on *networks and relationships*. These arrangements are typically localized and the arrangements tend to be idiosyncratic and differ from local to local. Local business coalitions for health, large insurance operations, and regional health data organizations may compile this type of data but this information is likely to be incomplete and not comparable from site to site. Business coalitions may track networks within their service areas.

Sources of Health Behavior Data

The federal government is the major generator of data on health behavior. The annual Behavioral Risk Factor Surveillance System (BRFSS) survey is conducted in every state and over 90,000 persons respond to the survey annually. The survey collects data on such timely items as smoking, alcohol and drug use, seat beat use, and obesity, as well as other factors that might contribute to one's health risk profile.

In some states data may be provided for regions or down to the county level. States have the option of requesting a larger sample if desired.

The National Health Interview Survey (NHIS) also annually collects data on health behavior from a sample of the population. The NHIS is a primary source of data on health behavior in addition to data on the incidence/prevalence of health conditions, the injuries and disabilities characterizing the population, health services utilization, and a variety of other health-related topics. The NHIS is not geographically based so it is necessary to profile a targeted population based on its attributes and then construct an approximate health behavior profile.

The *Medical Expenditure Panel Survey* (MEPS), co-sponsored by the Agency for Healthcare Research and Quality (AHRQ) and the National Center for Health Statistics (NCHS), is designed to generate data on the types of health services Americans use, the frequency with which they use them, how much is paid for these services, and who pays for them. In addition, MEPS provides information on health insurance coverage.

Health analysts may want to consider some of the national consumer databases that have been developed in their search for data on the community. Experian and Acxion, to mention two, are national data companies that maintain data on virtually every household within the United States. While the information is used primarily by marketers seeking to target individuals and households with certain characteristics—an activity that planners may have reason to consider—the data repositories include substantial amounts of data on demographics, lifestyles and consumer behavior.

There are also a few surveys sponsored by commercial data vendors that contain data useful for health planning. These organizations sponsor nationwide surveys every year or two that may include as many 100,000 households. Through these surveys, data are collected on health status, health behavior, and healthcare preferences. Certain market research firms (e.g., Nielsen, Simmons, Experian) collect health-related data as part of their consumer surveys, and public opinion pollsters may also collect data on health and healthcare. Some of the data collected in this manner is considered proprietary and is generally not available except to clients. Other vendors make data available for purchase to the general public

For many types of goods and services, an understanding of the psychographics or lifestyle characteristics of the target population is essential. Lifestyle clusters in a population often transcend (or at least complement) that population's demographic attributes. Psychographics can be linked to the attitudes, perceptions, and expectations of the target population as well as to its propensity to purchase certain products. Although use of psychographic analysis in healthcare has lagged behind other industries, health professionals are finding a growing number of applications for this approach, and more healthcare data are being incorporated into psychographic segmentation systems.

Analysts can choose from a handful of different psychographic segmentation systems for use in partitioning the market area by lifestyle. For example, the MOSAIC system developed by Experian assigns one of 71 lifestyle clusters to most households in the United States. Knowing the assigned psychographic cluster of a household opens the door to a variety of other useful information in addition to available lifestyle attributes.

Sources of Health Services Utilization Data

The federal government is the major source of data related to health services utilization. Primarily through the National Center for Health Statistics, the federal government maintains a number of on-going surveys that deal with hospital utilization, ambulatory care utilization, nursing home and home health utilization, medical care expenditures, and other relevant topics. The National Institutes of Health and the CDC also conduct surveys, although more episodically, that generate data of interest to health analysts.

A number of organizations have been formed in recent years that focus specifically on health services utilization data, while others have established formal sections that deal with health data within their broader context.

The *Medical Expenditure Panel Survey* (MEPS), noted above, is designed to generate data on the types of health services Americans use, the frequency with which they use them, how much is paid for these services, and who pays for them. In addition, MEPS provides information on health insurance coverage.

The National Association of Health Data Organizations (NAHDO), brings together disparate parties from the public and private sector who have an interest in health data. The National Association of County and City Health Officers (NACCHO) has become very active in terms of access to health data for local planning purposes.

Many state governments require that hospitals report utilization data to a state-wide database and subsequently make this information available to the public. This may be carried out by a state agency or contracted with some other entity. The amount of detail and the ability to link the data to a geography varies widely.

Issues with Traditional Health Data

Having outlined the major data components for traditional health needs assessments, it might be worthwhile to summarize their shortcomings prior to addressing more relevant data categories.

Issues with Epidemiological Data

Since there is no central repository of incidence and prevalence data, it is difficult to determine the level and nature of the morbidity characterizing a population. The process of determining morbidity patterns is a complex one and faces many challenges. There are two ways in which this is carried out. The reported cases method of assessing morbidity level holds much promise in that every official case must be recorded somewhere to make it qualify as a case. However, reported cases are just that—only cases that have been reported to healthcare entities. Thus, many individuals with clinically identifiable conditions are never diagnosed and never become part of the morbidity record. For those that are reported, there is no mechanism for compiling data from disparate sources.

The community survey method represents an attempt to overcome the deficiencies of the reported cases method and to generate an estimate of "true" prevalence. The National Health Interview Survey and the Behavioral Risk Surveillance System are the primary examples of community surveys. This method provides a different perspective from the reported cases method, although it is not possible through community surveys to generate the level of detail that can be produced through analysis of reported cases. Nevertheless, much of what we know about population health has been derived from community surveys.

Neither method is sufficient to provide the total picture when it comes to morbidity. It is necessary to use both methods in order to develop a more complete understanding of current morbidity patterns. The major drawback to using reported cases as the basis for the numerator, however, is inherent in the process itself. Reported cases represent cases that have been both diagnosed and entered into an appropriate data bank. Many cases are never diagnosed, especially for such conditions as mental disorders (for which much subjectivity is involved in the diagnostic process). In fact, the "known" cases of many diseases represent only the tip of the iceberg. For some conditions, more cases may go undetected than detected. Further, reporting is less than complete and is often selective.

The use of mortality as a metric in assessing health status has become less important over time. There are relatively few deaths today, and problems in establishing cause of death make the data that are available suspect. Further, the correspondence between mortality and morbidity has become diminished. Because of the preponderance of chronic disease within the US population, death certificates are less and less likely to capture the underlying disease. Chronic diseases typically do not kill people, but they die instead from some complication (of diabetes, AIDS or cancer, for example). This is not to say that mortality analysis cannot provide insights into morbidity patterns, but that the situation is much more complicated than in the past, and analysts require a better understanding of disease processes (and the vagaries of death certificates) today.

It can be argued that traditional metrics actually measure "sick status" as opposed to "health status." Mortality is increasingly downplayed since the emergence of chronic disease has created a disconnect between stated cause of death what the deceased were actually suffering from. While such information is not unimportant, it is felt that the focus on the deficiencies in community health status divert attention from the factors that keep people well and restore them to health after a healthcare episode.

Even if reasonably accurate data were available on the incidence and prevalence of disease, it would still be argued that such clinically related data are not true indicators of health status, since the do not reflect the perspective of the community under study. Realistically, community residents do not think in terms of death rates (or even morbidity rates for that matter) when considering what constitutes a health problem. They are much more likely to identify conditions that affect their everyday lives—the life circumstances that involve a lack of food, housing, safety and so forth.

Further, focusing on traditional epidemiological measures involves a downstream emphasis that describes the population after health conditions emerge. The population health model calls for a more proactive approach that moves upstream and assesses health risks rather than health conditions that are already a *fait accompli*. Finally, a reliance on traditional epidemiological data places over-emphasis on the healthcare system and its ability to contribute to community health improvement. The assumption is that these negative metrics reflect a failing of the healthcare system when that may not be the actual explanation for observed patterns.

Because of the historical focus of the CDC on communicable diseases, chronic diseases are generally not officially tracked as part of the public health agenda. This situation creates a serious void in the ability to monitor chronic conditions that now account for the bulk of morbidity within the US population. Although our knowledge of these conditions has been advanced through survey research on the part of the National Center for Health Statistics, information derived from sample surveys limits our understanding of the epidemiology of chronic conditions and, hence, the system's ability to monitor their prevalence.

Issues with Health Behavior Data

There are a number of issues related of data on health behavior. What we know about the health behavior of US residents is derived from community surveys. Based on these surveys, it is possible to estimate the proportion of the population engaged in various healthy and unhealthy activities. However, there is no consistent source of data on health behavior and, even if there were, there are conceptual and methodological issues to be considered.

Traditional health needs assessments are likely to view health behavior at the individual level. This assumes that individuals are making health behavior choices of their own volition and that their actions should be viewed in isolation. This conventional perspective flies in the face of the population health model, which would contend that decisions related to health behavior are not made in a vacuum but are influenced by the social context. It could be argued that health behavior—like health status—arises out of the social and cultural environment and reflects the operation of the social determinants of health.

Issues with Health Services Utilization Data

The issues related to data on health resources are numerous. The inventory of health-related resources is increasingly being downplayed by proponents of a population health approach. As a practical matter, the question is raised as to the extent to which the presence of formal health services represents an appropriate measure or predictor of health status. Policy analysts attempting to promote community health improvement have long grappled with the relationship between resource availability and community health status. It is felt by many that the emphasis on formal health facilities and services implies that any deficiencies in community health status are a result of deficiencies within the structure or operation of the healthcare system.

One reason that the use of utilization data in community health assessments is considered suspect is the fact that treatment patterns vary widely from one geographic area to another. Box 10.7 discusses this issue.

> **Box 10.7: Geographic Variation in the Treatment of Health Conditions**
> Healthcare analysts long ago realized that significant variation exists in the utilization of health services from community to community. This is significant in that utilization (i.e., the number of reported cases) may be used as a proxy for the morbidity level. As early as the 1970s research revealed that the rate of procedures performed even in adjacent states varied to a degree not explained by population differences. The rate of performance of procedures could range from 10% of the population in some markets to 50% in others. These studies suggest that the level of health services utilization is less a function of disease prevalence than a reflection of the characteristics of the medical community and practice patterns of local physicians.
>
> Typical of the findings on this issue are the results of a study that compared the cities of Boston and New Haven in terms of their health services utilization patterns. While the two cities are similar in terms of the factors that *should* determine the use of health services, they differed dramatically on virtually every indicator of health services utilization. The hospital admission rate, for example, was nearly twice as high in Boston as in New Haven. Furthermore, residents of Boston were much more likely to be hospitalized for various acute and chronic conditions than residents of New Haven. The average annual per capita expenditure on healthcare in Boston was twice that of New Haven. However, the comparative utilization patterns were not always consistent. Certain procedures were performed much more frequently in Boston but others more frequently in New Haven.
>
> It is now realized that a number of factors account for these seemingly inexplicable differences. A major factor is the variation in physician practice patterns from community to community. In some communities it is standard practice to treat a problem with surgery; in others the standard calls for less invasive treatment. In some communities, conventional medical wisdom calls for hospitalization for certain diagnostic tests and procedures, whereas in others it is customary to handle such cases on an outpatient basis.
>
> Other factors contributing to differential utilization rates include the relative supply of facilities and services. There is pressure, for example, to fill

(continued)

> **Box 10.7** (continued)
>
> hospital beds if they are available and to use technology in which the organization has invested. In contrast to other industries, competition in healthcare often drives up both utilization levels and costs, thereby accounting for an additional degree of variation. Even the presence of a medical school may influence both the level of utilization and types of procedures performed. Increasingly, the level of managed care penetration is a significant factor influencing utilization rates.
>
> Given these variations, how does the analyst know the appropriate level of utilization? Is the reported level of utilization high, low, or what should be realistically expected? Of course, one way to address this is to use some standard rate of utilization such as the utilization rates developed by the National Center for Health Statistics based on national surveys. These rates provide useful benchmarks, but because most analyses focus on local markets, how appropriate are they for the community in question? There is no easy answer to this dilemma. The analyst must be able to gain enough knowledge about the local healthcare environment to make reasonable assessments about the level of utilization and the extent to which this reflects differences in actual prevalence rather than variations in medical practices.
>
> Source: Wennberg and Cooper (1999).

Summary

The traditional approach to conducting a community health needs assessment reflects the historical orientation of the healthcare system. A variety of categories of data must be considered in performing an assessment. Demographic variables are significant since the profile of the population in question and often serve as proxies for other health metrics. The categories include *biosocial* variables (age, sex and race/ethnicity) and *sociocultural* variables (income, education, marital status, occupation and other socially assigned attributes) that reflect one's position within the social structure. The conventional approach was developed primarily by epidemiologists, so it is not surprising that these assessments rely heavily on epidemiological data, particularly morbidity and mortality data.

The tendency has been to rely on traditional epidemiological measures that may or may not reflect the community's perspective on health issues. Health needs assessments should be supplemented by often neglected metrics on such health issues as behavioral health and substance abuse, dental health, disability and domestic violence. Traditional assessments emphasis the availability of formal health resources as measure of system quality and view utilization levels as proxies for health status. They seldom consider community health assets that may be independent of the formal healthcare system.

Because of the variety of data involved a wide variety of sources must be accessed. The federal government is a major source for many of the types of data that are required. State and local governments may also be sources of some data. Various health-related organizations (e.g., American Medical Association, American Hospital Association) can be sources of relevant data, and commercial data vendors and consumer marketing companies may also contribute some data.

There are issues with regard to each source of data. The demographic data required are relatively straightforward but there are a number of issues with the epidemiological data. Chief among these is the concern that morbidity and mortality metrics may not accurately reflect health status and, in any case, are more focused on "sick status" than "health status". An over-reliance on the availability of data on health resources implies that the way to address any health challenge is by tweaking the system. Further, the manner in which utilization levels are interpreted raises more questions than answers.

Key Points

- Traditional health needs assessments require a wide variety of data that must be current and geographically appropriate.
- Demographic data have been a mainstay of health needs assessments since these data often serve as a proxy for health-related metrics.
- Epidemiological data have been the mainstay of health needs assessments (with an emphasis on morbidity and mortality data).
- Traditional health needs assessments place inordinate emphasis on the attributes of the formal healthcare system and the adequacy of health-related resources.
- Utilization levels are determined for various services, and these are often considered indicators of health status.
- Because of the range of data involved in a health needs assessment, a wide variety of data sources must be tapped.
- The federal government is a major generator of much of the data required for health needs assessments.
- There are a number of issues related to the various categories of data but a major concern is that the metrics used are measuring "sick status" and not "health status".
- There is also concern that conclusions about health status are being imposed externally by health professionals and do not reflect the perspective of those in the community.

References

Chaudhry, S., Jin, L., & Meltzer, D. (2005). Use of a self-report-generated Charlson comorbidity index for predicting mortality. *Medical Care, 43*(6), 607–615.

Romero-Corral, A., Somers, V. K., Sierra-Johnson, J., Thomas, R. J., Collazo-Clavell, M. L., Korinek, J., Allison, T. G., & Batsis, J. A. (2008). Accuracy of body mass index in diagnosing obesity in the adult general population. *International Journal of Obesity, 32*(6), 959–956.

Paradise, J., & R. Garfield. (2013). *What is Medicaid's impact on access to care, health outcomes, and quality of care? Setting the record straight on the evidence.* Downloaded from URL: http://kff.org/report-section/what-is-medicaids-impact-on-access-to-care-health-outcomes-and-quality-of-care-setting-the-record-straight-on-the-evidence-issue-brief/.

Thomas, R. K. (2016). *In sickness and in health: Disease and disability in contemporary America.* Springer.

Wennberg, J. E., & Cooper, M. M. A. (Eds.). (1999). *The Dartmouth atlas of health care.* American Hospital Association.

Additional Resources

American Hospital Association (*AHA* Guide) at https://ams.aha.org/eweb/DynamicPage.aspx?WebCode=ProdDetailAdd&ivd_prc_prd_key=40a14b40-6a53-4f4c-bdad-fbd84f9e0f63.

American Medical Association (Physician Master File) at https://www.ama-assn.org/about/masterfile/ama-physician-masterfile.

Centers for Disease Control and Prevention (Behavioral Risk Factor Surveillance System) at cdc.gov/brfss.

Centers for Disease Control and Prevention (*Morbidity and Mortality Weekly Report*) at https://www.cdc.gov/mmwr/index2021.html.

Centers for Medicare and Medicaid Services at www.cms.gov.

Health Resources and Services Administration (Area Resource Files) at https://data.hrsa.gov/topics/health-workforce/ahrf.

National Center for Health Statistics (various surveys) at cdc.gov/nchs.

National Center for Health Statistics (*Health, United States*) at https://www.cdc.gov/nchs/hus/index.htm.

Substance Abuse and Mental Health Services Administration at www.samhsa.gov/cmhs.htm.

US Census Bureau (American Community Survey) at www.data.census.gov.

US Department of Health and Human Services (Directory of Health and Human Services Data Resources) at https://aspe.hhs.gov/directory-health-and-human-services-data-resources.

Chapter 11
Data Needs for the Population Health Model

> *Any organization adopting a population health approach must know more about the consumer in its service area than ever before. Not only must traditional health data be accessed but data from sectors of society not typically considered must be gathered. In order to address the social determinants of health, analysts must be able to access data on housing, education, food access, transportation, criminal justice and other sectors that are typically not included in the standard health needs assessment. This chapter introduces the reader to these categories of data and provides a comparative analysis of a traditional community health needs assessment and a population health assessment.*
>
> In this chapter, the reader will:
>
> - Learn about the non-conventional types of data required for a population health analysis
> - Find out about the sources of these non-conventional types of data
> - Be exposed to the barriers to acquiring data for a population health analysis
> - Learn the difference between a traditional community health needs analysis and a population health analysis

Introduction

The population health model calls for an innovative approach to the information required for assessing community health status and implementing a population health initiative. The information required to support a population health model is significantly broader than that required for traditional health analyses. To be effective, the population health approach requires an unprecedented and in-depth understanding of the attributes of the service area population. Healthcare organizations have been slow to expand the scope of the data utilized and, even today, many healthcare organizations are content with compiling internal data on the characteristics of their existing clients with little concern for external data. This situation was noted by the Institute of Medicine (2011) a decade ago:

> "[N]o coordinated, standard set of indicators exist to assess and improve the health of the community". To the extent that indicators do exist "these distal indicators are typically based on data collection systems developed in isolation and far removed from data on their underlying causes...[T]he proliferation of these fragmented and heterogeneous indicator sets can cause confusion, overwhelm busy decision-makers, impair valid community-level comparisons, and contribute to an inefficient use of limited resources.

Nature of Relevant Data

There are a number of attributes characterizing the data to be considered in conducting population health analyses. A consideration of these attribute is relevant in order to understand the types of data utilized in population health needs assessments.

Perspective

Data are never compiled in a vacuum and the question of *whose* data perspective we are recognizing must be addressed. Health professionals are notorious for imposing their perspectives on groups within the population when it comes to their health status. Yet, when consumers are asked what they see as the health problems most affecting their communities, their answer are likely to be much different from those assumed by the healthcare system. Indeed, the health problems identified may not even be health problems but may be such factors as domestic violence, toxic environments or unsafe housing. At the community level, the underlying causes of observed health problems may be more relevant than the observed pathological states. A shift in perspective is required in conducting a population health assessment.

Individual vs. Community

Health-related metrics can be used to profile individuals or whole populations. The most common measures of population health, mortality or morbidity rates, are derived from counts of individuals, which are then aggregated up to a population level in the form of incidence and prevalence rates. However, proponents of a population health approach would contend that societal morbidity is more than the sum of its constituent parts. In fact, it could be argued that, in communities that exhibit persistently poor health status, something of a "subculture of ill-health" emerges that fosters poor health rather than inhibits it. This perspective would contend that health problems cannot be understood at the individual level but that a holistic approach is required that takes into consideration not only the affected individuals but the environments that contribute to morbidity.

A health status measure should reflect the attributes of the group independent of the attributes of the individuals that comprise it. This reflects the sociological precept that the characteristics of groups arise *sui generis* out of the interaction that takes place among group members and between the group and its environment. This would explain, for example, why poor health status persists within a particular community decade after decade regardless of who moves into the community or the fact that one's ZIP Code of residence is thought to be the best predictor of one's health status (Roeder, 2014).

Level of Data Collection

Data can be collected at a variety of levels of aggregation. While it has been commonplace to obtain data on individuals and households, data at this level are not very useful for health needs assessment, particularly within the population health model. At that level, one is more concerned with data related to life circumstances than to the social determinants of health. Typically, data at the individual or household level are summed or averaged in order to develop a group metric. While there is nothing wrong with this simple approach, it violates the notion that health and illness are products of the group and not the sum of the attributes of individual group members or households. While this manner of data generation is straightforward, it is not in keeping with a population health approach.

Data can also be viewed at what Morgenstern (1995) termed the environmental level. Environmental indicators record factors external to the individual, such as air and water quality. These indicators can be recorded at the individual or at the community level. The distinguishing characteristics of Morgenstern's environmental health indicators is that they have no obvious analogue at the individual level. These are indicators that reflect the attributes of communities that exist independent of the sum of the parts.

Finally, there is a level that we might refer to as global health measurement, reflecting the overall characteristic of the community that are beyond the control of individual community members. This would include such factors as crime rates, disease prevalence, educational levels, and so forth. Most of the emphasis within a population health model would be at this level since it speaks to community health.

Qualitative vs. Quantitative

In the past, researchers and managers have been enamored with quantitative research and statistical analyses. In recent years there has been a resurgence of interest in qualitative research, especially with the emergence of the population health model. Researchers hail qualitative research for the richness of detail it provides and prefer it (over quantitative) in situations in which opinions, choices, and perceptions are sought. Focus groups and interviews with naturally occurring groups are conducted on a regular basis to supplement quantitative research.

Admittedly, qualitative methods have their limitations. They cannot be subjected to statistical analysis nor can they be generalized and applied to other populations. Their contributions are limited to generating broad conclusions and hypotheses. In this sense, they can serve as a guide for designing quantitative research initiatives.

Researchers today recognize the value of both quantitative and qualitative approaches. They may be conducted simultaneously to obtain data using one approach that can supplement the other. Both approaches have evolved over the years, and surveys are no longer composed of closed-ended, yes/no questions; they now pose open-ended questions that encourage respondents to volunteer more detail. The use of both qualitative and quantitative data allows the researcher to triangulate the findings for better-informed conclusions. Case Study 11.1 discusses the application of quantitative and qualitative research to a community health initiative.

> **Case Study 11.1: Applying Quantitative and Qualitative Research To a Community Health Initiative**
> On the advice of a consultant, a network of faith-based clinics opened a new clinic in a low-income, predominantly African-American community. This community had once received widespread acclaim for its level of home ownership, the stability of its households, and the achievements of its residents. After one year of operation, the clinic still was not receiving the support it expected from the local community. Area residents were not taking advantage of the services offered by the clinic, even though demand clearly existed. The network's marketing department designed and sent a sample survey to 200

(continued)

Case Study 11.1 (continued)

households of the community's 3000 households. It conducted in-depth interviews with key informants, who either lived in the area or had a long history of working with its residents. It facilitated focus groups and carried out observational research—all involving local residents.

Findings from the sample survey essentially reinforced the results of the previous market analysis: Respondents reported a high level of morbidity (particularly chronic diseases), a high level of psychiatric morbidity and substance abuse, and a low level of treatment or medical intervention. In addition, more health problems and greater unmet needs were revealed than anticipated.

Observational research added critical layers of information. While the community had a high rate of home ownership, it also had many empty, dilapidated, or abandoned single-family dwellings; trash-filled vacant lots; and crumbling buildings (including the low-rated elementary and high schools). Furthermore, residents had little or no social interaction, even among neighbors. Few adults walked and talked on the streets, and few children played outside. The sight of residents sitting on their porches or working in their yards was rare. Even vehicular traffic was light. The churches that dotted virtually every corner had low attendance and did little community outreach. Many grocery stores and restaurants had boarded up their doors and moved out, creating a "food desert."

The in-depth interviews and focus groups helped qualify the findings from the sample survey and observations. The observed social dysfunctions were primarily rooted in a decline in the quality of housing, which encouraged detachment from the community. Longtime residents felt marginalized, isolated from their neighbors, and afraid to leave their homes. The community's educational system, once the pride of the neighborhood, faltered partly as a result of young families leaving the area.

The analysts concluded that the observed health problems were symptoms of a bigger problem. Faced with so many environmental concerns, the residents accorded their medical conditions and general health low priority. As a result of the disintegration of face-to-face interactions and word-of-mouth promotion between neighbors, most people were unaware that a new clinic had been built in the area. Leaders of the network and the clinic realized that at least some of these underlying issues must be fixed before the community could focus on its health problems.

The combined quantitative and qualitative research methods applied in this case, as well as the triangulation of the findings, did not yield a solution. However, integrating the two perspectives enabled the community health clinic to peel back the layers to reveal social and health issues that needed immediate—even urgent—attention.

Data Categories for Population Health Assessments

In support of the population health model, data must be collected on a wide range of topics that historically have not been linked to the health of the population. The recognition of the social determinants of health status has opened the door to the acquisition of data on a wide range of topics historically ignored by healthcare organizations. While most analyses include data on the demographic and socioeconomic characteristics of the service area population, additional information is now required on the lifestyles of consumers, their social context and cultural milieu, and the life circumstances that have implications for health status and health behavior. In keeping with the population health approach, this information is not collected for individuals per se but for groups within the population. So, it's not so important to know that John Doe has certain characteristics but that one hundred John Does in ZIP Code 99999 have those characteristics in common.

Even more radical is the notion that data must be collected on topics previously thought to have no implications for health status. Data on attributes like income, educational level and employment status for the target population would continue to be collected, but now data on the social and physical environment, the availability of affordable and adequate housing, employment options and job training opportunities, access to affordable and healthy food, access to green spaces and recreational activities, access to transportation, and exposure to crime and violence must be considered. The significance of this type of information has been highlighted as it has become increasingly obvious that no level of medical care can overcome poverty, environmental toxicity, malnutrition and the health implications of a stressful environment.

The categories of non-health-related data generally parallel the social determinants of health discussed in Chap. 6. The data associated with each category are described below. This list of metrics is not intended to be exhaustive and, in fact, is generally limited to those attributes for which data are available with some level of granularity.

Economic Instability

Economic success is a primary value in American society, and financial status has an inordinate impact on the health status and health behavior of members of various groups. Income is the indicator that most directly measures material resources. Income can influence health by its direct effect on living standards, and while we typically think of income as an individual or family attribute, it is the economic status of various population subgroups that has relevance for population health. Most health status indices, in fact, include the poverty level as a component, and this information becomes more critical when conducting a population health assessment.

The primary metrics associated with economic instability revolve around *income* and associated attributes. Data are available at a relatively granular level for various measures of income. These include total household income and family household income broken into relevant intervals, along with the median household income and median family household income. This information can be broken out for various racial and ethnic groups and is available down to the census block group level.

Data are also available on the *poverty* population, with poverty rates presented for households, individuals and children separately. The extent of poverty is reported (e.g., 100% of federal policy level, between 100% and 150%, etc.), and, as with the income data, information on poverty level by race and ethnic group is also available. Some independent organizations have developed methodologies for tracking poverty over time for various geographies in the United States.

Another dimension of economic security to be considered is source of income. This attribute can be examined in a couple of different ways. One trait associated with income is one's occupation. These data, also available at a granular level, indicate the type of job for which compensation is obtained. The fact that disadvantaged populations are generally relegated to low-paying, dead-end jobs has important implications for their economic stability. This distinction also has implications for the range of benefits available to workers in different jobs that contribute to the level of economic security.

An additional dimension of economic status that has attracted attention is *wealth* as opposed to income. The historical focus on income (i.e., compensation received in a particular year) has drawn attention away from the fact that the real economic discrepancy is not in terms of income—although that is significant—but in terms of accumulated wealth. The fact that one portion of the population has accumulated disproportionate wealth and most of remainder has accumulated virtually little wealth is a major contributor to the disparities that exist in society.

Although economic attributes have been singled out for special attention, the link between economic status and virtually all of the other categories of non-health-related data are affected. As each of these categories is examined below, the impact of poverty on other attributes will be clearly seen.

Neighborhood and Physical Environment

A growing body of research suggests that the best predictor of health and well-being is a person's ZIP Code of residence (Roeder, 2014). The impact of the conditions characterizing the community in which one lives, works and plays on health status cannot be overstated. Not only does the environment have an immediate effect on the health status of residents but its impact can last for years to come and even have multi-generational effects (Chetty et al., 2014).

This category of data focuses on the physical environment and its implications for the health status of the population. (Both the social environment and housing stability are discussed below). In this regard considerable emphasis has been placed on measuring pollution levels and other aspects of the physical environment that may have implications for health status.

Concern over legacy lead pipe plumbing has been revived in view of some high-profile situations that have recently come to light. The fact that the United States is facing serious water deficiencies in various areas is shocking. However, it is not shocking that these environmental crises are virtually all concentrated in low-income, minority communities. As such, they contribute to the on-going environmental crisis—and low health status—associated with these communities.

Another attribute associated with the physical environment is access to open space, green space and other recreational opportunities. An association has been found between access to green space and health status and, as with most other resources, green space is in short supply within disadvantaged neighborhoods. The high-density, urban neighborhoods where disadvantaged populations mostly reside do not lend themselves to extensive open space, and safety concerns may prevent residents from accessing even these limited resources.

Housing Access and Quality

Housing is an important determinant of health, and access to adequate, affordable housing can affect how healthy a person is. People spend most of their time indoors, especially young children, who are particularly vulnerable to threats in the home environment. As a result, housing adequacy is long been recognized as a public health issue.

Substandard housing affects multiple dimensions of health, and the federal government assesses conditions in selected cities on an annual basis. While the assessment of the quality of housing may not be available nationwide, various local governments conduct assessments of the quality of housing. Variables that might be considered are the age of housing, access to various features, and value of housing relative to other housing options. Household size relative to the size of the housing unit is also a consideration.

Although lead levels in the blood of young children have been declining, recent incidents suggest that there may be a resurgence in lead poisoning and that the metrics used may understate the extent of the problem. Most lead exposure occurs in the home, particularly in homes built before 1978 that often contain lead-based paint and lead in the plumbing systems. Lead surveillance is primarily a local matter, but the age of the housing stock provides an indicator of the potential for lead-related health threats.

Transportation

Patterns of physical activity are influenced by the physical and built environments, and transportation plays a role in this. Most Americans take access to transportation for granted but, for a large part of the population, this is a constant source of stress.

Transportation may not often be associated with health conditions but it affects community health along a number of dimensions. There is growing consensus that the US transportation system can be harmful to our health and well-being (Robert Wood Johnson Foundation, 2012). Motorized transportation modes dominate in our society, leading to increased air pollution, traffic crashes, and decreased physical activity. Major highways often run through or adjacent to low-income neighborhoods that are more likely to have minority residents and be disproportionately affected by poor air quality and noise pollution. Young children are particularly affected.

Health and aging researchers measure some or all of the "five As of access": availability, accessibility, accommodation, affordability, and acceptability (Arcury et al., 2005; Sagrestano et al., 2014). Many of the measures employed address one or more dimensions of transportation insecurity as we define it, but no consistent measure is used across these studies. Instead, measures are often tailored to the subpopulation of interest, making it difficult to compare findings across populations and health-related outcomes as well as between health-related domains and other domains.

Proximity to a major roadway places residents at higher risk for asthma and other respiratory illnesses, cardiovascular disease, pre-term births, and premature death. A recent survey of the studies on the effect of traffic emissions on pregnancy outcomes has linked exposure to emissions to adverse effects on gestational duration and possibly intrauterine growth (Pereira et al., 2010).

Our current transportation system contributes to physical inactivity—each additional hour spent in a car per day is associated with an increase in the likelihood of obesity. On the other hand, use of public transportation is associated with greater physical activity. Walking or bicycling as a form of transportation or walking to public transportation stations, such as bus stops, also count toward meeting the daily physical activity recommendations. Analysis by federal agencies found that there is a significant reduction in mortality associated with active transportation.

Transportation barriers are often cited as barriers to healthcare access. Transportation barriers lead to rescheduled or missed appointments, delayed care, and missed or delayed medication use. These consequences may lead to poorer management of chronic illness and thus poorer health outcomes. A synthesis of the literature on the prevalence of transportation barriers to healthcare access (Syed et al., 2013) found that access to transportation is an important barrier, particularly for those with lower incomes and the under-insured or the uninsured.

Patients with transportation barriers carry a greater burden of disease which may, in part, reflect the relationship between poverty and transportation availability. This situation has become more obvious with the movement of disadvantaged populations into America's suburbs (Kneebone & Garr, 2010). While there are some advantages to suburban living over inner-city living, access to transportation is not one of them. The "suburbanization of poverty" has had the effect of decreasing access to health facilities and services.

Education

The relationship between educational attainment and health status has been well documented, and educational attainment has long been considered a component of any health status index. The aspects of education that might have relevance for population health include access to educational opportunities (including job training), educational enrollment, educational attainment, graduate and education continuation rates and related data preferably provided for various demographic categories. Other structural factors to be considered are the location, size and characteristics of educational institutions at all levels. Fortunately, there are a number of sources of data available related to education.

The relationship between educational level and mental illness, like that for physical illness, appears to be fairly clear cut. Adults with less than a high school education report the highest rates of sadness, hopelessness and worthlessness while those with at least a bachelor's degree report the lowest rates. Further, the poorly educated are more likely to report feelings of nervousness and restlessness. As the level of education increases, there appears to be an increase in the prevalence but a decrease in the severity of disorders. The better educated appear to be more characterized by neurotic conditions, while the less educated appear to be more frequently psychotic. The presence of psychiatric symptoms can exacerbate stress which in turn can generate physical symptoms.

The level of disability exhibits a clear pattern with regard to educational attainment (National Center for Health Statistics, 2020). An analysis of data from the National Health Interview Survey found an inverse relationship between educational levels and chronic conditions, limitation of activities, and number of bed days for disability.

The pattern with regard to mortality also resembles that exhibited for income. The death rate for the poorly educated is much higher than for those with higher educational achievement. According to NCHS data, the risk of mortality for those with a high school education is 60% higher than that for those with a graduate degree (University of Pennsylvania, 2020). Indeed, recent research indicates an increase in mortality among poorly educated US citizens (Olshansky et al., 2012). The poorly educated are likely to be characterized by lifestyle-related deaths such as homicides and accidents. Education, in fact, has been shown to demonstrate a stronger association with mortality than does income (Rogers et al., 2000).

Infant mortality, once a leading cause of death, has been virtually eliminated from the groups with the highest educational levels, with the poorly educated accounting for the bulk of infant deaths. The correlation between educational level and infant mortality rates is reflected in differences in low birth-weight babies and premature births for those at different educational levels. Babies born to women who did not complete high school are almost twice as likely to die in their first year than babies born to women who did finish high school.

As with income, the relationship does not necessarily reflect the level of education per se but the differential consequences of varying educational levels. Those with less education are likely to be more affected by financial insecurity, poor housing conditions, and unsafe environments, all contributing to an increase in morbidity levels.

Food Insecurity

Food insecurity refers to the inability to afford nutritionally adequate and safe foods. Most adults living in food-insecure households report being unable to afford balanced meals, concern about the adequacy of their food supply, running out of food, and cutting the size of meals or skipping meals, all of which have implications for health status. During the past two decades policy makers and those responsible for conducting research have come to appreciate the connection between food insecurity and the conditions, manifestations, and ramifications of ill health. Among other things, the implication is that hunger, in addition to being a symptom of food insecurity, is also a part of the panoply of conditions that signal compromised health status (Schroeder, 2016).

There is strong evidence that food deserts are correlated with high prevalence of overweight, obesity, and premature death as supermarkets traditionally provide healthier options than convenience stores or smaller grocery stores. Additionally, those with low income may face barriers to accessing a consistent source of healthy food. This in turn is related to negative health outcomes such as weight gain, premature mortality, asthma, and activity limitations, as well as increased healthcare costs. While some episodes of food insecurity may be of short duration, the dietary changes associated with food insecurity may persist over extended periods due to repeated food shortages (Seligman et al., 2010).

Where people live has a dramatic effect on their health and access to affordable and healthy food. Residents who live far away from grocery stores and cannot access healthy foods are considered to live in "food deserts." Since the availability of supermarkets is associated with socioeconomic status (Cummins & Macintyre, 2005), low-income and minority neighborhoods have fewer chain supermarkets and produce stores (Powell, 2007). The result is less variety and poorer quality of healthy foods in low-income neighborhoods (Sloane et al., 2003). The only available restaurants may be "fast food" establishments. Higher consumption of fast foods is associated with a decrease in nutrient intake and diet quality and an increase in energy intake, weight gain, and insulin resistance (Pereira et al., 2005).

A lack of access to affordable healthy foods has laid the groundwork for the current epidemic of obesity. Obesity underlies the growing diabetes epidemic, with all the co-morbid disorders that entails: heart disease, kidney failure, leg amputations, and blindness. Healthcare for obese individuals costs more than for normal-weight individuals, and the costs increase with increasing levels of obesity. The annual health-care costs for people who are extremely obese are almost twice those of normal-weight people.

The population health model looks at environmental conditions that contribute to the obesity epidemic through their effects on food consumption. The supersizing of cheap sources of energy-dense food and the proliferation of fast-food outlets pit healthy food choices against convenience and getting "the most bang for your buck." The food industry's marketing of foods that exploit evolutionarily programmed human preferences for sugar and fat affects food preferences and their associated caloric intake. There is particular concern about the marketing of food like sweetened cereals, beverages, and snack foods to children (Kumanyika & Grier, 2006).

Community and Social Context

Health status is influenced by the social environments of neighborhoods. This includes the characteristics of the social relationships among their residents, including the degree of mutual trust and feelings of connectedness. A supportive community has been found to contribute to good health while communities that foster isolation, disassociation, and lack of social support are detrimental to health.

A society with wide gaps between rich and poor produces low levels of social cohesion which is important for coping with stress. One way of examining this situation is by examining the social networks that exist within the defined community. Some of these data may be derived from an assessment of community health assets. The existence of social organizations and service organizations that may serve to encourage networking should be noted, along with any community "gathering places." Ultimately, however, some primary research may be required in order to identify the extent to which social networks exist and function within the targeted community.

Some other indicators related to social context that may be considered are included under the education category and may include such factors as school enrollment, dropout rates, and proportion of subsidized lunches. These indirect indicators are likely to define the level of community cohesiveness. Some private organizations have combined certain of these metrics to create a social needs index. Participation in the labor force and employment rates (as noted above) also provide clues to the nature of the social context.

Public safety is a major consideration when it comes to community stability, and the relationship between an unsafe community (even if only the perception exists) and health status has been clearly documented. Evidence suggests that individuals' sense of neighborhood safety is associated with the extent to which they participate in and interact with their community (de Jesus et al., 2010). Studies examining the role of neighborhood factors on health demonstrate that higher levels of safety are associated with higher respondent perceptions of social cohesion and better health outcomes. This research demonstrates that individuals' connectedness with their communities is vital to their health and well-being.

Social network structure tends to vary by socioeconomic status (SES), and the social networks of those with lower incomes tend to be more place-based, be homogeneously low income, contain more close relationships, and involve more overlapping relations. Conventional wisdom suggests that lower-income populations are more relation-oriented since this is about the only resource available to them. For example, Child (2016) examined the social networks in a low-income neighborhood and found that those who lived in these neighborhoods, rather than being involved in more intense and strong relationships, tended to have weaker relationships than those in middle income areas. Thus, even existing relationships may be too weak to offer beneficial social support, and these relationships are made even more tenuous due to frequent changes of residence.

Residential Segregation

Perhaps the most significant aspect of the community context is the persistent (and in some cases increasing) residential segregation exhibited by many communities. Although this phenomenon was not cited specifically in the Kaiser framework, it has come to be seen as a major consideration with regard to health status. Segregation is a fundamental cause of differences in health status between African Americans and whites because it shapes socioeconomic conditions for blacks not only at the individual and household levels but also at the neighborhood and community levels. Although other racial and ethnic groups may report similar poverty levels, the degree of segregation experienced by African Americans is unparalleled. In fact, the 2016 *County Health Rankings* report added a new measure on residential segregation to illustrate the extent to which populations are isolated from the larger society.

Although most overtly discriminatory policies and practices promoting segregation, such as separate schools or seating on public transportation or in restaurants based on race, have been illegal for decades, segregation caused by structural, institutional, and individual racism still exists throughout US society. The removal of discriminatory policies and practices has impacted overt acts of racism but has had little effect on structural racism resulting in lingering structural inequalities. Residential segregation is a key determinant of racial differences in socioeconomic mobility and, additionally, can create social and physical risks in residential environments that adversely affect health. Although this area of research is gaining interest, structural forms of racism and their relationship to health inequities remain under-studied.

Residential segregation remains prevalent in many areas of the country and may influence both personal and community well-being. Residential segregation of black and white residents is considered a fundamental cause of health disparities in the US and has been linked to poor health outcomes, including mortality, a wide variety of reproductive, infectious, and chronic diseases, and other adverse conditions. Structural racism is also linked to poor-quality housing and disproportionate exposure to environmental toxins. Individuals living in segregated neighborhoods often experience increased violence, reduced educational and employment opportunities, limited access to quality healthcare and restrictions to upward mobility.

An investigation of segregation also sheds light on the racial differences in some health outcomes that have strong environmental components. African Americans are much more likely than whites to be victims of all types of crime, including homicide, and several studies have found that segregation is positively associated with the risk of being a victim of homicide for blacks. Irrespective of racial status, the homicide rate was strongly patterned by SES. These dramatic racial differences may reflect an important area effect, and Sampson's research on the causes of urban violence clearly suggests that the elevated homicide rate for African-Americans is a consequence of residential segregation (Peterson & Krivo, 1993). Residential segregation also contributes to racial differences in drug use.

Racial residential segregation also leads to unequal access for most blacks to a broad range of services provided by municipal authorities. Political leaders have been more likely to cut spending and services in poor neighborhoods, in general, and African American neighborhoods, in particular, than in more affluent areas. Poor people and members of minority groups are less active politically than their more economically and socially advantaged peers, and elected officials are less likely to encounter vigorous opposition when services are reduced in the areas in which large numbers of poor people and people of color live.

Crime and Criminal Justice

The criminal justice system is another contributor to health status that was not included within the Kaiser framework. Factors associated with crime have a significant impact on a community in two important ways: the level of crime to which community residents are exposed and the extent of involvement of the population with the criminal justice system.

Crime is a major factor in actual and perceived community safety. Members of low-income, minority populations are particularly at risk for victimization. In addition to the direct effect of a burglary, robbery or assault—which may have an impact on health status—the stress associated with such events introduces another factor that contributes to general ill-health.

Epidemiologic studies have confirmed that jail and prison inmates have a higher burden of chronic diseases such as hypertension, asthma, and cervical cancer than the general population (Binswanger et al., 2009). Furthermore, inmates are particularly at risk for substance use disorders, psychiatric disorders, victimization, and infectious diseases, including hepatitis C, HIV, and tuberculosis. Despite the prevalence of poor health status among both minorities and inmates, the effect of criminal justice involvement on population health disparities has been largely overlooked in research on population health disparities. Probationers and parolees, who represent the largest proportion of criminal justice involved populations, suffer from inadequate access to care and risk deterioration in health status and death (Binswanger et al., 2012).

Prisons are overcrowded with people who have mental illness, drug addictions and little education, and they generally receive inadequate therapy for their conditions. Half of all people in prison are parents, with their families suffering the consequences. The average prison sentence is nearly 10 years, and prisoners are often inappropriately cared for while there. After release, few options exist within their communities, further reducing the likelihood of successful rehabilitation.

In addition to health effects on criminal justice-involved individuals, the system is likely to impact the health of families and communities, predominantly in urban areas (Binswanger et al., 2012). The adverse effects of criminalization of drug users on health involve decreased access to health benefits, housing, and employment, as well as subsequent impacts on families and communities. Rates of sexually transmitted diseases and teenage pregnancy have been shown to be associated with community incarceration rates. Urban neighborhoods whose inhabitants have high rates of incarceration and many returning inmates experience a phenomenon similar to "forced migration" which disrupts social, family, and sexual networks and has secondary effects on the health of the community. For instance, community members find new sexual partners when prior partners go to prison.

Sources of Data for Population Health Assessments

The growing recognition of the impact of social determinants on the health status of the population and increased interest in community health needs assessments has generated demand for types of data not historically considered within the purview of healthcare analysts.

Because data on social determinants is scattered over a wide range of sources, there have been increasing efforts to aggregate relevant data on one platform. An example of that is the PolicyMap application (Farris, 2020). PolicyMap is an online data and mapping tool that enables government, healthcare, non-profit, and academic institutions to access to a extensive variety of data sets from public and private sources. Since the indicators are linked to geography, it is possible to generate integrated data sets with a high level of granularity. A lot remains to be done in terms of harnessing available data and generating more detailed information, but this represents a start in establishing a one-stop-shop for data related to social determinants. The sections below describe some of the sources for categories of data relevant to population health analyses.

Sources of Data on Economic Instability

The federal government is the major source of data related to economic activity and the financial status of the population. The US Department of Commerce is a major generator of data on income, employment and wealth. The Census Bureau within the Department is the leading source of data on income, poverty and welfare benefits. Under the auspices of the American Community Survey, these data are available down to the census block group level.

Data on employment status is available from Census Bureau surveys at a fairly granular level. This information addresses labor force participation (by sex and by racial and ethnic group) and indicates the unemployment rate for various categories of workers. The federal government also closely tracks employment and unemployment as do most states.

Data on income received from a source other than a job are available from federal reports, with information provided on benefits received from the Social Security Administration, unemployment compensation, various welfare programs, food and housing subsidies and so forth. Details are available on the characteristics of those receiving non-work-related subsidies from state agencies.

Sources of Data on the Neighborhood and Physical Environment

The federal government is the major source of data on the status of neighborhoods and the physical environment. The extent to which the physical environment contributes to ill-health is tracked by a various of agencies—mostly federal but including a number of state agencies. The Department of Housing and Urban Development collects extensive data on neighborhood conditions, and the Environmental Protection Agency and various other agencies collect data on air quality, water quality and the extent of pollution. Various federal agencies track the availability of green space and make that information available to the public. Information on the location of "brown fields" and "superfund sites", as well as other sources of pollution, are available from federal regulatory agencies.

Sources of Data on Housing Access and Quality

The primary source of data on *housing accessibility and quality* is the US Department of Health and Human Services (HUD). The American Housing Survey (AHS) is sponsored by the Department of Housing and Urban Development (HUD) and conducted by the US Census Bureau. The survey is the most comprehensive national housing survey providing current information on the size, composition, and quality of the nation's housing and measuring changes in our housing stock as it ages. HUD's housing affordability database reports changes in housing affordability for families and individuals (both owners and renters) at different price levels, changes in affordability by demographic category, and reasons why people cannot afford a house.

Various local governments conduct assessments of the quality of housing. Variables that might be considered are the age of housing, access to various features, and value of housing relative to other housing options. Household size relative to the size of the housing unit is also a consideration. Residential density levels may also be reported.

The Housing Vacancies and Homeownership database provides current information on rental and homeowner vacancy rates and characteristics of units available for occupancy. These data are used extensively by public and private sector organizations to evaluate the need for new housing programs and initiatives. In addition, the rental vacancy rate is a component of the index of leading economic indicators and is used by the economic forecasters to gauge the current economic climate. Rental and homeowner vacancy rates and homeownership rates are available for the US, US regions, states and for the 75 largest Metropolitan Statistical Areas.

This national housing survey assesses, among other factors, the extent to which housing contributes to ill-health. The survey provides up-to-date information about the quality and cost of housing in the United States and major metropolitan areas. The survey also includes questions about:

- The physical condition of homes and neighborhoods,
- The costs of financing and maintaining homes, and
- The characteristics of people who live in these homes.

Planners, policy makers, and community stakeholders use the results of the AHS to assess the housing needs of communities and the nation. These statistics inform decisions that affect the housing opportunities for people of all income levels, ages, and racial and ethnic groups.

The availability of affordable housing is an issue of increasing concern and there are various approaches to determining the level of affordability. The National Association of Realtors is a private organization that provides certain data on affordability (geared primarily to the real estate industry). The RealtyHop Housing Affordability Index analyzes both proprietary and ACS Census data to provide an index of housing affordability and homeownership burden across the 100 most populous cities. Median home prices are calculated using over 300,000 listings in the RealtyHop database over the month prior to publication. The following statistics are used to calculate the index:

- Median household income from the US Census
- Median for-sale home listing prices via RealtyHop data
- Local property taxes via ACS Census data
- Mortgage expenses, assuming a 30-year mortgage, 4.5% interest rate, and 20% down payment.

The American Community Survey includes limited data on housing down to the census block group level. This includes data on the age and condition of housing as well as turnover and vacancy rates.

Sources of Data on Transportation

Data on *transportation* is relatively limited, although the US Department of Transportation (DOT) does maintain and disseminate data on access to private vehicles and to public transportation. The American Community Survey provides data on household access to vehicles, commuting patterns, distance to work and use of public transit. The Environmental Protection Agency (EPA) provides data on distance to transit stops.

The federal government also provides some detail on access to transportation at the household level. It collects data on access to a vehicle, means of transport to work, and average commute time. The National Household Travel Survey (NHTS) is another source of data on travel by US residents. This inventory of travel behavior includes trips made by all modes of travel (private vehicle, public transportation, walking and cycling) and for all purposes (e.g., travel to work, school, recreation, and personal/family trips) State transportation agencies often provide state-level data to supplement national resources.

Data on travel for specific demographic groups involves an analysis of the travel behavior of commuters, school children, millennials, the elderly, and immigrant and low-income groups. Data are also generated on travel patterns in terms of age, gender, mode use, auto occupancy and time of day.

Sources of Education Data

The federal government is a major source of educational data. Beginning with the Census Bureau, data are collected and disseminated for educational enrollment and educational attainment by level of education, broken down for various demographic groups. Other federal agencies provide data on school enrollment and graduation, as well as information on the number and quality of educational institutions. Information may be provided for individual schools and/or school districts. Separate data are available relative to public schools and private schools.

Federal agencies collect and report information on the academic performance of the nation's students, as well as the literacy level of the adult population. The National Assessment of Educational Progress (NAEP) is the primary assessment tool for the National Center for Education Statistics (NCES) for measuring what American elementary/secondary students know with regard to academic subjects. This NCES program also assesses the proficiency of adults in performing basic literacy and mathematical tasks through the National Assessments of Adult Literacy

(NAAL). NCES also participates in international assessments. Other information available on students includes:

- Characteristics of students in various educational institutions
- Student performance statistics
- Schools with high proportion of disadvantaged students and subsidized lunches

Data related to the structure of operation of schools includes:

- Accreditation status
- Expenditures per student
- Faculty qualifications

Data are also available on poorly performing schools and teacher shortage areas. Separate data sets are available on Head Start programs and other early childhood education activities.

Information is also available on the status of post-secondary education individuals and on the availability of job training programs.

Sources of Data on Food Insecurity

Federal agencies (most notably the Department of Agriculture) have turned increasing attention to the issue of food security, conducting various surveys and surveillance activities and establishing relevant databases. For various geographic areas (and, in some cases, for a specific location) information is available related to access to healthy foods and grocery stores and the extent to which the defined area is a "food desert." Data are also maintained on participation in federal food subsidy programs (e.g., SNAP and WIC). The federal Food Access Research Atlas provides point-based data on access to healthy foods.

A variety of private agencies have also become involved in monitoring food security and are making data available related to access to food and the existence of food deserts. The County Health Rankings measure of the food environment accounts for both proximity to healthy foods and income. This measure includes access to healthy foods by considering the distance an individual lives from a grocery store or supermarket, locations for healthy food purchases in most communities, and the inability to access healthy food because of cost barriers. The Food Environment Index ranges from a scale of 0 (worst) to 10 (best) and equally weights two indicators of the food environment:

1. Limited access to healthy foods estimates the percentage of the population that is low income and does not live close to a grocery store. Low income is defined as having an annual family income of less than or equal to 200% of the federal poverty threshold for the family size. Living close to a grocery store is defined differently in rural and nonrural areas; in rural areas, it means living less than 10 miles from a grocery store whereas in nonrural areas, it means less than 1 mile.

2. Food insecurity estimates the percentage of the population that did not have access to a reliable source of food during the past year. A two-stage fixed effects model was created using information from the Community Population Survey, Bureau of Labor Statistics, and American Community Survey to estimate food insecurity.

The Food Security Index (FSI) is a multidimensional measure capturing "uncertain, insufficient, or unacceptable availability, access or utilization of food" due to a lack of financial resources (National Research Council, 2006). Rather than attempting to measure the content of what people eat, the FSI was explicitly designed to *directly* "measure food insecurity based on the way people actually experience it.

Sources of Data on Community and Social Context

The federal government is the primary source of data on community and social context. Many of the agencies already referenced contribute to the body of knowledge related to this category of social determinant. The Department of Housing and Urban Development, for example, provides detailed information on the extent of subsidized housing found in a community. Other sources report on housing turnover and housing vacancy levels, considered measures of housing stability. Other federal (and some local) sources track the level of homelessness. In an effort to address social context issues federal agencies and some private organizations have created social vulnerability indices.

To the extent that health risks reflect the social context of a community, a wide range of metrics related to health behavior and subsequent health risks are available from the federal government and some state governments. Examples include the CDC's Behavioral Risk Factor Surveillance System and the NCHS' National Health Interview Survey. However, the level of granularity and even the topics covered vary from state to state.

A category of data included in a population health assessment is community health assets. Traditional community health needs assessments have focused on formal healthcare resources and ignored community health assets. This information is considered essential for a population health assessment. Data on community health assets are not likely to be readily available (unless a previous study has been carried out), so primary research is likely to be required. Box 11.1 addresses the important issue of community health assets.

Sources of Data on Residential Segregation

Tracking the diversity of our society is crucial to understanding the shifting demographics of race and ethnicity in the United States. ESRI's Diversity Index captures the racial and ethnic diversity of a geographic area in a single number, 0 to 100. The

> **Box 11.1: Identifying Community Health Assets**
> Community health assets are resources that may not be considered part of the formal health care system but, nevertheless, are perceived by community residents as contributing to the population's health. The notion of community health assets arose out of Third World contexts in which formal healthcare resources were lacking or non-existent. Health analysts sought to determine how these populations dealt with health problems in the absence of formal health services. They found that members of these groups identified other resources as "community health assets", and this notion was ultimately incorporated into population health analyses. One other "asset" that should be considered is access to the Internet. This is increasingly being considered a minimal requirement for maintaining a adequate level of social involvement. This notion of community health assets fits well into a model that attempts to focus on health rather than illness.
>
> Community health assets include a wide range of institutions, programs and personnel that would not typically be considered health assets. Community residents may see such "institutions" as social service agencies, community development agencies and community centers as health assets. Churches and other faith-based organizations may be seen as health assets and this may even include funeral homes. Interestingly, barber shops and beauty parlors are often considered health assets in that they are important gathering places for members of some minority groups and serve as a conduit for information (including health-related information). The significance of these organizations has been recognized in that a number of pilot health education programs have been based a barber shops and beauty parlors.

Diversity Index allows for efficient analysis and mapping of seven race groups that can be either of Hispanic or non-Hispanic origin—a total of 14 separate race/ethnic groupings. Although immigration has largely contributed to gains in diversity over the past four decades, there are new forces driving diversity in America. More than half of all children born in the United States are minorities, defined as any race/ethnicity other than non-Hispanic white. Minorities accounted for 30.9% of the population in 2000 and were expected to make up 40.4% of the population by 2019. That reduces the majority (non-Hispanic whites) share of the population from 69% to less than 60%. The transition to a "majority-minority" population is expected around 2040. When viewed through a generational lens, the differences in diversity by age are unmistakable.

The Diversity Index from ESRI represents the likelihood that two persons, chosen at random from the same area, belong to different race or ethnic groups. Ethnic diversity, as well as racial diversity, is included in our definition of the Diversity Index. If an area's entire population belongs to one race group or one ethnic group, then an area has zero diversity. An area's diversity index increases to 100 when the population is evenly divided into two or more race/ethnic groups.

A residential segregation index has been developed by County Health Rankings in recognition of the impact of segregation on health status. Its values ranges from 0 (complete integration) to 100 (complete segregation). The index score can be interpreted as the percentage of either black or white residents that would have to move to different geographic areas in order to produce a distribution that matches that of the larger area.

Sources of Data on Crime and Criminal Justice

The primary source of data on crime at the national level is the federal government, and the Federal Bureau of Investigation has overall responsibility for monitoring trends in various types of crimes. Although detailed data are collected and reported by the FBI, this information is of limited usefulness from a population health perspective. First, participation in the crime reporting database is voluntary. Most police departments participate in it, but many do not. Second, the data are presented only down to the county level. Since most community assessments will be conducted in search of more granularity federal crime data may be of little use. The County Health Rankings also present crime statistics but these too are only down to the county level.

X A second and potentially more useful source of crime data is private crime monitoring systems. SpotCrime is a crime data aggregator. This application maps crime incidents, plots them on Google Maps, and delivers alerts via email, Facebook, Twitter, SMS, RSS and a multitude of other platforms.

X Radford/FGCU Serial Killer Research

Population Health Data Challenges

The population health model mandates a new approach to measuring health status and acquiring the data necessary for implementing community health improvement initiatives. This creates challenges that go beyond the already substantial barriers to accessing timely, granular and detailed data. The issues faced by those attempting to obtain health data from disparate sources and integrating them in a manner that supports efficient analysis and data mining are well known. Population health proponents are a long way from being able to effectively profile a community in terms of its health status utilizing the full range of attributes to be considered. Any effort toward the implementation of a population health approach must be cognizant of the shortcomings that exist with regard to data management and the subsequent barriers likely to hinder the implementation.

A number of practical barriers exist that, while not unknown with regard to traditional data collection activities, are more of a challenge when it comes to population health analyses. The following issues need to be addressed in order to develop adequate data resources to support a population health model.

Granularity Analysts performing traditional community health needs assessments have had to settle for data at a high level of geography—in most cases no more granular than the county level. As a result, CHNAs have been restricted to analyses for fairly large geographical units—usually at the county level but occasionally at the ZIP Code level. This has meant that a fairly broad brush is used to paint the picture of health status and health service needs. This limitation reflects the lack of public health data for lower levels of geography exacerbated by the fact that public health officials are reluctant to release data for smaller geographic units. Although there are situations in which the "community" corresponds with the county, a ZIP Code, or a grouping of ZIP Codes, it has become well established that communities do not neatly follow formal geographic boundaries. Health departments—a source of much of the data required for a population health analysis—are resistant to providing detailed data in general and particularly providing data below the county level.

To effectively implement a population health analysis, the analyst requires data at a lower level of geography, and those conducting population health analyses tend to be much more aggressive in delineating meaningful boundaries that reflect a coherent community. This approach is suffers from a lack of data for small geographic areas but, as shown below, the focus on the social determinants of health rather than traditional epidemiological data means that data from non-traditional sources must be accessed in order to carry out a population health assessment. Thus, while mortality rates may not be available at or below the ZIP Code level, it is possible to identify housing conditions, food deserts, transportation access issues, crime rates and other factors—including access to health services—for lower levels of geography. The marshaling of these types of data allows for the disaggregation of large geographical units into meaningful subunits for analysis.

Timeliness All analysis utilizing health-related data face the issue of data timeliness. In most cases, the data required for population health analyses must be collected at one level and compiled at another—resulting in delays in data distribution. A prime example involves the National Center for Health Statistics (NCHS) and its processing of vital statistics data. Birth and death certificates, for example, must be collected at the county level where they are processed to a greater or lesser degree and then submitted to the state health department. The state health department compiles the certificates for all of its counties and, when that compilation is complete, submits the certificates for the entire state to the NCHS. The NCHS then compiles certificates from each of the states and processes them into a national database. Only then is it possible for the NCHS to analyze the data and disseminate the findings. While this may be an extreme example, the process across the federal government and state governments is not that much different.

Accessibility Regardless of the quality of the data it is not useful unless it can be accessed. The federal government and many state governments have made great strides in making data available to the public. However, there are still challenges in obtaining access to certain categories of data, and this is particularly the case if you are seeking data below the county level. As noted above, data generated by local health departments are characterized by limited accessibility due to privacy concerns. Data from other sources may be inaccessible because of its format or storage method. In some cases extensive data may exist but not in the desired from. Some information may be maintained as point data and will have to be assigned to a geographical identifier in order to be useful. Other data may be available for a school district that is not co-terminus with other geographic boundaries. Clearly, a lot of work is going to be required to develop a repository of data for use in population health analyses.

Data Gaps Population health analyses require a wide range of data, including many types of data not collected previously. While standard demographic and epidemiological data are likely to be readily available and often at an appropriate level of granularity, much of the data desired for population health analyses has not been traditionally collected and may be difficult to find. This includes the non-traditional health-related data desirable for population health analyses on topics such as mental illness and substance abuse, dental health, obesity and domestic violence to name a few. Additional challenges exist when it comes to data on the social determinants of health. These will typically exist outside the comfort zone of healthcare analysts and may be a challenge to find and access. Data on housing stability, food insecurity, crime and safety, transportation and a host of other topics is widely dispersed and, when accessible, may not lend itself to integration with other data sets.

Projectability Traditional community health assessments may make an effort at projecting future health conditions, health service needs and utilization, but most of their emphasis is on past trends and current conditions. A population health approach is much more future oriented and more aggressive in identifying at-risk populations and projecting their conditions into the future. Data on the social determinants of health, for example, do not always lend themselves to projection techniques and some creativity may be required in order to generate the data needed to look downstream and develop proactive intervention initiatives.

Emphasis There are other challenges as well beyond the practical ones identified above. Traditional CHNAs have focused on "sick status" while a more contemporary approach would focus on "health status". The intent has historically been to identify conditions (e.g., mortality rates, morbidity rates) that indicate how unhealthy the population is. A population health approach, while not ignoring standard assessment metrics, seeks to determine what is healthy about the population. This involves the identification of the factors that contribute to good health (e.g., community health assets) and then determine the contribution they make to community health improvement.

A defining feature of traditional CHNAs is their emphasis on shortfalls in healthcare resources in the community. The reasoning is that the mere presence of formal healthcare services represents assets for the community. Yet, we now know that the presence of facilities and practitioners within a geographic area does not: (1) assure access; (2) assure utilization if access is available; or (3) contribute to improved community health status if facilities are available and accessed. Population health assessments, on the other hand, are sensitive to health resources that, while not being noted by public health officials, are recognized by the community. These "health assets" may include social service programs, community development corporations, faith-based organizations, and community associations, to name a few. Even such unlikely "facilities" as barber shops and beauty salons may be considered health assets by community residents. This approach involves a shift in data emphasis from typical resource inventories to the inclusion of a much wider variety of data

Finally, there needs to be a shift in emphasis from data imposed from the outside to data generated by the community. It has been noted that epidemiological data and the conclusions that they generate reflect the perspectives of epidemiologists and not the perspective of members of the community being served. Epidemiological data are readily available and, hence, a ready target for data analysts. However, as noted elsewhere, there are issues especially with using mortality data for purposes of health status assessment. The use of morbidity data is even more questionable given issues surrounding the generation of morbidity data and the fact that known cases for various conditions are likely to represent an undercount. Ultimately, community residents must be the ones to determine the main health problems and that is a task that is likely to require primary research.

Transitioning from CHNA to PHA

Community health needs assessments (CHNA) have historically been conducted by healthcare organizations in order to determine the health status of their communities. CHNAs have primarily been conducted by government agencies and not-for-profit organizations although many for-profit organizations may have reasons to conduct a CHNA. The CHNA represents a systematic method of determining the health status and unmet healthcare needs of a population and changes required to address these unmet needs. These assessments can take various forms and are typically conducted for health planning purposes. They involve both quantitative and qualitative approaches for collecting data to determine priorities that must balance clinical, ethical, and economic considerations of need.

Now—at least for certain hospitals—conducting a CHNA is not an option as the Affordable Care Act requires not-for-profit hospitals to conduct a comprehensive assessment at least every 3 years. Even providers who have routinely conducted community health assessments are not likely to be in compliance with the provisions of the Act. Tax-exempt hospitals must demonstrate an understanding of the healthcare needs of the total community (even those segments that it does not serve), identify gaps in services (even those that it does not provide), and formulate a plan for addressing any gaps that have been identified.

As originally conceived, CHNAs have the following attributes (Wright et al., 1998):

- Health needs assessment is the systematic approach to ensuring that the healthcare system uses its resources to improve the health of the population in the most efficient way
- The CHNA involves epidemiological, qualitative, and comparative methods to describe the health problems of a population; identify inequalities in health and access to services; and determine priorities for the most effective use of resources
- The health needs to be assessed are those that can benefit from healthcare or from wider social and environmental changes
- Successful health needs assessments require a practical understanding of what is involved, the time and resources necessary to undertake assessments, and sufficient integration of the results into planning and commissioning of local services

Ultimately, a health needs assessment provides the opportunity for:

- Describing the patterns of disease in the local population and the differences from regional or national disease patterns;
- Learning more about the needs and priorities of their patients and the local population;
- Highlighting the areas of unmet need and providing a clear set of objectives to work towards meeting these needs;
- Deciding rationally how to use resources to improve the local population's health in the most effective and efficient way; and
- Influencing policy, interagency collaboration, and research priorities.

Importantly, health needs assessments also provide a method for monitoring and promoting equity in the provision and use of health services and addressing inequalities in health.

The Changing Context for Community Assessments

A number of developments are influencing the CHNA process and pointing to the need for a different approach. The population being assessed is undergoing considerable change that may affect the assessment process. Among the developments are the continued aging of the population as the last of the baby boomers enter their senior years. The aging of the population, of course, has resulted in an increasingly female population. Perhaps even more significant is the increasing racial and ethnic diversity of the US population. Non-Hispanic whites are rapidly becoming a minority as various racial and minority groups—most notably Hispanics—outpace the white population in growth. This increasing diversity complicates the aging picture in that members of most racial and ethnic groups tend to be much younger than their non-Hispanic white counterparts.

Families and households have been experiencing a second "demographic transition" as non-traditional households come to dominate and fewer Americans are getting married and even fewer are having children. The marital status/household structure configuration reflects differences between the older non-Hispanic white population and the younger populations comprising various racial and ethnic minorities.

These developments have been accompanied by changes in the population's disease profile. The acute conditions of the past have been displaced by the chronic conditions that affect a more mature population. The "diseases of civilization" represent the predominant health problems today even to the point that young children are exhibiting health conditions restricted to the elderly in the past. Add to these the "diseases of despair" that have been recently identified that are contributing to the changing morbidity and mortality profiles.

Driving much of the change in patient characteristics and health problems is contemporary disease etiology. Few conditions today are a result of biological organisms or genetic factors. Instead, the primary etiological factors have become lifestyles and the vagaries of unhealthy physical and social environments. A major factor in this regard is the role played by the social determinants of health status. It is increasingly conceded that observed health problems are really symptoms of underlying social pathology—the true causes of disease. Thus, housing instability, food insecurity, polluted neighborhoods, unsafe communities, lack of education and other "external" factors are blamed for the level of ill-health.

Because of the changes noted above and the failure of late twentieth century healthcare to improve community health, there is growing interest in population health assessments (PHAs). As an approach that assesses health from a population rather than a patient perspective, this represents an opportunity to develop a better understanding of the health status of populations—whether they are patients or not—and an innovative approach to improving a population's health status.

This approach focuses on social pathology rather than biological pathology and addresses conditions within the environment and policy realms. While an underlying assumption is that a population health approach aims to improve health status by focusing on the healthcare needs and resources of *populations* not individuals, it does not rule out specific patient-based medical treatment but views healthcare as only one component of a health improvement initiative.

A PHA uses population-based indicators to describe, prioritize and address specific health-related issues within economic, social, racial, or environmental domains. It focuses on community-based solutions at the health system, environment/infrastructure, education or policy level. Fig. 11.1 depicts the population health assessment model.

There is little agreement as to the attributes of the population health model, just as there is no consensus with regard to the term's definition. However, the following attributes—each with implications for health needs assessments—are thought to distinguish the population health assessment from the traditional community health needs assessment..

Recognition of the Social Determinants of Health Problems Social factors are powerful determinants of health status (and health services utilization). An emphasis on understanding the social determinants of health is critical to the population

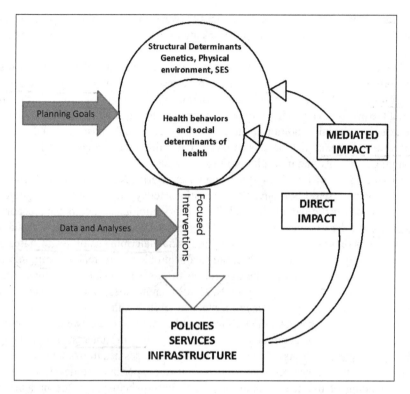

Fig. 11.1 Population Health Assessment Model. (Source: Deprez & Manchester, 2018)

health model, and the importance of social pathology over biological pathology must be recognized. Depending on the source it could be argued that social determinants account for 40–60% of the variation in health status among subgroups of the population. If social factors are considered the root cause of observed health problems, any health improvement initiative should take these factors into consideration.

Focus on Populations* (or Subpopulations) Rather than Individuals Application of the population health model involves measuring the health status of the total population rather than simply assessing clinical readings for individual patients and combining them into an aggregate health status index. This assumes that a population's health status is not simply a reflection of the health status of its members but exhibits attributes that are characteristic of the population independent of the attributes of its members. It should be noted that meaningful subpopulations should be identified in order to focus on the social context characterizing targeted populations.

Shift in Focus Away from Patients to Consumers As the healthcare industry was evolving in the late 1900s, "patients" came to be seen as "consumers". This trend was driven by baby boomers who wanted the benefits of quality care as patients coupled with the efficiency, convenience and value that they had come to expect as consumers. This represented a significant conceptual leap for healthcare providers and moved the focus to potential patients (i.e., consumers) rather than only existing patients. This perspective shifts the focus to the total population.

Health Status Measured at the Community Level A community-based (participatory) understanding of what the critical health issues are is a prominent feature of population health. While some argue that community health status represents the sum total of the health status of the individuals within the community, a population health approach would posit the existence of a state of health that exists independent of the health of the individuals who make up the population. This would explain the fact that certain communities exhibit persistent health problems over time regardless of who resides in the community. Even personal lifestyles might be thought to reflect the influence of the social groups with which the individuals are affiliated.

Geography as a Predictor of Health and Health Behavior There is increasing recognition of the importance of the spatial dimension in the distribution of health and ill-health. One of the most significant—and some would say disturbing—findings from decades of health services research is that the utilization of health services varies in terms of geography. Where one lives is a powerful determinant of the kind and amount of medical care received. Rates for various procedures may vary by as much as a factor of 10, reflecting such conditions as local practice patterns, insurance coverage, availability of services and consumer lifestyles.

Innovative Ways of Measuring Health Status The ways in which health status has historically been measured depend on indicators that have relevance for health professionals. Not surprisingly these indicators represent a biomedical bias. Any assessment of health status should reflect the perspectives of the community rather than those imposed externally by health professionals. The problems identified through community input are not likely to correspond with those recognized by the healthcare establishment. Even the public health department's criteria for assessing health issues may differ from those held by the general public.

Addressing the Problems Not the Symptoms As the impact of social factors on health status has become documented, the argument is increasingly being made that the health conditions exhibited by a population are not the *problems* per se but are *symptoms* of underlying problems. Thus, the morbidity levels exhibited by various populations are a reflection of the social determinants of health and illness that are, in effect, the true problems. The presence of disease can thus be seen as the manifestation of these underlying conditions. This perspective is supported by research that suggests that disadvantaged populations are likely to identify as "health problems" such factors as lack of food, inadequate housing, and unsafe streets.

Critics of the US healthcare system point out that we have been treating these symptoms while not addressing the true cause of the problems. Putting a band-aid on the wound is of limited usefulness if the underlying infection is not addressed, and an approach that addresses symptoms without affecting a true cure is clearly ineffective when it comes to improving population health. This explains the fact that there is no correlation between health resources expended and health status. Further, it is now acknowledged that better access to health insurance does not guarantee access to care and that access to care does not assure utilization of services. Finally, utilization of services does not necessarily foster better patient outcomes and by itself clearly does not contribute to improved population health.

Similarities Between CHNAs and PHAs

There are a number of attributes that CHNAs and PHAs have in common. Both are comprehensive in their approach, including the entire population within the community and addressing the full range of health issues. Both recognize the importance of considering the total population while addressing relevant subpopulations and their attributes. The importance of disaggregating data and conducting analysis at the lowest level of geography possible is recognized by both. Similarly, both employ a broad notion of what constitutes health issues in that they attempt to assess not only physical health but to the extent possible mental and spiritual health (although, admittedly, the population health assessment goes further in this regard).

To this end, both CHNAs and PHAs compile comparable data to establish a baseline for comparative analysis. This involves the collection of data on the demographics of the population (and relevant subpopulations), its morbidity characteristics, and its mortality patterns. Both types of assessment attempt to determine the health status of the population and do this using proxy variables to supplement direct measures.

CHNAs and PHAs both rely on the core sets of data that are thought to define health status and health behavior. These data are generated primarily through the efforts of local health departments on the one hand and through reporting of activities by healthcare providers on the other. Despite the deficiencies in both sources of data, they represent the primary options for obtaining data to define the attributes of the community's population. Both approaches also rely to a certain extent on synthetic data in that any plans should be future oriented.

Both types of assessments involve an inventory of the health-related resources available to the population under study. Thus, an assessment is made of the available facilities, personnel, equipment, programs and services within the community. With CHNAs the emphasis is more likely to be on the *quantity* of services rather than their *quality*, relying on availability rates to determined adequacy (e.g., ratio of primary care doctors to population).

Finally, both CHNAs and PHAs attempt to measure the utilization of services by community residents. The emphasis historically has been on the use of formal healthcare resources such as hospitals, clinics and other sources of clinical or custodial care. Utilization rates for various types of resources have typically been calculated to determine the level of health behavior within the target population. While some attention is paid to informal and non-traditional types of health behavior, with the CHNA less aggressive in seeking out the elusive metrics for this type of health-inducing activity.

Both approaches ultimately employ gap analysis in order to assess the variance between identified needs and available resources. While any subsequent plans should consider the totality of issues related to the health of the community and the proposed responses, both pay particular attention to any shortfalls in resources or mismatches between the observed needs and the resources offered to address these gaps.

Differences Between CHNAs and PHAs

Despite the similarities that can be cited between CHNAs and PHAs, at the end of the day they represent qualitatively different approaches to the same task. There are conceptual differences between the two approaches and practical differences related to types and sources of data, analytical techniques and importantly the approach to improving community health.

A critical distinction between CHNAs and PHAs is the fact that CHNA's focus on "sick status" while PHAs focus on "health status". The intent of the CHNA is to identify the conditions (e.g., mortality rates, morbidity rates) that indicate how unhealthy the population is. This standard approach is reflective of the medical model underlying it and the conviction that factors amenable to modification by the healthcare system should be the focus. PHAs, on the other hand, while not ignoring standard assessment metrics, seek to determine what is healthy about the population. Thus, community "health assets" are likely to be identified. What, for example, are conditions that reflect positively on the health of the population? Even the most disease-prone population is likely to exhibit some positive attributes.

A defining feature of CHNAs is their emphasis on shortfalls in healthcare resources in the community. The reasoning is that the mere presence of formal healthcare services represent assets for the community. Yet, we now know that the presence of facilities and practitioners within a geographic area does not: (1) assure access; (2) assure utilization if access is available; or (3) contribute to improve community health status even if facilities are available and accessed. PHAs, on the other hand, are sensitive to health resources that, while not being noted by public health officials, are recognized by the community. These "health assets" may include social service programs, community development corporations, faith-based organizations, and community associations, to name a few. Even such unlikely "facilities" as barber shops and beauty salons may be considered health assets by community residents.

CHNAs are more focused on developing a "snapshot" of the current situation that describes the population at a point in time, while the PHA is more future oriented in its approach. The PHA's emphasis on the social determinants of health enable a more prospective approach to health status determination, one that anticipates future developments with implications for the population's health status.

The differences are more than a matter of the time horizon emphasized but reflect a basic contrast between the two approaches. The CHNA is content to establish a current baseline based on somewhat weak data and project past trends into the future. While the PHA does not eschew this methodology, the conceptual approach is much different. Instead of extending past trends into the future, the PHA approach identifies factors in the current environment that are likely to have implications for the future. The emphasis is on the social determinants of health with the notion that current housing instability, food insecurity, unemployment level, and transportation access, among other factors will be contributors to future health status. Thus, the PHA places more emphasis on factors in the environment and the extent to which they portend a healthy or unhealthy future for the affected population.

Historically, CHNAs have been restricted to analyses of large geographical areas—usually at the county level but occasionally at the ZIP Code level. This has meant that a fairly broad brush was used to paint the picture of health status and health service needs. This limitation reflects the lack of public health data for lower levels of geography exacerbated by the fact that public health officials are reluctant to release data for smaller levels of geography. Although there are situations in which the "community" corresponds with the county or one or a grouping of ZIP Codes, it has become well established that communities do not neatly follow established geographic boundaries.

Those conducting population health analyses tend to be much more aggressive in delineating meaningful boundaries that reflect a coherent community. This approach is still faced with the lack of data for small geographic areas but, as shown below, the focus on the social determinants of health rather than traditional epidemiological data means that other types of data from non-traditional sources must be accessed in order to carry out a PHA. Thus, while mortality rates may not be available at or below the ZIP Code level, it is possible to identify housing conditions, food deserts, transportation access issues, crime rates and other factors—including access to health services—for lower level of geography. A different data perspective allows the disaggregation of large geographical units into meaningful subunits for analysis.

A final difference between CHNAs and PHAs relates to the types of recommendations that the respective approaches might generate, recommendations that reflect previously noted differences. CHNAs are more likely to frame recommendations within the context of the healthcare delivery system. Operating on the assumption that "more is better", there is a tendency to treat the healthcare system as a hammer and see any gap as a nail. Thus, the answer to most identified problems is more facilities, personnel and/or services. The PHA, on the other hand, is more likely to recognize the limitations of the healthcare delivery system in addressing identified problems. While the judicuous deployment of health resources within the community is certainly an objective, less faith would be placed in the ability of these resources to address identified issues.

CHNAs are more likely to turn to traditional public health initiatives as a major component of any efforts at amelioration. While many of these efforts to address the factors that affect populations are worthwhile, they still represent a health system solution to to a non-health situation. Even then, many public health programs are geared toward changing individual behavior rather than influencing group behavior. The CHNA is more likely to recommend health education programs, for example, that attempt to change the behavior of individuals.

The PHA, on the other hand, is more likely to be focused on population-oriented solutions that take a "wholesale" approach to health problems rather than focusing on individuals. The focus of PHAs on the social determinants of health mandates a solution that attempts to address the root causes of health problems. Rather than focusing on specific health problems, the intent is to create a healthier overall environment. The assumption here is that people are not healthy because they receive good healthcare but because they are healthy enough to never need it.

Finally, while both CHNAs and PHAs recognize the importance of policies in establishing a context for community health improvement, the CHNA is more likely to limit its policy recommendations to the healthcare arena. The PHA, on the other hand, would take a broader approach to examine policies within a number of sectors of society. It is one thing to monitor pollutants in the environment and recommend mitigative actions (CHNA approach), it is another to lobby for policy changes that would have a major impact on the release of pollutants in the environment. Policies related to spheres such as education, housing, criminal justice, transportation and healthcare among others are more likely to be considered in the recommendations of a population health assessment.

Summary

The population health model calls for an innovative approach to the information required for assessing community health status and implementing a population health initiative. The information required is significantly broader than for a traditional health needs analysis. The population health approach requires an unprecedented and in-depth understanding of the attributes of the service area population and is responsive to the assessment mandates of the Affordable Care Act. In determining population health data needs a number of issues must be considered, such as the level of aggregation and the role of qualitative versus quantitative data. The data requirements for a population health analysis include the data accessed for a traditional health needs analysis, although those data categories are downplayed in favor of data that reflect the social determinants of health. This approach calls for information drawn from other sectors besides healthcare and includes data on economic conditions, housing stability, food security, transportation, criminal justice and other sectors of society. The data required for these categories supported of population health analyses are scattered over a wide range of sources, requiring at this point a certain level of research effort. In some cases, primary research might be required—as in the case of community health assets. Agencies of the federal government are the best sources for much of the data related to the social determinants of health, with state and local governments sometimes supplementing these sources. Increasing numbers of private and public organizations are compiling relevant data in response to the demand for information on social determinants. The implementation of a population health assessment is qualitatively different from the traditional health needs analysis, with the former distinguished from the latter in terms of purpose, perspective, emphasis, assumptions and types of recommendations among other attributes. While there are increased efforts to generate and disseminate data for population health analysis issues remain with regard to data timeliness, granularity and specificity.

Key Points

- The current environment calls for an innovative approach to community health needs assessment
- While much of the data used for a traditional needs assessment can still be used, a different interpretation may be required
- The primary difference in terms of data is the emphasis in the population health model on data unrelated to health and healthcare
- The focus is of the PHA is on data that provide insight into the social determinants of health
- This model requires data from sectors such as education, housing, transportation, environment and criminal justice
- These data are scattered over a wide range of organizations and some effort is required to identify their locations
- The federal government is a major source of much of the data related to the social determinants of health
- Various private and public organizations are increasing their emphasis on data related to social determinants
- There are increasing attempts at aggregating data for population health analyses but these are in the early stages
- Some primary research may be required as in the case of identifying community health assets
- There is a qualitative difference between the traditional health needs assessment and a population health assessment
- These two approaches differ in terms of purpose, perspective, emphasis and types of recommendations among other factors
- Communities attempting to address community health needs must adopt a population health approach to be effective in improving community health status

References

Arcury, T. A., Gesler, W. M., Preisser, J. S., et al. (2005). The effects of geography and spatial behavior on health care utilization among the residents of a rural region. *Health Services Research, 40*(1), 135–155.

Binswanger, I. A., Krueger, P. M., & Steiner, J. F. (2009). Prevalence of chronic medical conditions among jail and prison inmates in the USA compared with the general population. *Journal of Epidemiology and Community Health, 63*(11), 912–919.

Binswanger, I. A., Redmond, N., Steiner, J. F., et al. (2012). Health disparities and the criminal justice system: An agenda for further research and action. *Journal of Urban Health, 89*(1), 98–107.

Chetty, R., et al. (2014). Where is the land of opportunity? The geography of intergenerational mobility in the United States. *The Quarterly Journal of Economics, 129*(4), 1553–1623.

Child, S. (2016). *Social capital and social networks: The importance of social ties for health among residents of disadvantaged communities.* Unpublished dissertation. https://scholarcommons.se.edu/etd/3848

Cummins, S., & Macintyre, S. (2005). Food environments and obesity—Neighbourhood or nation. *International Journal of Epidemiology, 35*(1), 100–104.

De Jesus, M., Puleo, E., Shelton, R. C., et al. (2010). Associations between perceived social environment and neighborhood safety: Health implications. *Health & Place, 16*(5), 1007–1013.

Deprez, R., & Manchester, C. (2018). Population health assessment: Methods for diagnosing and fixing the health of communities. *Maine Policy Review, 17*(7), 51–59.

Farris, D. (2020). Policy Map. *Journal of the Medical Library Association, 108*(1), 158–160.

Institute of Medicine. (2011). *Leading health indicators for healthy people 2020: Letter report.* Downloaded from URL: https://pubmed.ncbi.nlm.nih.gov/24983065/

Kneebone, E., & Garr, E. (2010). *The suburbanization of poverty: Trends in Metropolitan America, 2000 to 2008.* Downloaded from URL: https://www.brookings.edu/wp-content/uploads/2016/06/0120_poverty_paper.pdf

Kumanyika, S. K., & Grier, S. (2006). Targeting interventions for ethnic minority and low-income populations. *The Future of Children, 16*(1), 187–207.

Morgenstern, H. (1995). Ecologic studies in epidemiology: Concepts, principles, and methods. *Annual Review of Public Health, 16*, 61–81.

National Center for Health Statistics. (2020). *Health: United States 2019.* National Center for Health Statistics.

Pereira, M. A., Kartashov, A. I., Ebbeling, C. B., et al. (2005). Fast-food habits, weight gain, and insulin resistance (the CARDIA study): 15-year prospective analysis. *Lancet, 365*, 36–42.

Pereira, G. et al. (2010). *Residential exposure to traffic emissions and adverse pregnancy outcomes.* Downloaded from URL: http://sapiens.revues.org/966?gathStatIcon=true

Peterson, R. D., & Krivo, L. J. (1993). Racial segregation and black urban homicide. *Social Forces, 71*(4), 1001–1026.

Powell, L. M. (2007). Food store availability and neighborhood characteristics in the United States. *Preventive Medicine, 44*, 189–195.

Robert Wood Johnson Foundation. (2012). *Health policy snapshot public health and prevention: How does transportation impact health?* Downloaded from URL: http://www.rwjf.org/content/dam/farm/reports/issue_briefs/2012/rwjf402311

Roeder, A. (2014). *Zip code better predictor of health than genetic code.* Downloaded from URL: http://www.hsph.harvard.edu/news/features/zip-code-better-predictor-of-health-than-genetic-code/

Rogers, R. G., Hummer, R. A., & Nam, C. B. (2000). *Living and dying in the USA: Behavioral, health and social differentials of adult mortality.* Academic.

Sagrestano, L. M., Clay, J., Finerman, R., et al. (2014). Transportation vulnerability as a barrier to service utilization for HIV-positive individuals. *AIDS Care, 26*(3), 314–319.

Schroeder, B. (2016). *Health and food security.* Downloaded from URL: http://www.resilience.org/stories/2011-02-01/health-and-food-security

Seligman, H. K., Laraia, B. A., & Kushel, M. B. (2010). Food insecurity is associated with chronic disease among low-income NHANES participants. *Journal of Nutrition, 140*(2), 304–310.

Sloane, D. C., Diamant, A. L., Lewis, L. B., et al. (2003). REACH Coalition of the African American Building a legacy of health project improving the nutritional resource environment for healthy living through community-based participatory research. *Journal of General Internal Medicine, 18*, 568–575.

Syed, S. T., Gerber, B. S., & Sharp, L. K. (2013). Traveling towards disease: Transportation barriers to health care access. *Journal of Community Health, 38*(5), 976–993.

University of Pennsylvania. (2020). *The increasing mortality gap by education*. Downloaded from URL: https://budgetmodel.wharton.upenn.edu/issues/2020/7/6/mortality-gap-by-education#:~:text=Summary%3A%20Over%20the%20last%20two,18%20percent%20lower%20mortality%20rate

Wright, J., Williams, R., & Wilkinson, J. R. (1998). Development and importance of health needs assessment. *British Medical Journal, 316*(7140), 1310–1313.

Additional Resources

American Community Survey (annual) at www.data.census.gov.

American Psychological Association. (2013). *Diagnostic and Statistical Manual IV.*

ESRI Diversity Index at URL: http://downloads.esri.com/support/whitepapers/other_/2015_USA_ESRI_Diversity_Index_Methodology.pdf.

National Center for Health Statistics at www.cdc.gov/nchs.

National Research Council publication, *The aging population in the twenty-first century: Statistics for health policy*. Downloaded from URL: https://www.ncbi.nlm.nih.gov/books/NBK217737/.

Policy Map at www.policymap.com.

Chapter 12
The Role of the Community in Population Health Improvement

In this chapter, the reader will:

- Learn why the community (not the healthcare system) should be responsible for community health
- Appreciate the role that policy contributes to community health
- Be exposed to the concept of "collective impact" and its significance
- Learn about efforts on the part of communities to improve health status
- Find out about some useful techniques for promoting community health improvement

It is increasingly recognized that contemporary health problems and their solutions have their roots in the community. Past efforts focusing on observed health problems are now seen as attempts to treat the symptoms without addressing the underlying causes of ill-health. Many now concede that the healthcare system has limited ability to contribute to community health improvement and that the community—however constituted—must drive the population health movement. This chapter addresses the importance of the community in this regard and reviews actions that communities can take toward population health improvement.

Introduction

It is increasingly recognized that contemporary health problems and their solutions have their roots in the community, yet it is hard to break our dependency on the healthcare delivery system and the tremendous resources at its disposal. Based on past successes it is not surprising that many—particularly health professionals—continue to place unmerited faith in the system's ability to improve community health. While the past accomplishments of medical science are unarguable, the question arises as to how effective the healthcare system is today even in the clinical sphere. The deficiencies characterizing the system have been enumerated elsewhere, and except for the implementation of life-saving procedures, the current benefits of the healthcare system for improving community health status are arguably limited.

There are a number of reasons why the healthcare system is not in a position to lead the population health effort and, in fact, may not be in a position to make a significant contribution to it. A major limitation of the healthcare system is its restricted range of vision. The healthcare system holds a fairly narrow view of health status and the factors considered in its assessment. Yet the population health approach requires an expansive perspective.

Healthcare providers are not trained for and often have little capacity to address the non-medical health issues of their own patients—much less those of the total population. While some engage in health promotion, health education and related prevention activities, the focus is usually on the clinical management of specific health conditions affecting a defined population. At the end of the day, the problems to be addressed are not the health conditions focused on in the past. Those are symptoms of deeper problems that are beyond the purview of the healthcare system.

Health professionals are unlikely to have much exposure to representatives of the entities that could provide a broader perspective. Indeed, it was not unusual in the past for health professionals to scoff at the idea that these factors influenced the types of problems they were seeing. Few hospital administrators or doctors would say that out loud today, but the insular nature of medical practice is hard to overcome. With the exception of emergency department providers, clinicians know very little about the conditions in the community that affect their patients before they show up nor do they know what happens to their patients after they walk out the clinic door. They do know that many of these patients show up with the same problems a couple of months later.

A major contention of the population health movement is that ill-health is not an attribute of individuals but of populations. While the healthcare system—primarily through public health—can have some impact at the group level, its approach is mechanistic rather than organic. Public health aside, the focus is on "fixing" the problems of group members rather than manipulating the social factors that influence group health status.

Problems that originate in the community call for a community-based response. As with allopathic medicine, the challenge is to identify the cause of the malady and then take measures to counteract the effect of that cause. The population health approach not only replicates this approach at the societal level but responds through a multi-pronged attack on the roots of health problems.

Why Not Community?

Well before the emergence of the population health movement astute observers pointed to social pathology as a progenitor of ill health. Even though forward-thinking professionals and policy makers may have appreciated this at some level, it was still believed that a healthcare system was in place to address these issues. It was easy for civic leaders to argue that it was not their problem.

Even among those who appreciated the role of the community it was felt that healthcare was too complex for non-professionals to understand much less impact. It did not help that the medical profession had spent decades promoting the notion that only medical doctors can understand health issues and bring about any remedies. Today, however, physicians are more likely to concede that they are not confident in their ability to address their patients' social needs. They admit that they have no control over diet, fitness and even transportation to allow their patients to receive health and social services (Robert Wood Johnson Foundation, 2011).

One factor that has often prevented a community-wide approach to population health has been the tendency of health problems to affect often "invisible" populations within society. If most of the population appears hail and hardy, there is a tendency to overlook the minority that exhibits the most severe health problems. Indeed, it is easy to blame the victim in such circumstance while overlooking the contribution of social factors to the situation. A lack of data for small geographic areas may contribute to this situation in that the "average" metric for a county (typically the lowest level of geography for which data are available) is likely to mask the fact that some subgroups may exhibit very unfavorable health indicators. (Take for example the county that reports an infant mortality rate of 10/1,000 live births. While this in its own right would be considered unfavorable, it masks the fact that the rate for the white population is 5/1,000 while that for the black population is 15/1,000—a rate comparable to some third-world countries.

One other factor that has prevented communities from aggressively addressing the factors that contribute to health status is the often-fragmented nature of community resources. Different "kingdoms" may exist in the housing, education, healthcare and criminal justice systems for example. Even within a particular sector, units may operate as "silos." Each area has its own issues and challenges that, it is felt, occupy its attention and prevent multi-sector collaboration. In a period of financial entrenchment, different spheres vie for scarce resources, a situation that encourages competition rather than collaboration. Further, the data generated in these different spheres typically exist in silos that are not and perhaps cannot be interfaced. The ability to share data is a prerequisite for an effective population health initiative and the inability to do so is a major barrier to community health improvement.

Community entities may have fairly clear-cut notions about the community's health problems, problems that are not likely to correspond with those identified by the healthcare establishment. In fact, it is not unusual—and not surprising—for public health agencies to hold different views of health problems than both the medical establishment and the general public. It is notable that some health departments are reassessing their priorities based on input from consumers. This is thin gruel, of course, in that the public health community should be—but is not—leading the charge for population health.

Why the Community?

It has become increasingly clear that the community as a whole, rather than the healthcare system is the logical entity for promoting a population health approach and this is true for several reasons. The population health model assumes that health problems arise from conditions in the community and, in this regard, represent collective rather than individual problems. The cause of the bulk of identified problems reflects social pathology, structural factors and/or policy-related issues, all generated by and in the community. An evaluation of county health rankings by the University of Wisconsin indicates that the greatest opportunities for making a sustainable impact on the health of a population lie in the 80% of factors outside the realm of clinical care. At the end of the day, as Dan Buettner notes, "people may get sick as individuals, but they get healthy as a group" (Minnesota Public Radio, 2015).

The "chain of causation" is embedded in the community and the ability to trace the causes of health problems back to their roots is imperative. As a simple example, take the case of a community characterized by a high prevalence of diabetes. At one step removed, it can be argued that much of adult-onset diabetes can be attributed to obesity and, clearly, the increase in the prevalence of this disease corresponds to the increase in obesity exhibited by US society. Taking another step back, it could be argued that the increase in obesity is driven by poor dietary practices that involve not too much food but too much of the wrong types of food. Thus, the obesity epidemic can be traced to a significant extent back to the food insecurity affecting much of the population. Food insecurity, of course, is an inevitable consequence of poverty. When faced with a lack of income the availability of food is likely to be affected.

We are now several steps removed from the health problem itself and we could actually take it a step further and example the causes of poverty for the affected community. In some cases, it could be a result of a lack of job opportunities or, at the very least, a lack of jobs in locations accessible to those needing jobs. Or, alternatively, it could reflect not a lack of jobs but a lack of job skills within the affected population. In all three of these cases, there is little individuals can do to address the situation.

Representatives of the "community", however it is defined, may not be fully aware of the epidemiological profile of its population and may feel this should be left to the healthcare system. Even so, they *are* typically aware of many if not most of the sources of its health-related problems. They may not immediately connect social and environmental conditions to health status, but its agencies do know about toxic environmental sites, unsafe housing, concentrations of poverty, defects in the educational system, food deserts, deteriorating infrastructure, and the the factors limiting educational achievement in school children. Thus, the housing authority has some sense of the health problems facing its residents (indeed, some have on-site health services), the impact of inadequate housing on the health of residents, and even the implications of frequent moves due to housing insecurity. The school system will be aware of the health problems facing its students with most schools having on-site nursing services as well as programs for special needs students. A high proportion of public school children are on prescribed drugs and the schools have been in the forefront of identifying the childhood obesity epidemic. Employers are increasingly aware of the health status of their employees. An unhealthy workforce is damaging to productivity and runs up the cost of employer-sponsored health insurance. The proliferation of employee health programs has led to a greater appreciation for the health status of employees and what this means for the company's bottom line.

An advantage that the community has over health professionals lies with its ability to take a comprehensive view of the condition of its citizens. This ability arises from two sources: (1) the requirement for government agencies to cover a wide range of aspects of civic life and (2) the combined knowledge of representatives of non-health entities within the community. In considering the social determinants of health status, such factors as educational opportunities, job options, adequate housing and a variety of other factors that come under the purview of local government are notable. Further to the extent that the social and physical environments are major contributors to health status, it is the community through local government that has responsibility for these factors. The final component, public policy, is also in the realm of local government to a significant extent.

The fact that the various sectors of the community have an understanding of the health-related issues affecting their sphere of influence is a positive thing. At the same time, however, this could retard efforts at examining the big picture of health problems within the community. If different agencies are focusing on their respective issues in isolation, it is unreasonable to expect any collective impact benefits. This also means that the data related to health issues exist in silos within the various sectors. For example, the health problems associated with children in public housing may not be linked to the health problems identified by the school system or the failure of the public transportation system to provide access to pediatric services for these same children.

Although this fragmentation of responsibility represents a challenge, at the end of the day it is ultimately the community as a whole that has the ability to overcome this and take a comprehensive view of the situation. The civic leaders of the community are in a position to connect the dots better than any parties operating in the trenches. Not only are local politicians in a position to see the big picture (if they so choose) they are also in a position to encourage efforts toward collective impact that will cross sectoral boundaries.

The Affordable Care Act recognizes this and emphasizes the importance of public input into the community health needs assessment process. It could be argued that the community should actually drive this process while seeking input from the local healthcare system rather than the other way around. Community entities have a much broader view of the health status of the population and interface with those who do not or cannot access the healthcare system as well as those who do. Clearly, a community-based participative research approach is required to identify the "true" level of health as perceived "on the ground".

Importantly, many of the entities that need to be involved not only report to the power structure of the community but may depend on the community for its funding. If various departments and agencies can be seen as components of an integrated system, it is possible to encourage cross-sectoral cooperation. The community should have the leverage in fact to demand the coordination of activities toward the its collective goals. Thus, joint ventures between the public health department, the school system and the public housing authority, as just one example, could be expected to have a collective impact that no one agency can affect.

It is frequently argued that such a comprehensive approach requires a level of funding that is impractical in times of governmental financial retrenchment. Even the healthcare system with its extensive resources falls far short of achieving its ends. At the same time, however, all of the entities that should be participating in a community-wide effort toward improved population health have allocated resources. If the totality of the budgets allocated across the agencies for even a modestly sized community are considered, the amount of resources is considerable. Given that many of the agencies are already addressing health issues in one manner or another on their own, it is not unreasonable to think that joint initiatives could yield a higher "rate of return" on their health-related efforts.

Because population health improvement requires action on multiple determinants—including medical care, health behaviors, and the social and physical environments—no single entity can be held accountable for achieving improved outcomes (Kindig & Isham, 2014). Healthcare organizations, government, schools, businesses, and community organizations all need to make substantial changes in how they approach health and how they allocate resources.

Improving total population health requires partners across many sectors—including public health, health care organizations, community organizations, and businesses—to integrate investments and policies across all determinants.

The various arguments presented above for the role of the community in advancing population health can eventually be linked to the community's role in setting policy. There is virtually no sector within the community that the political structure does not affect in one way or another through its policies. Governmental policies provide the context for operations for every sector of society. Obviously public health policies have a major impact on the health conditions of the community, and health insurance-related policies have an impact on the ability of citizens to obtain care. The impact of the Affordable Care Act has been significant for the communities that were able to expand Medicaid coverage compared to those who were not able to.

The policy implications go well beyond healthcare and, in fact, are more impactful on population health in arenas not traditionally associated with health. The examples are almost limitless in this regard. Local policies related to business determine where different businesses locate (e.g., differential taxation), labor costs (e.g., local minimum wage), and tax incentives (e.g., for employer-sponsored health insurance). Policies exist at various levels within the community—from broad-reaching structure-related policies (e.g., support for urban sprawl) down to very specific policies such as regulations with regard to the animals that can be maintained in residential areas. Box 12.1 discusses the concept of collective impact.

> **Box 12.1: Collective Impact**
> Collective Impact is a framework established to tackle deeply entrenched and complex social problems. It is an innovative and structured approach to making collaboration work across government, business, philanthropy, non-profit organizations and citizens. The Collective Impact approach is premised on the belief that no single policy, government agency, organization or program can solve the increasingly complex social problems faced by society. This approach calls for multiple organizations or entities representing different sectors to downplay their own agendas in favor of a common agenda, shared measurement and alignment of effort.
>
> Collective effort is needed by sectors not accustomed to working together and by stakeholders who may not be aware of how their actions affect population health. In addition, incentives and new public and private resources (both knowledge and funding) must be created to ensure that plans are implemented.
>
> With collective impact innovative, social value-creating activity occurs both within and across the nonprofit, government, and business sectors. Unlike traditional collaborations or partnerships, collective impact initiatives have centralized infrastructure—known as a backbone organization—with dedicated staff whose role is to help participating organizations shift from acting alone to acting in concert.
>
> The collective impact movement can be traced to Kania and Kramer (2011) who first wrote about collective impact in the *Stanford Social Innovation Review*. They identified the five key elements described below:
>
> 1. A common agenda for change including a shared understanding of the problem and a joint approach to solving it through agreed upon actions.
> 2. Collecting data and measuring results consistently across all the participants ensures shared measurement for alignment and accountability.

(continued)

> **Box 12.1** (continued)
> 3. A plan of action that outlines and coordinates mutually reinforcing activities for each participant.
> 4. Open and continuous communication across the many players to build trust, assure mutual objectives, and create common motivation.
> 5. A backbone organization(s) with staff and specific set of skills to serve the entire initiative and coordinate participating organisations and agencies.
>
> According to Kania and Kramer, evidence of the effectiveness of this approach is still limited, but enough examples exist to suggest that substantially greater progress could be made in alleviating many of our most serious and complex social problems if nonprofits, governments, businesses, and the public were brought together around a common agenda to create collective impact. Funders and nonprofits overlook the potential for collective impact because they are used to focusing on independent action as the primary vehicle for social change.
> Source: Collaboration for Impact (2016)

Community Preparation

Since few communities across the nation have taken the lead role in population health, few communities are prepared for this responsibility. Hence, there are a number of steps that should be taken to position a community for coordinating the various components involved in a population health improvement effort.

First, the community needs to reframe health status as a community problem rather than a problem for the healthcare system. Everything else flows from this premise. It must be recognized that healthy communities lead to healthy individuals not the other way around. A key tenet of a population health approach is that health status is a measure of community health, not combined individual health. This shifts the responsibility away from personal choice on the part of individuals to decision-making on the part of the community and its component agencies. This thinking radically shifts the "blame" for health problems from the citizens to the community.

The community must be in a position to trace the causes of health problems back to their origins. This is another concession that the community must make and it must be prepared to follow the trail wherever it leads. This is not an exercise that civic leaders are used to carrying out. Such an approach takes a certain mindset and the ability to sort through the information and draw conclusions concerning causality. This can also become problematic if the trail leads back to influential actors within the community. One can imagine that identifying a leading real estate executive as a promoter of illness-inducing slum housing, the police department as failing to provide health services to its jail inmates, or the school system as promoting unhealthy foods because a school official has a relationship with a food service vendor is easily embraced. Even within the political structure itself it may be that policies are identified that have been promulgated by an official at the behest of a vested interest in the community. Serious ethical issues may arise when the sun shines on various activities that are the antithesis of positive health improvement but involve vested interests within the community.

The community must agree to "own" the problem given that the community in this model is the progenitor of ill-health. It is hard to face the fact that the community is the source of its own problems, that even well-meaning initiatives may have unintended consequences that retard population health improvement, or that policies promulgated by local government are contributors to on-going health problems. Serious self-reflection is required and may require someone outside the local power structure to analyze the situation, identify the source of the community's problems, and be willing to point the finger wherever necessary. The community must be willing to accept its responsibility in this regard.

Finally, the community must start by identifying its assets. Building on work in resource-poor Africa, various parties have attempted to take a more positive approach to the issue of population health improvement by focusing on assets rather than liabilities (Cutts, 2014). The question was raised as to how impoverished third-world communities with virtually no formal healthcare resources address issues of health and well-being. This led to the study of community assets and the role they play in managing the population's health. One result of this line of inquiry was the conclusion that a variety of assets can be and are leveraged in pursuit of community health in such situations. When the asset mapping approach was applied in the United States it was found that disadvantaged communities have a different perspective on what constitutes a health asset, with residents identifying a wide range of entities that they feel contribute to health and well-being. One of the by-products of this initiative was the development of the notion of "leading causes of life" (Gunderson & Pray, 2009). This turned the conventional view of the nature of health status on its head and provided a framework useful for the application of the population health model.

Steps in Community Involvement

There is little guidance as yet with regard to the steps communities should take in advancing a population health agenda. Some of the most innovative work along these lines has been carried out by Insightformation based on its experience with various communities around the nation (Barberg, 2020). This organization has identified six practical steps for developing and implementing a collaborative strategy for advancing population health.

1. Establish the Urgency and Commitment to Collaborate on Selected Health Issues

   Most people and organizations are busy, so it is unlikely that they will make the necessary effort if they don't see both the importance and urgency of action. It is important to clearly establish the "burning platform" that will make people realize that failing to act is more dangerous than the uncertainty and effort of working towards a solution. In many communities, short lists of priority issues are defined in the community health needs assessments conducted by non-profit hospitals and the community health assessments led by public health departments. CHNAs and CHAs often engage many different stakeholders and create consensus on three to six priority health issues; they also provide data that supports their decision to pick these issues.

2. Introduce New Concepts, Techniques and Tools for Managing a Community Strategy

Once there is a shared understanding of the need for urgency and requisite levels of teamwork to address specific priority health issues in a community, the next step is to establish support for the adoption of the concepts, techniques and tools necessary for this higher level of collaboration. The real power of collaboration is harnessed when participating organizations are able to combine their efforts and resources in mutually-beneficial and mutually-reinforcing ways that go beyond the sum of their previous isolated efforts. Organizations that aspire to work together in community-wide population health improvement efforts can benefit from understanding and adopting key points of the collective impact approach.

3. Engage the Coalition in Co-Creating a Strategy Map

Once there is a consensus on the need for a common agenda, the coalition leaders should engage a diverse team in the development of a Strategy Map. There is no one "right" way to collaboratively develop a Strategy Map, but many principles can be embraced to enhance the success of the effort. The Strategy Map should focus on the *changes* that the community will be working to achieve, not the current actions or ongoing operations. The sequential order in which a shared population health strategy is created and implemented is very important. It is best to build a consensus on the framework of objectives (the Strategy Map) *before* wrestling with the details of the measures, targets and actions. Establishing a consensus on the objectives makes it easier to gain an agreement on the shared measures, targets and actions that organizations will use to implement the strategy.

4. Distribute the Work of Strategy Execution

To achieve the necessary progress on the broad range of mutually-reinforcing changes that make up the strategy, it is important to distribute the workload among multiple working groups that can focus on subsets of the overall strategy. The use of well-designed Strategy Maps and strategy management techniques can help people avoid being overwhelmed by complex population health issues. It is not necessary for all the partnering organizations to become experts in the theory and techniques of strategy management. As long as the people who are providing "backbone support" understand how to structure and manage the details of a large integrated strategy, everyone else can benefit from that structure. Once people appreciate the basic concept of the strategy map, they can focus their efforts on working on their smaller parts of the larger puzzle and be confident about how they are contributing to the overall strategy.

5. Adopt Shared Strategy Measures and a Shared Measurement System

Most funders and boards have placed increasing emphasis on measurement in recent years. Yet, as more and more time gets consumed by developing measures and gathering data, it is questionable whether the emphasis on measurement is proving to be as helpful as was once thought. Our recent experience suggests that to effectively support the successful implementation of the population health model, communities should adopt important changes in the way measures are typically developed and used. Since significant improvements in population health outcomes will generally require a large number of different actions by different organizations, this approach tends to engender a huge number of very different measures. Requiring measures of success for each action reinforces the emphasis on accountability as a key to a successful population health initiative.

6. Harness, Align, and Monitor the Actions

The previously described techniques are intended to improve the success of the aligned actions that lead to the desired changes and outcomes. Without the actions, strategy implementation remains a hollow hope even if you are measuring and evaluating every part of a well-crafted strategy. In previous steps, the actions are intentionally separated from the objectives and measures. But once the strategic framework is in place and there is a preliminary plan for measurement, the work on actions can begin.

Achieving population health goals is expected to require several years of effort, with most major changes to population health outcomes taking between five and ten years to accomplish. The fact of the matter is we are only now seeing community-wide efforts to address the social determinants of health, and it will be some time before a recipe for successful amelioration of the many challenges facing efforts toward population health improvement.

Hoping to create shorter-term accountability for long-term actions or goals, some funders are asking for detailed work plans with annual or quarterly tasks. Instead of work plans, funders and coalition leaders should rely on the strategy framework and strategy measures to manage the long-term picture, while allowing for "emergence" in how the community innovates and continually adds aligned actions to accomplish the well-defined objectives in their part of the Strategy Map. Case Study 12.1 provides an example of the application of these principles to advance population health.

Case Study 12.1: Communities of Hope
Communities of HOPE is a holistic program for social change started in the Detroit metro area. Communities of Hope is focused on meeting the health, educational, employment, and entrepreneurial development challenges facing the community. The organization seeks to strategically leverage a community's purchasing power while forming effective partnerships with local socially responsible businesses. These profits are then applied to the areas of need identified through case studies and surveys.

The program addresses the root causes of some of the biggest challenges facing US communities today, all of which are particularly concentrated and intertwined in an urban cycle of poverty in government affordable apartment communities. These key targeted problem areas include: preventable chronic diseases (diabetes, heart disease, etc.); overall poor health for low-income populations; low high school graduation rates; poverty and economic hardship; substance abuse and smoking; isolation and poor relationships; and crime and gang activity.

In order to effectively combat these large social issues the program is based on several new and unique innovations that address both root causes and intertwined factors in order to create a holistic approach. Some of the key innovations include:

- Transforming the property management firms to take on a role of coordinating and supporting the development of strong, supportive communities that help their residents improve their lives and collectively create a positive culture to sustain the changes;
- Leveraging the property management firm's existing assets (buildings, communication, concentration of residents, information, purchasing power, etc.) that can greatly enhance the efficiency and effectiveness of the programs of other non-profit organizations;
- Engaging the residents in an organized way to actively participate in the co-creation of a positive community for them to live, leveraging their talents and cooperation by providing mechanisms for people to be able to help each other and the apartment community;
- Leveraging state-of-the-art strategic management tools and technologies that bridge the gap between a bold vision and the myriad of details that go into the execution of the strategy for achieving that vision, enabling much more effective engagement of a broad spectrum of organizations and individuals;
- Establishing innovative cooperative food purchasing and delivery programs to overcome current destructive equilibrium with regard to food purchasing practices where low-income individuals depend on food stamp programs to purchase foods, yet they live in "food deserts" where the pri-

(continued)

Case Study 12.1 (continued)

  mary stores that accept food stamps are liquor stores, gas stations, convenience stores, dollar stores or other fringe retailers that typically sell very unhealthy food;
- Providing low income families and seniors with cutting-edge, scientifically-designed nutritional products (at affordable prices) that can replace junk food in the diets of residents, thereby improving their ability to perform in school, work and life, enhancing their well-being, and reducing the occurrence of both current and long-term health problems;
- Developing an internal economy based on blending financial management training, micro-entrepreneurship (with on-site shared business centers, mentoring and marketing support), asset-building programs, gainsharing, and other innovations to help residents increase their financial security and self-sufficiency;
- Establishing relationships with private and charter schools in order to establish reinforcing environments that help create a culture that supports educational success both at school and at home;
- Changing the unhealthy equilibrium where property management firms typically respond to HUD programs in ways that waste resources, isolate residents, diminish the quality of life, and destroy—rather than create—value;
- Harnessing "mass collaboration" through the use of leading-edge strategic management tools and technologies to align the efforts of many non-profit and government organizations whose current efforts are seriously undermined by fragmentation and unnecessary duplication.

The initial work in Detroit is expected to improve the lives of several thousand people in over 25 apartment communities managed by Premier Property Management, LLC. (PPM). As property management firms, non-profit organizations and government agencies copy successful practices of this model around the country, the impact can truly transform the state of affordable housing in the United States.

The ground-breaking concept of a "Community Balanced Scorecard" is being used to engage partners in defining strategy maps for each of the 16 Levers of Change. These strategy maps address specific ways that the Levers of Change can be implemented to achieve the strategic themes. The process of developing the strategy maps helps to identify and develop ways of overcoming obstacles and will serve as a structure for breaking down major issues into specific objectives that different organizations can address. The logic of the strategy map—supported by the three-dimensional cascading capabilities of the InsightVision software—can allow for strategic alignment among many different organizations, mutual accountability, and strategic performance management.

> **Case Study 12.1** (continued)
>
> The first area for results to be evident has been in the radical transformation of the culture of Premier Property Management, LLC. This change of culture was seen as an essential driver of the other changes in both the community and corporate strategy maps that define the Communities of HOPE strategy. Within several days of launching the new strategy to the entire company (beyond the Theme Team members that had helped to develop the Theme strategy maps), employees engaged in a dramatic volunteer effort to clean, paint and landscape two of the properties most in need of help.
>
> Source: Communities of Hope (2021).

Community Health Business Model

The development of a community health business model has been suggested as a framework for promoting population health (Kindig & Isham, 2014). Business models represent the core aspects of a business, including its purpose, offerings, strategies, infrastructure, organizational structure, trading practices, and operational processes and policies. While such models are usually developed by individual firms in the corporate sector, some that are suitable for application in the health business arena are available from entities in business, government, and the nonprofit sector.

A community health business model must go beyond narrow interests to involve many sectors and organizations that can command sufficient resources or control the actions required for improving health outcomes. According to Kindig and Isham the business model concept should include the following elements:

1. All stakeholders from relevant sectors that can affect the population's health must be engaged in the process, as no single stakeholder has the resources to achieve, or can be accountable for, improved health in communities.
2. The community health business model must operate in a transparent manner and engage and report its progress to the general public.
3. A leadership structure needs to be designed and implemented.
4. Common purpose needs to be established. To do so, the benefits of improved health to the community must be identified and aligned with the benefit to be gained by individual stakeholders. Common purpose for these partnerships would address improved health for the community and depend on the identification of effective strategies that get to that overall goal. Those strategies would need to consider the particular state of health and availability of resources in each community.
5. Resources, including required skills, financial resources, and infrastructures, need to be identified.
6. Collective and in-kind evidence-based interventions that are directed at the overall purpose of improving community health and that are consistent with the iden-

tified community health improvement strategies must be established and implemented collectively and in each sector by the partners.
7. Economic incentives need to be identified to shape collective and individual stakeholder actions that are consistent with the overall purpose of improved community health and with the identified community health improvement strategies.
8. The state of health in each community needs to be assessed and monitored on an ongoing basis to inform the efforts of the community health partnership. The effectiveness of the community health improvement strategies and the progress of the evidence informed interventions need to be measured and assessed.
9. The lessons learned from each cycle of effort must be incorporated into the continuous redesign and improvement of the community business model for health improvement. Successful community health business models across the country will also require the commitment, supportive policies, and infrastructures of state, regional, and federal levels of government to assign the appropriate national context to the importance of health improvement, provide incentives for that improvement in communities, and provide information against which a community may evaluate its success relative to other communities.

An innovative approach to the application of a community health business model is represented by the emerging social impact investment movement. Box 12.2 describes the social impact investment phenomenon.

Box 12.2: Social Impact Investment
Poverty, homelessness, crime, and unemployment continue to plague even the wealthiest of nations. Imagine it was possible to leverage trillions in private capital and bring the same level of focus and entrepreneurial dynamism that we see in the private sector? What if these efforts could be applied to meet the pressing needs for better schools, more job opportunities, improved public services, safer streets? In answer to this question social impact investing has emerged as a means of investing in efforts that not only provide a return on investment but also target specific social needs.

Started in the mid-1960s, the idea of professionally-managed venture capital (VC) partnerships had nearly evaporated by late 1970s. Then the US government implemented several changes that sparked the resurgence of this industry. Among the policy changes were clarifications to ERISA's "Prudent Man" rule that allowed pension funds to make VC investments, and a safe harbor rule making it clear that VC managers wouldn't be considered plan fiduciaries. In just two years, VC investments went from virtually zero to more than $5 billion. And this capital helped unleash waves of innovation. Now we are poised to see the same happen with social impact investing.

(continued)

Box 12.2 (continued)

Around the world, there are stories of how impact investments are meeting needs in areas as diverse as childhood education, clean technology, and financial services for the poor. And last year, New York State, Social Finance and Bank of America Merrill Lynch teamed up to launch a "social impact bond" designed to cut New York City's seemingly insoluble recidivism problem. The $13.5 million raised will extend the proven approach of the Center for Employment Opportunities. If the Center meets targets for reducing recidivism rates, investors stand to earn up to a 12.5% return. Recently, J.P. Morgan and the Global Impact Investing Network studied 125 major fund managers, foundations, and development finance institutions and found $46 billion in sustainable investments under management. Some estimate that the impact investment market could grow to $3 trillion. And as the more socially conscious millennial generation of entrepreneurs build impact-driven businesses, it is expected that the supply of impact investment opportunities will vastly expand.

A recent report released by the Social Impact Investment Taskforce outlines comprehensive policy steps that should be taken to realize the potential. Among them: regulators should once again review ERISA rules for pension funds to make it clear that plan managers can consider social, targeted economic, or environmental factors in investment decisions because they affect the long-term financial performance of their investments.

Employers have a rich history of philanthropy, but they also have a stake in a healthy and productive future workforce. The National Business Coalition on Health, a nonprofit, purchaser-led group, is just one example of business leaders encouraging partnerships between businesses and other local stakeholders. The involvement of business with healthcare and public health is often focused on reducing healthcare costs and improving employee productivity. As important as these factors are, we believe that many other factors contribute to better health, providing a strong rationale for an even wider role for business in making the communities in which they operate healthier. This role can be rooted in core business objectives far beyond corporate social responsibility. This has been driven by the recognition that any benefits of an employee program can be negated if that same workforce lives in unhealthy communities, employer investments can be seriously compromised. Better community health can contribute to the corporate bottom line in many ways beyond reducing healthcare costs. These include: attracting and retaining talent, engaging employees, supporting human performance, ensuring personal safety, supporting manufacturing and service reliability, ensuring sustainability, and managing brand reputation (Kindig et al., 2013).

This trend represents somewhat of an extension of the role traditionally played by charitable foundations. Many private foundations, such as the California Endowment and the Robert Wood Johnson Foundation, are

(continued)

Box 12.2 (continued)

increasingly focused on developing comprehensive neighborhood pilot strategies for health improvement. Similarly, community social service agencies can play—and are playing—increasingly critical organizational and financial roles in catalyzing health business models at the community level. Part of the mission of United Way Worldwide, for example, is to galvanize and connect individuals, businesses, non-profit organizations and governments to create long-term social change that produces healthy, well-educated and financially stable individuals and families. Some communities have historical patterns of substantial philanthropy that could be emulated elsewhere in support of a community health business plan.

Policy-Setting and Population Health

Of the acknowledged three components of community health improvement—clinical care, environmental modification, and policy formulation—policy is the most likely to be neglected. This is not to say that health-related policies are ignored. Indeed, they are often prominent factors affecting the healthcare system (but not necessarily health status). It is policies affecting other areas that are often overlooked. The primary reason for this is the disconnect that typically exists between the recognized issues of other sectors and health conditions.

If policy changes are critical to improving health status, it is the community that must orchestrate these changes. Recent local efforts to change policies related to farmers markets, mobile produce markets and community gardens are examples of policy changes that are expected to contribute to the improvement of health status via better access to healthy foods (Centers for Disease Control and Prevention, n.d.).

There are two different approaches that might be taken with regard to policy. First, a community can promulgate a broad based community-wide policy that is meant to relate to all sectors within the community. An example that has already been implemented in several communities is a health-in-all-policies approach. Described in a previous chapter, this policy would mandate that the health impact of any decision, program or sector-specific policy be analyzed in terms of its impact on the health of the community. Another example would be a policy that directed all government agencies to consider the impact of their actions on other agencies and encouraging cross-sector collaboration for collective impact. Improved community health would presumably not be the only outcome of this with other non-health benefits anticipated.

Short of—or in addition to—establishing community-wide policies expected to have a global impact, communities may focus on priority health issues. Most communities have carried out studies of the most serious health needs, with public health departments typically identifying critical health issues and local healthcare systems (now under ACA mandate) identifying unmet health needs. The priorities identified here, of course, represent the perspective of the formal health care system.

Additional input should be garnered from representatives of the community whether consumers or representatives of non-health-related organizations have perspectives that need to be taken into consideration. If obesity, for example, is identified as a priority health issue, a policy(s) could be adopted for use community wide to address this problem.

As ever, the devil is in the details when promulgating policies of this type, and most communities are not used to making such broad-based pronouncements. They also are likely to confront entrenched interests and established "kingdoms" that are not easily influenced. Fortunately, there are a number of organizations that have been established to assist communities in carrying out such policies. (See "Additional Resources" at the end of the chapter.)

The second approach involves sector-specific policy formulation that involves more of a tailored approach than the community-wide model. This approach reflects the health-in-all-policies model but is more proactive in that it seeks to establish health-inducing policies on the front end rather than assessing the impact after a policy or program has been proposed. Thus, the question is not "What is the likely impact of this policy/program on health" but "What policy(s) can be enacted that will contribute to the improved health of the population affected by this sector?"

Many school systems across the nation have enacted policies aimed at improving the deteriorating health of their students. Many have established formal school health programs that include activities such as expanded physical education activities, healthier cafeteria meals, removal of soft drink and candy machines and health education instruction. The employee health programs established my many employers represent another example, and some churches have developed comprehensive health enhancement programs for not only their members but the surrounding communities. One could envision these types of activities being initiated in other sectors as well.

Policies can be both prescriptive and proscriptive, with the respective approaches having their plusses and minuses. Prescriptive approaches may involve financial incentives, whereby material rewards accrue to individuals or organizations in exchange for acting in a particular way. Proscriptive policies typically involve negative incentives, with some type of "penalty" associated with "undesirable" behaviors. Regulatory mandates, such as laws requiring seat belt use in vehicles and limiting smoking in public spaces, are appropriate. However, such mandates are often viewed as coercion and can be controversial. It is therefore unlikely that population health objectives will be fully achieved through regulation

One of the functions of policy is to provide guidance for the allocation of resources. Past policies have dictated, for example, that inordinate healthcare resources but devoted to clinical care with lesser amounts allocated for prevention and public health. Yet, a population health approach would emphasize social service resources at the expense of investment in clinical care. This entrenched pattern is likely to be difficult to overcome because of the financial incentives currently in place. The research community has lagged behind in generating the knowledge needed to guide the allocation of resources toward improved population health. It is not yet known what factors contribute most to community health improvement, limiting the ability to make informed decisions regarding the allocation of resources. Limited guidance is available because of the lack of knowledge on the impact of policies across small units of population, such as communities and counties. The impact of investment in each health factor area (health behaviors, clinical care, social and economic factors, and the physical environment) must be better understood in order to derive a base level of investment needed to achieve health benchmarks (Kindig & Mullahy, 2010). There are some models for determining the appropriate allocation of resources utilized in other countries that are further along in addressing the social determinants of health status.

Barriers to Community Leadership

As with many an innovative movement its champions begin to realize there are barriers to the consummation of the movement's goals—some of which are totally unanticipated. Arguably, there is no barrier that cannot be overcome. However, it is important that proponents of community leadership in population health improvement be forewarned of the challenges. Three key barriers are discussed below.

The data-related challenges for the implementation of a population health approach have been previously alluded to. The issues surrounding health-related data are well documented with fragmentation, incompleteness, timeliness and consistency being common deficiencies. Importantly, from a population health perspective, the lack of geographic granularity is a major impediment for the in-depth analyses required to obtain the data necessary to support a population health model.

With the population health model, however, the serious barrier relates to non-health-related data. As previously noted, when it comes to data related to the environment, the economy, the educational system, housing, food security and criminal justice among others, the federal government represents the most comprehensive source of data. These data of course are distributed in silos over a wide range of agencies, each with its own approach to data generation, management and dissemination. Further, despite some efforts to disseminate place-based data (e.g., the EPA maps of toxic wastes), little information is available below the county level and, in some cases, not even at that level. Even resource-rich states are challenged by the difficulty in locating usable data, a lack of resources among public agencies to upgrade information technology systems for making data more usable and accessible to the public, and a lack of enterprisewide coordination and geographic detail in data collection efforts (Casper & Kindig, 2012). Some communities have good data on healthcare access and quality while their attention to social and environmental factors is underdeveloped. Enormous variation is seen across the country in such profiles, but it is likely that a reasonable number of representative situations exist for most communities and counties in this regard.

A second barrier is the lack of evaluative research on the effectiveness of different approaches to population health improvement. The challenges faced in the successful implementation of initiatives related to population health improvement demand that proponents focus on those policies and programs that have been shown to be effective. Yet there is no doubt that the evaluation of policies and programs is an oft neglected function. For this reason little information is available with regard to the types of initiatives that work best in various situations. There is incomplete evidence of the effectiveness of different programs and policies, particularly regarding cost-effectiveness. It is not clear which level of investment in a particular determinant or factor is optimal, when diminishing return sets in, or when resources should be moved to other areas of concern. In particular, the available evidence relative to different types of outcomes, particularly disparity reduction is sorely missing (Kindig & Isham, 2014).

One final consideration is the lack of accountability that exists in the emerging population health environment. Given that in the ideal community-based population health configuration the "actors" are spread across the public and private sectors (government, businesses, school systems, community organizations and the healthcare system among others), there is no one actor or agent accountable and responsible for such broad population health outcomes as mortality, morbidity, and disparities.

While public health is charged with assuring the conditions that make us healthy, local public health agencies find it increasingly difficult to carry out their own essential services much less support a population health initiative. While some suggested mechanisms such as a public health "system", public-private partnerships, health outcomes trusts, and an integrator function for healthcare organizations, none of these mechanisms have been established beyond theory or taken to scale. Obstacles to systematic transformation include not only the inherent tension between "bottom up" local community approaches and more centralized "top-down" planning perspectives, but also communities' unique strengths and challenges across a broad spectrum of health-related issues.

The bottom line is that no one-size-fits-all formula exists to guide population health improvement through resource allocation and activities across multiple sectors and multiple levels. Communities must identify the configuration of collaborators that best fits their situation. Each sector must appreciate how improving population health contributes to its primary mission within the realm in which it operates. Each sector must also work toward the economic alignment of its business model with the community health business model. There is no doubt that new or realigned resources will be required if our population health improvement efforts are to be accelerated.

A key point made above relates to the necessity of establishing a dedicated organization to guide the planning, development, implementation and evaluation of the population health initiative. With one organization essentially having the responsibility for managing the population health enterprise, this provides a place where the buck can stop. The responsibility would rest squarely on the shoulders of those whose sole job is to advance community health using a population health model.

Summary

The healthcare system has limited ability to contribute to community health improvement and the community—however constituted—must drive the population health movement. It is increasingly recognized that contemporary health problems and their solutions have their roots in the community, yet it is hard to break our dependency on the healthcare delivery system and the tremendous resources at its disposal. There are a number of reasons why the healthcare system is not in a position to lead the population health effort and, in fact, may not be in a position to make a significant contribution to it. Yet, it is easy for civic leaders to argue that it was not their problem. Even among those who appreciate the role of the community, it is often felt that healthcare is too complex for non-professionals to understand much less impact.

It has become increasingly clear that the community as a whole, rather than the healthcare system, is the logical entity for promoting a population health approach and this is true for several reasons. The population health model assumes that health problems arise from conditions in the community and, in this regard, represent collective rather than individual problems. The cause of the bulk of identified problems reflects social pathology, structural factors and/or policy-related issues, all generated by and in the community. An advantage that the community has over health professionals lies with its ability to take a comprehensive view of the condition of its citizens. This ability arises from two sources: (1) the requirement for government agencies to cover a wide range of aspects of civic life and (2) the combined knowledge of representatives of non-health entities within the community. The civic leaders of the community are in a position to connect the dots better than any parties operating in the trenches.

There are a number of steps that should be taken to position a community for coordinating the various components involved in a population health improvement effort. First, the community needs to reframe health status as a community problem rather than a problem for the healthcare system. Everything else flows from this premise. The community must be in a position to trace the causes of health problems back to their origins. The community must agree to "own" the problem given that the community in this model is the progenitor of ill-health.

Collective effort is needed by sectors not accustomed to working together and by stakeholders who may not be aware of how their actions affect population health. In addition, incentives and new public and private resources (both knowledge and funding) must be created to ensure that plans are implemented. The development of a community health business model has been suggested as a framework for promoting population health. A community health business model must go beyond narrow interests to involve many sectors and organizations that can command sufficient resources or control the actions required for improving health outcomes. Policy changes are critical to improving health status, and it is the community that must orchestrate these changes.

Key Points

- Contemporary health problems (and their solutions) have their roots in the community.
- The healthcare system is not in a position to lead the population health movement, yet civic leaders are reluctant to take the lead in community health improvement.
- The fragmentation that often characterizes community resources is a barrier to community involvement.
- At the same time, community leaders are in a better position to take a comprehensive view of the situation.
- Although adequate funding may be available within the community, its may be hampered by competition for scarce resources.
- The main benefit of a community approach is the opportunity to generate collective impact through multi-sector collaboration.
- There are a number of steps a community should follow to prepare itself for a leadership role with regard to improving community health.
- A community health business model is important for getting all parties on the same page.
- Of the three components to community health improvement, policy is the area that is most relevant for the community.
- Cross-sector collaboration on the formulation of policy is critical.

References

Barberg, B. (2020). *Starter guide to implementing population health strategies.* Downloaded from URL: https://static1.squarespace.com/static/576aec9ed2b8579bb7ce3e26/t/5932c5d617bffcb21f65860b/1509736305169/Starter+Guide+to+Implementing+Population+Health+Strategies.pdf.

Casper, T., & Kindig, D. A. (2012). Are community-level financial data adequate to assess population health investments? *Preventing Chronic Disease, 9,* 120066.

Centers for Disease Control and Prevention. (n.d.-a). *State initiatives supporting healthier food retail: An overview of the national landscape.* Downloaded from URL: http://www.cdc.gov/obesity/downloads/Healthier_Food_Retail.pdf.

Cohen, R., & Bannick, M (2014). Is social impact investing the next venture capital. *Forbes.* Downloaded from URL: https://www.forbes.com/sites/realspin/2014/09/20/is-social-impact-investing-the-next-venture-capital/#7709c1e046a4.

Collaboration for Impact. (2016). *The collective impact framework.* Downloaded from URL: http://www.collaborationforimpact.com/collective-impact/.

Communities of Hope. (2020). *What we do.* Downloaded from URL: https://communitieshope.org/services/

Communities of Hope. (2021). *What we do.* Downloaded from URL: https://communitiesofhope.com/about-coh/what-we-do/

Cutts, T. (2014). Community Health Assets Mapping Partnership (CHAMP). *Stakeholder Health.* Downloaded from URL: https://stakeholderhealth.org/champ-cutts/.

Gunderson, G., & Pray, L. M. (2009). *Leading causes of life: Five fundamentals to change the way you live your life*. Abingdon Press.

Kania, J., & Kramer, M. (2011). Collective Impact. *Stanford Social Innovation Review*. Downloaded from URL: https://ssir.org/articles/entry/collective_impact.

Kindig, D. A. (2017). *Improving population health (blog)*. Downloaded from URL: https://uwphi.pophealth.wisc.edu/publications/other/blog-collection-final-2014-04-05.pdf.

Kindig, D. A., & Isham, G. (2014). Population health improvement: A community health business model that engages partners in all sectors. *Frontiers of Health Services Management*, 30.4 (Summer), 3–20, 56–57.

Kindig, D. A., Isham, G., & Siemering, K. Q. (2013). *The business role in improving health: Beyond social responsibility*. Discussion paper, Institute of Medicine. Downloaded from URL: http://iom.edu/Global/Perspectives/2013/TheBusinessRole.

Kindig, D. A., & Mullahy, J. (2010). Comparative effectiveness—Of what? Evaluating strategies to improve population health. *JAMA, 20*(8), 901–902.

Minnesota Public Radio. (2015). *Dan Buettner on lifestyle and longevity: The blue zones*. Downloaded from URL: http://www.mprnews.org/story/2015/10/05/mpr_news_presents.

Robert Wood Johnson Foundation. (2011). *Health care's blind side: Unmet social needs leading to worse health*. Downloaded from URL: http://www.rwjf.org/en/library/articles-and-news/2011/12/health-cares-blind-side-unmet-social-needs-leading-to-worse-heal.html.

Additional Resources

Association for Community Health Improvement: www.healthycommunities.org.

Center for Community Health and Development (University of Kansas): Community Tool Kit at URL: https://ctb.ku.edu/en.

Centers for Disease Control and Prevention—Health Impact Assessment from URL: https://www.cdc.gov/healthyplaces/hia.htm.

Centers for Disease Control and Prevention—Parks and Trails Health Impact Assessment Toolkit from URL: https://www.cdc.gov/healthyplaces/parks_trails/default.htm.

Centers for Disease Control and Prevention—Transportation Health Impact Assessment Toolkit from URL: https://www.cdc.gov/healthyplaces/transportation/hia_toolkit.htm.

Costanza, K. (2015). Investing with health in mind. *Crosswalk*. Downloaded from URL: https://medium.com/bhpn-crosswalk/investing-with-health-in-mind-f9a07416d7f1.

Insightformation.: https://www.insightformation.com/insightvision/.

University of Cambridge—Integrated Transport and Health Impact Modelling Tool from URL: https://www.mrc-epid.cam.ac.uk/research/research-areas/public-health-modelling/ithim/.

University of Wisconsin—What Works for Health from URL: http://whatworksforhealth.wisc.edu/.

CPSIA information can be obtained
at www.ICGtesting.com
Printed in the USA
LVHW081631140322
713410LV00004B/242